THE
RENIN-ANGIOTENSIN
SYSTEM

ADVANCES IN EXPERIMENTAL MEDICINE AND BIOLOGY

THE RENIN-ANGIOTENSIN SYSTEM

Edited by

J. Alan Johnson and
Ralph R. Anderson

University of Missouri at Columbia
Columbia, Missouri

SPRINGER SCIENCE+BUSINESS MEDIA, LLC

Library of Congress Cataloging in Publication Data

Midwest Conference on Endocrinology and Metabolism, University of Missouri—
Columbia, 1978.
The renin-angiotensin system.

(Advances in experimental medicine and biology; v. 130)
"Proceedings of the Fourteenth Midwest Conference on Endocrinology and Metabolism, held at the University of Missouri at Columbia, Missouri, September 28—29,
1978."
Includes index.
1. Angiotensin — Congresses. 2. Renin — Congresses. I. Johnson, Joseph Alan, 1931-
     II. Anderson, Ralph Robert, 1932-   III. Title. IV. Series.
QP572.A54M52 1978   612'.4   80-17962

ISBN 978-1-4615-9175-7   ISBN 978-1-4615-9173-3 (eBook)
DOI 10.1007/978-1-4615-9173-3

Proceedings of the Fourteenth Midwest Conference on Endocrinology and
Metabolism held at the University of Missouri, Columbia, Missouri,
September 28-29, 1978 and sponsored by:

> University of Missouri - Columbia
>   Graduate School and Office of Research
>   University Assembly Lectures
>   College of Agriculture
>   College of Veterinary Medicine
>   Department of Veterinary Medicine
>   and Surgery
>   Department of Veterinary Pathology
>   Veterinary Medicine Diagnostic Laboratory
>   School of Medicine
>   Department of Medicine
>   Department of Pathology
>   Department of Pharmacology
>   Department of Physiology
>   Division of Biological Sciences
>   Dalton Research Center
>   Sinclair Comparative Medical Research Farm
> Harry S. Truman Memorial Veterans Administration Hospital
> Merck and Company, Inc.
> The Upjohn Company

© 1980 Springer Science+Business Media New York
Originally published by Plenum Press, New York in 1980
Softcover reprint of the hardcover 1st edition 1980

CONFERENCE CHAIRMAN

Ralph R. Anderson, Ph.D., Professor of Dairy Husbandry, University of Missouri - Columbia.

PROGRAM CHAIRMAN

J. Alan Johnson, Ph.D., Associate Professor of Physiology, University of Missouri - Columbia.

PLANNING COMMITTEE

John D. David, Ph.D., Associate Professor of Biological Sciences, University of Missouri - Columbia.

C. William Foley, Ph.D., Professor of Veterinary Anatomy and Physiology, University of Missouri - Columbia.

Leonard R. Forte, Ph.D., Associate Professor of Pharmacology, University of Missouri - Columbia.

John M. Franz, Ph.D., Associate Professor of Biochemistry, University of Missouri - Columbia.

James Green, Ph.D., Professor of Anatomy, University of Missouri - Columbia.

Murray Heimberg, M.D., Ph.D., Professor, Chairman of Pharmacology, University of Missouri - Columbia.

David M. Klachko, M.D., Professor of Medicine, University of Missouri - Columbia.

Harold Werner, M.D., Assistant Professor of Medicine, University of Missouri - Columbia.

Walter T. Wilkening, Ph.D., Director of Conferences and Short Courses, University of Missouri - Columbia.

Warren L. Zahler, Ph.D., Associate Professor of Biochemistry, University of Missouri - Columbia.

SPEAKERS

Luciano Barajas, M.D., Professor, Department of Pathology, University of California at Los Angeles, Harbor General Hospital, Torrance, California.

David W. Cushman, Ph.D., Senior Research Fellow, Squibb Institute for Medical Research, Princeton, New Jersey.

Robert E. McCaa, Ph.D., Professor, Department of Physiology and Biophysics, University of Mississippi School of Medicine, Jackson, Mississippi.

Alan Moore, Ph.D., Norwich-Eaton Pharmaceuticals, Norwich, New York.

Hiroko Nishimura, M.D., Associate Professor, Department of Physiology and Biophysics, University of Tennessee Center for the Health Sciences, Memphis, Tennessee.

Michael J. Peach, Ph.D., Department of Pharmacology, University of Virginia, Charlottesville, Virginia.

Ian A. Reid, Ph.D., Associate Professor, Department of Physiology, University of California at San Francisco, California.

Leonard T. Skeggs, Ph.D., Director, Hypertension Research Laboratory, Veterans Administration Medical Center, Cleveland, Ohio.

John E. Zehr, Ph.D., Associate Professor, Department of Physiology and Biophysics, University of Illinois, Urbana, Illinois.

MODERATORS

John Bauer, M.D., Associate Professor, Department of Medicine, University of Missouri - Columbia.

C. Stephen Brooks, M.D., Assistant Professor, Department of Medicine, University of Missouri - Columbia.

James O. Davis, M.D., Chairman, Professor, Department of Physiology, University of Missouri - Columbia.

Ronald H. Freeman, Ph.D., Assistant Professor, Department of Physiology, University of Missouri - Columbia.

DISCUSSANTS

Davis, J. O., Department of Physiology, University of Missouri - Columbia.

Freeman, R. H., Department of Physiology, University of Missouri - Columbia.

Goetz, K. L., St. Luke's Hospital, Kansas City, Missouri.

Jawadi, M. H., University of Kansas, Wichita, Kansas.

Klachko, D. M., Department of Medicine, University of Missouri - Columbia.

Miller, R. P., Eli Lilly and Co., Indianapolis, Indiana

Poisner, A. M., Department of Pharmacology, University of Kansas School of Medicine, Kansas City, Kansas.

Ray, W. J., Department of Physiology, University of Missouri - Columbia.

Rowe, B., University of Tennessee Center for the Health Sciences, Memphis, Tennessee.

Wang, B. C., St. Luke's Hospital, Kansas City, Missouri.

Williams, G. M., Squibb Institute for Medical Research, Princeton, New Jersey.

PREFACE

The Fourteenth Midwest Conference on Endocrinology and Metabolism, held at the University of Missouri - Columbia on September 28th and 29th, 1978, brought together several prominent researchers who are authorities on various aspects of the renin-angiotensin system. Each speaker presented an in-depth coverage of a topic related to his own area of expertise, including recent findings from his own research laboratory. Following each presentation there was a general discussion of the material by the speaker and the audience. These presentations and the ensuing discussions are summarized in these published Proceedings.

Traditionally the Midwest Conferences on Endocrinology and Metabolism have emphasized breadth as well as depth of coverage of the selected topic; the present Conference is no exception. Perusal of the titles of the presentations will reveal that the Conference dealth with many different facets of the renin-angiotensin system, including the biochemistry, anatomy, physiology, and comparative endocrinology of this hormonal system, plus special areas of consideration such as angiotensin receptors, angiotensin-converting enzyme, the control of renin release, angiotensin and aldosterone secretion, and the role of the renin-angiotensin system in the central nervous system. The selection of the renin-angiotensin system as the topic for the present conference was very timely because of the many noteworthy advances in this area in recent years, many by the participants in the Conference.

The Editors are very appreciative of the excellent manuscripts which the speakers provided for these Proceedings. We also thank the Moderators and the staff of Conferences and Short Courses for their help in organizing and presenting this Conference. Also, the Editors and the Planning Committee are very grateful for the financial support of the sponsors of the Conference.

J. Alan Johnson

Ralph R. Anderson

CONTENTS

THE BIOCHEMISTRY OF THE RENIN-ANGIOTENSIN SYSTEM

L. T. Skeggs, F. E. Dorer, M. Levine, K. E. Lentz, and
J. R. Kahn

Departments of Medicine and Surgery
Veterans Administration Medical Center and
Departments of Biochemistry and Pathology
Case Western Reserve University
Cleveland, OH 44106

OUTLINE

I. HISTORY OF THE RENIN-ANGIOTENSIN SYSTEM

Renin, the primary, rate-limiting substance of the renin-angiotensin system, was discovered by Tigerstedt and Bergmann (1898).
It is easily extracted from kidney tissue, where it is present in
very large amounts. Direct intravenous injection of crude preparations into experimental animals produces a very dramatic increase
in blood pressure that may last for an hour or more.

Despite its early discovery, the real importance of renin was
not appreciated until after the work of Goldblatt in 1934. In a
classic series of experiments, Goldblatt produced hypertension in

experimental animals, showed that the hypertension possessed a
humoral basis, and proved that it was of renal origin (Goldblatt,
Lynch, Hanzal, and Summerville, 1934; Goldblatt, 1947; Goldblatt,
1948). Goldblatt, as a pathologist, was impressed by the presence
of arterio- and arteriolosclerosis which he found in the kidneys
of hypertensive patients coming to autopsy. He believed that the
stenosing effect of this disease might reduce the blood flow through
the kidneys and thus be the cause of essential hypertension. In a
deliberate effort to duplicate this situation experimentally, he
designed a silver clamp and applied it to the main renal arteries
of dogs. He discovered that a moderate reduction of blood flow
produced by this method resulted in a form of persistent arterial
hypertension that closely resembled the human form of the disease.
Constriction of only one renal artery in the dog with the other
kidney untouched, however, produced an increase in pressure that
usually declined to normotensive levels in a few weeks. This form
of hypertension is now known as two-kidney hypertension. Although
this form of hypertension is not persistent in the dog, it apparently
does persist in rats and also in man. Goldblatt found that constriction of both renal arteries or of just one artery, the opposite
kidney being removed (one-kidney hypertension), produced a form of
hypertension which might last for many years.

Goldblatt went on to show in later experiments that the hypertension produced by the constriction of the renal arteries has a
humoral basis. He found that the elevation in pressure which follows
the constriction of the artery could not be prevented by complete
sympathectomy, destruction of the spinal cord by pithing, or by
transplantation of the clamped, denervated kidney to the neck. He
also showed that the hypertension was abolished if the renal veins
were ligated, the animal becoming normotensive and eventually suc-
cumbing to uremia. It seems certain that this form of hypertension
is caused directly or indirectly by a humoral substance or substances
released by the clamped kidney. This important work of Goldblatt led
immediately to a search for the humoral agent responsible for the
elevation of pressure in hypertension. It is natural that it led
directly to a rediscovery of renin, which had been known for such a
long time (see Figure 1).

Two different groups of workers soon found that renin was not
a direct pressor or vasoconstrictor substance. Thus, Page and Helmer
(1940) in this country, and Braun-Menendez, Fasciolo, LeLoir, and
Muñoz (1940) in Argentina, found that renin acted on a substance
present in plasma to produce a heat-stable, short-acting vasoconstrictor substance. Page and Helmer named the new substance "angiotonin" while Braun-Menendez and his group used the term "hypertensin".
Many years went by, with investigators throughout the world divided
into two schools, each with its own terminology. Finally, after a
period of many years, at a meeting at the University of Michigan in

Asp-Arg-Val-Tyr-Ile-His-Pro-Phe-His-Leu-Leu-Val-Tyr-Ser-R

RENIN SUBSTRATE, a glycoprotein, molecular weight about 58,000 contained in the plasma.

> RENIN, an enzyme produced by the juxtaglomerular cells of the kidney and released into the general circulation via the renal vein.

Asp-Arg-Val-Tyr-Ile-His-Pro-Phe-His-Leu + Leu-Val-Tyr-Ser-R

ANGIOTENSIN I, a decapeptide with no direct pressor action.

> CONVERTING ENZYME, contained in the lung, acts on the decapeptide in the plasma as it passes through the pulmonary circulation. Also present in plasma and other tissues. Requires chloride ion for activation.

Asp-Arg-Val-Tyr-Ile-His-Pro-Phe + His-Leu

ANGIOTENSIN II, causes contraction of arteriolar smooth muscle. The most powerful directly pressor substance known. Has other indirect actions mediated through the adrenal cortex.

Figure 1. Relationships of the renin-angiotensin system. (From Skeggs, Dorer, Kahn, et al., Am. J. Med. 60: 737-748, 1976).

1961, Drs. Page and Braun-Menendez agreed to call the new substance "angiotensin".

Although renin and angiotensin were the only two substances known to originate in the kidney, there were a number of workers who questioned whether they might be the mediators of hypertensive disease in humans or in experimental hypertension in animals. Thus, it seemed very important to us to show that angiotensin was actually present in the blood of animals with experimental hypertension. In our laboratory, the blood of hypertensive dogs was subjected to dialysis in an artificial kidney in the hope that angiotensin, which was thought to be a small molecule, might pass through the membrane. The dialysate was collected, concentrated, and tested for pressor activity in the rat. Although the method was exceedingly clumsy, the results provided the first demonstration of the presence of angiotensin in the blood of animals with experimental hypertension (Skeggs, Kahn, and Shumway, 1951).

We later developed a method for the assay of angiotensin in arterial blood samples. Large samples of arterial blood were drawn directly into alcohol from either humans with hypertension or animals with experimental hypertension. The alcoholic filtrate was purified, concentrated and tested for pressor activity in the rat (Kahn, Skeggs and Shumway, 1952). By this means we showed that the angiotensin levels in the blood of patients with malignant hypertension were very greatly increased, by as much as twenty times normal. In patients with benign essential hypertension, however, the blood angiotensin levels were elevated in only about one-half of the patients. The method was crude compared to present day methods employing radioimmunoassay; the results, however, were consistent with present day findings. The true importance of the work was that it convinced us and some others that renin and angiotensin might really be involved in some forms of hypertension, and that they deserved further study.

There were still other reasons to believe that renin was the mediator of experimental hypertension. It was demonstrated that the blood pressure of dogs with experimental hypertension could be lowered to normal by immunization with extracts of hog kidney containing renin. Inasmuch as the immunization evoked an antibody which neutralized not only hog but also dog renin, it was natural to believe that the reduction in pressure resulted from the neutralization of the dog's own renin by crossreaction with anti-hog renin antibody (Wakerlin, Bird, Brennan, *et al.*, 1953; Kremen and Walkerlin, 1955; Wakerlin, 1958). These results were confirmed by several other groups of workers and helped to convince many of us at that time that renin and angiotensin were the mediators of experimental hypertension (Helmer, 1958; Haas and Goldblatt, 1959; Deodhar, Haas, and Goldblatt, 1964; Hill, Chester, and Wisenbaugh, 1970). Thus it was that in the early 1950's work started in several laboratories directed towards purification, structural analysis and synthesis of angiotensin.

II. CHEMISTRY OF ANGIOTENSIN

The amounts of angiotensin present in the blood of animals with experimental hypertension are exceedingly small, far too small to provide a starting point for the isolation of the compound. In our own laboratories we found it necessary to prepare crude renin from hundreds of pounds of hog kidneys, and to react it with a renin substrate obtained from many hundreds of liters of horse plasma in order to obtain our first crude angiotensin, which was to be the starting point of our purification. The methods which we employed to purify angiotensin were relatively crude compared to the elegant methods which are available today. They consisted of extraction into butanol, adsorption onto and elution from alumina, and countercurrent distribution. The first pure angiotensin was isolated in our laboratory in 1954 (Skeggs, Marsh, Kahn, and Shumway, 1954a). Our amino acid analysis showed it to be a decapeptide containing nine different amino acids (Skeggs, Marsh, Kahn, and Shumway, 1955). Shortly thereafter, Peart (1956), in England, isolated and was first to observe the structure of an angiotensin that he obtained from bovine plasma which had been reacted with rabbit renin.

The amino acid sequence for both the hog and the bovine plasma angiotensin ultimately proved to be the same, with the exception that valine replaced the isoleucine in position 5 in the bovine compound. Somewhat later, Bumpus, Schwarz, and Page (1957) isolated angiotensin from the reaction of hog renin with hog plasma. In this case the amino acid sequence was the same as that derived from the hog renin and horse substrate combination. The amino acid sequence of human angiotensin has been reported to be identical to that of the horse and the hog (Arakawa, Nakatani, Minohara, and Nakamura, 1967).

Early in our purification of angiotensin we discovered that the substance actually exists in two different forms (Skeggs, Marsh, Kahn, and Shumway, 1954b). Both forms were equally pressor in the rat, but had completely different chemical properties. We soon discovered that plasma and the crude renin substrate we were using to prepare our angiotensin contained an enzyme that is chloride-activated and which we later called the angiotensin-converting enzyme. This enzyme acts upon the initial product of the renin reaction, angiotensin I, and converts it to angiotensin II. It was later learned that the converting enzyme removes the last two amino acids in the angiotensin I molecule as the dipeptide, His-Leu, resulting in the conversion of the decapeptide structure of angiotensin I to the octapeptide structure of angiotensin II (Lentz, Skeggs, Woods, *et al.*, 1956).

Only a short time after we had isolated angiotensin II and demonstrated its structural relationship to angiotensin I, the synthesis of the compound was announced (Rittel, Iselin, Kappeler, *et al.*, 1957). This was followed almost immediately by a second synthesis of the peptide (Schwarz, Bumpus, and Page, 1957).

Not long after this, we discovered that angiotensin I is actually inactive, and that the entire pressor effect of the renin-angiotensin system is due to the vasoconstrictor action of angiotensin II (Skeggs, Kahn, and Shumway, 1956). We found that angiotensin II was an extremely potent vasoconstrictor substance when it was perfused in a physiological salt solution through an isolated rat kidney. Under the same conditions, angiotensin I was virtually inactive. Similar results were obtained by Helmer (1957), who used rabbit aortic strips, and by Bumpus, Schwarz, and Page (1956), who found that angiotensin I had not more than 5% of the oxytocic activity of angiotensin II in the isolated rat uterus.

These results have been convincingly confirmed through the relatively recent discovery of converting enzyme inhibitors. These inhibitors, which were originally discovered in the venom of the South American snake, *Bothrops jararaca*, specifically inhibit the converting enzyme *in vivo* and block the pressor action of angiotensin I (Ferreira, Bartelt, and Greene, 1970; Ng and Vane, 1970).

It was discovered that angiotensin II had still another important function in addition to its action on smooth muscle. Davis and his group discovered, in cross-circulation studies in dogs, that a humoral factor is responsible for the release of aldosterone from the adrenal cortex (Davis, 1963). Shortly thereafter it was shown by two different groups of workers that the humoral factor stimulating the aldosterone release was angiotensin II (Laragh, Angers, Kelley, and Lieberman, 1960; Biron, Koiw, Nowaczynski, *et al.*, 1961). Thus, angiotensin II, in addition to being fifty times more powerful than norepinephrine as a pressor agent, acts through the adrenal cortex to cause retention of sodium and to produce extracellular fluid volume expansion.

It has been shown recently that a third form of angiotensin may play an important physiological role (Blair-West, Coghlan, Denton, *et al.*, 1971; Campbell, Brooks, and Pettinger, 1974; Goodfriend and Peach, 1975). The compound [des-Asp^1] angiotensin II (also called angiotensin III) may be generated by the action of the aminopeptidase, angiotensinase A, on angiotensin II. Alternatively, angiotensin III could be produced by the sequential action of angiotensinase A and the converting enzyme on angiotensin I. Both angiotensin III and angiotensin II have been shown to produce similar blood levels of aldosterone in the rat. However, angiotensin III has only about one-quarter of the pressor effect possessed by angiotensin II. Whether angiotensin III is produced in sufficient quantities to attain an appreciable blood level and to play a significant role in the renin system is not yet clear.

III.   CHEMISTRY OF RENIN SUBSTRATE

Following our work with angiotensin, we became very interested in finding some method of blocking the renin system *in vivo*. It seemed logical to us to attempt the inhibition of renin, which was the initial and rate-limiting component of the system. However, to design an inhibitor of renin required further knowledge of the structure and properties of renin and of its substrate. Our knowledge at that time of the chemistry of renin substrate was derived from a partial purification of hog renin substrate which had been accomplished by Green and Bumpus (1954) and from the very early work of Plentl, Page, and Davis (1943) who showed that the substrate was present in the alpha$_2$-globulin fraction of the plasma proteins.

The liver is the principal source of circulating renin substrate (Page, McSwain, Knapp, and Andrus, 1941). Nasjletti and Masson (1972) and Freeman and Rostorfer (1972) have demonstrated the synthesis of renin substrate by the isolated rat liver and by rat liver slices. The concentration of renin substrate in the plasma is increased by nephrectomy and decreased by adrenalectomy.

The starting material for our purification of hog renin substrate (Skeggs, Lentz, Hochstrasser, and Kahn, 1963) was derived from 50 batches of plasma having an aggregate volume of 3750 liters. Midway in the purification process the substrate was subjected to chromatography on DEAE-cellulose in a descending pH gradient. We were surprised to find that the active material was separated into three different forms in the elution patterns: A, B, and C, each appearing at a characteristic pH value. Two of these forms later were separated into two parts. Thus, a total of five major forms were identified: A, B_1, B_2, C_1, and C_2. All of the forms were found to be glycoproteins, having what appeared to be essentially the same amino acid composition. They differed in their content of sialic acid and hexosamine. Molecular weights of all of the forms were very close to 58,000. The reaction rates with renin of all of the forms appeared to be very similar, and all yielded the same angiotensin molecule.

More recently, renin substrate has been purified from human plasma (Eggena, Chu, Barrett, and Sambhi, 1976; Tewksbury, Premeau, and Dumas, 1976; Printz, Printz, and Dworschack, 1977; Dorer, Lentz, Kahn, *et al.*, 1978b) and has been shown to be a glycoprotein with 14% carbohydrate and a molecular weight similar to that of hog renin substrate (Tewksbury, Frome, and Dumas, 1978). Like hog renin substrate, the human renin substrate exists in multiple forms which can be demonstrated by ion-exchange chromatography or isoelectric focusing (Printz, Printz, and Dworschack, 1977; Lentz, Dorer, Kahn, *et al.*, 1978) (see Figure 2). These different forms are present in untreated plasma and do not appear to be artifacts produced by the isolation procedures. However, the forms of human renin substrate have lower isoelectric points and are unstable below pH 4.

The purification of hog renin substrate did not in itself bring us any closer to our goal of determining the enzymatic specificity of renin. The structural analysis of a protein with a molecular weight of 58,000 appeared to be an impossible task. It occurred to us that the specificity of most proteolytic enzymes is based upon one or two amino acid residues at most, and it seemed unlikely that the entire substrate molecule with a molecular weight of 58,000 would be necessary for the action of renin. Accordingly, we attempted the degradation of the protein substrate with various enzymes, hoping to find a smaller fragment which would be susceptible to the action of renin.

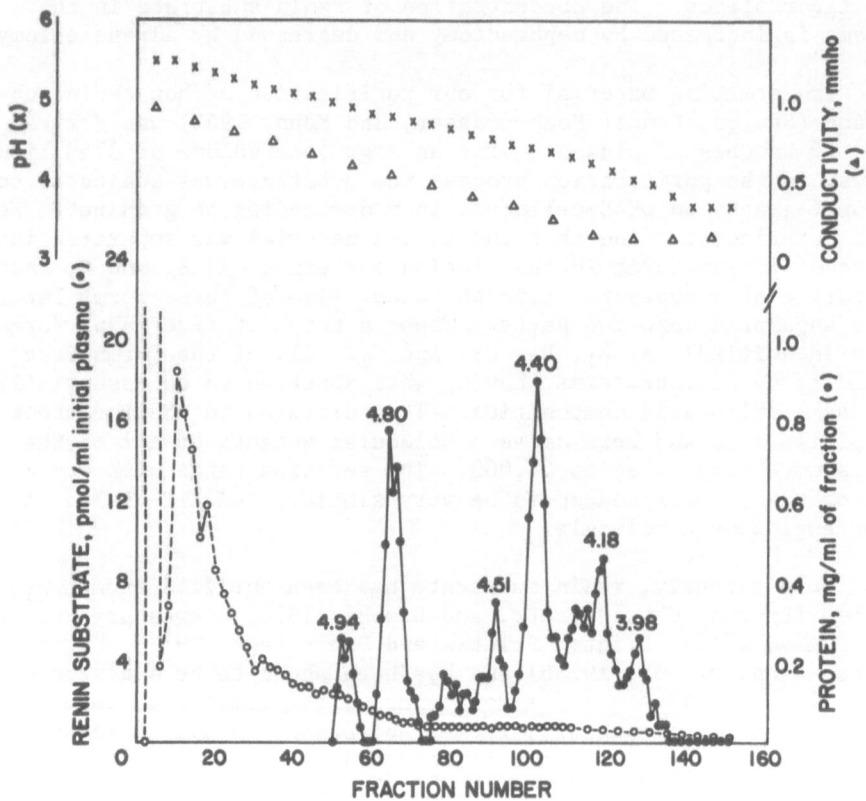

Figure 2.   Multiple forms of human renin substrate.   DEAE-cellulose
chromatography in a descending pH gradient of 5 ml of
plasma from a normal male.   (From Lentz, Dorer, Kahn,
et al., Clin. Chim. Acta 83: 294-257, 1978)

We were successful in finding that trypsin releases a peptide
from the protein substrate, which in turn is capable of yielding
angiotensin I upon incubation with renin (Skeggs, Kahn, Lentz, and
Shumway, 1957).   We isolated a total of 10 milligrams of this
peptide from a reaction of trypsin with 2840 grams of semi-purified
protein-renin substrate that had been obtained from over a thousand
liters of horse plasma.

Our structural analysis showed that the molecule consisted of a tetradecapeptide which contained the ten amino acids of angiotensin I plus four more on the carboxyl end of the molecule. Thus, the sequence proved to be that shown in Figure 3 (Asp^1---Ser^{14}). The finding of serine on the carboxyl terminal was very surprising, since this is not in accord with the enzymatic specificity of trypsin. However, we confirmed the structure by synthesis using classical methods entirely. The final synthetic product had 90% of the biological activity of the tetradecapeptide that had been isolated from natural sources (Skeggs, Lentz, Kahn, and Shumway, 1958).

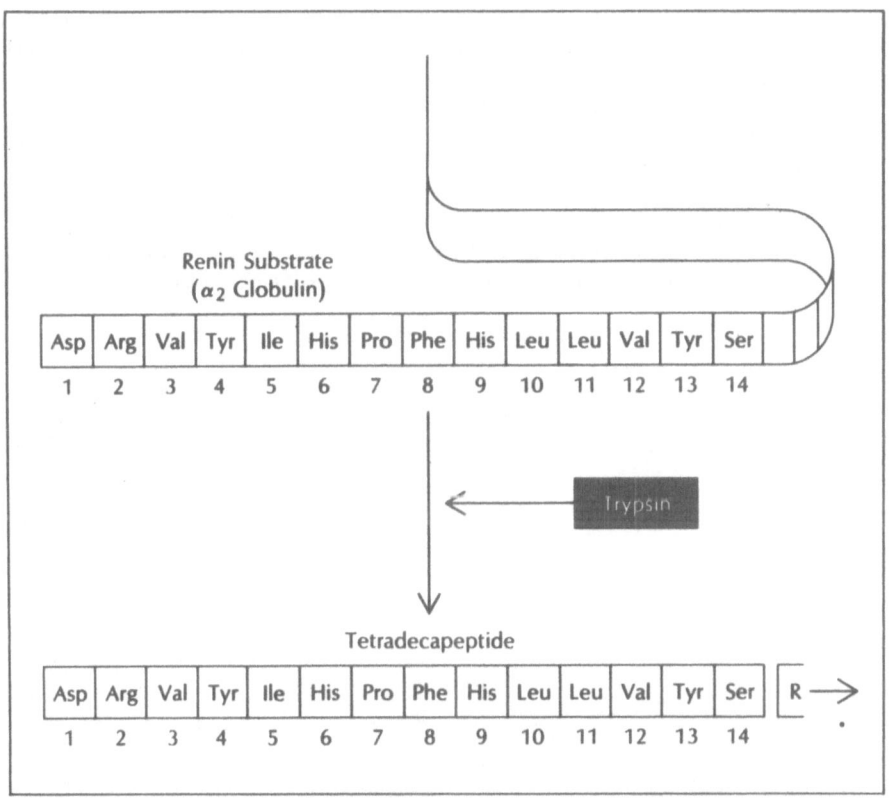

Figure 3. Formation of the tetradecapeptide renin substrate by partial degradation of plasma renin substrate with trypsin. (From Skeggs, L. T. Hospital Practice 9: 145-154, March, 1974)

Since renin was used to degrade the molecule for structural analysis, it was immediately obvious that the enzyme hydrolyzes the bond between the two leucyl residues in positions 10 and 11. In this manner, it liberates angiotensin I and a biologically inactive tetrapeptide, Leu-Val-Tyr-Ser, from the carboxyl end of the molecule. When renin acts on the naturally occurring substrate to produce angiotensin I, the inactive fragment consists of the tetrapeptide linked in some manner to the large residue for which no biological function is known.

It was soon learned that the specificity of renin was not based on a simple leucyl-leucine sequence and that instead the enzyme had very particular requirements. In order to elucidate these require- ments, we synthesized a large number of peptides which represented portions of the tetradecapeptide molecule (Skeggs, Lentz, Kahn, and Hochstrasser, 1968). Monitoring the rate of reaction of renin with these peptides presented various difficulties. The products of the reactions were biologically inactive, requiring a chemical method for determining reaction velocities. Furthermore, the peptides themselves had very limited solubility. The problem was solved by using continuous flow analysis and employing ultra-sensitive chem- ical methods for determination of the reaction rates (Figure 4). It was found that the maximum affinity of the enzyme for substrate (Lowest K_m value) was achieved only with the full tetradecapeptide

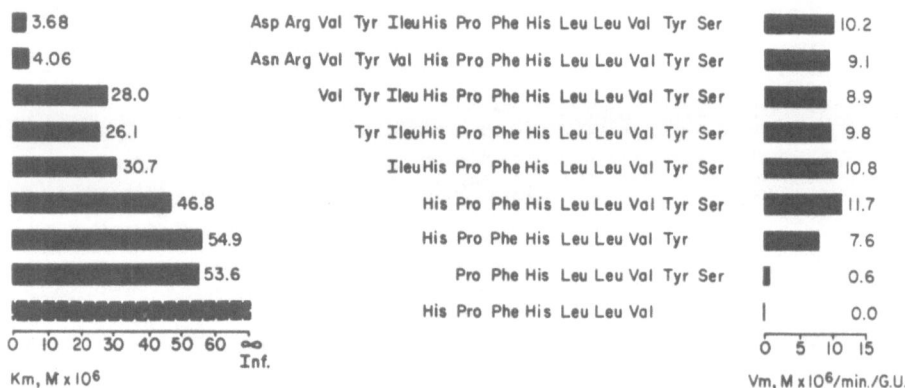

Figure 4.   *Kinetics of the reaction of renin with nine synthetic peptide substrates. Peptides were incubated with partially purified hog renin at pH 7.4. Initial velocities were measured by continuous flow analysis using the ninhydrin method. (From Skeggs, L. T. Hospital Practice 9: 145-154, 1974)*

molecule. Removing the aspartyl and arginyl residues from the N-terminal increased the K_m (and reduced its affinity) value more than eight-fold. A fairly moderate increase in K_m occurred when the next amino acids in the sequence (valine, tyrosine, isoleucine) were removed. It was confirmed that the smallest molecule reacting with renin at a practical rate was the octapeptide, His^6---Tyr^{13}. The octapeptide Pro^7---Ser^{14} also is attacked, although very slowly.

IV. CHEMISTRY OF RENIN

Renin has been the most difficult component of the system to purify. Our own efforts in this direction have been only partially successful. The problem is complicated by the fact that hog renin exists in more than one form. Thus, upon DEAE-cellulose chromatography in a descending pH gradient, four forms of renin were obtained (Skeggs, Lentz, Kahn, and Hochstrasser, 1967). Kinetic studies of all four forms showed similar reaction rates with purified hog substrate and with synthetic tetradecapeptide substrate as well. Human renin also may exist in several forms (Skeggs, Lentz, Kahn, *et al.*, 1972). A neutral extraction of human kidneys, followed by the use of DEAE-cellulose in a batch procedure, concentrated virtually all the active material into a single fraction. This material, upon DEAE-cellulose chromatography, yielded two major fractions which showed marked differences in charge. Whereas renin A passed quickly through the DEAE-cellulose column, renin B was bound firmly at low ionic strength and was eluted only after the sodium chloride concentration exceeded 0.1 M. Two minor forms, designated C and D, were also found. Additional forms of human renin were discovered by countercurrent distribution. Analysis by gel-filtration indicated a molecular weight of approximately 39,500 for all forms. Preparations were found to differ markedly in their relative rates of hydrolysis of the tetradecapeptide and natural substrate.

The final purification of hog renin was achieved by Inagami and Murakami (1977), who obtained a stable form of the enzyme from hog kidney by means of a 130,000-fold purification with a remarkable 19% yield. A major step in the purification was the use of a pepstatin affinity column followed by chromatography on Sephadex G-75, DEAE-cellulose, and CM-cellulose. Renin is strongly inhibited by pepstatin. This N-acylated pentapeptide (iso-valeryl-L-valyl-L-valyl-4-amino-3-hydroxy-6-methylheptanoyl-L-alanyl-4-amino-3-hydroxy-6-methylheptanoic acid) was isolated from actinomycetes (Umezawa, Aoyagi, Morishima, *et al.*, 1970). Although the inhibition is non-specific and occurs with acid proteases in general, it is remarkably effective with renin. Inagami and coworkers have used immobilized pepstatin to form a very effective affinity column for renin. They have used this column to very good advantage in the purification of hog and human renin.

The purification of human renin has presented formidable problems. The supply of human kidneys is limited and is of very poor
quality. The concentration of renin is very low and consequently
extracts have a low specific activity. Despite these problems,
Yokosawa, Inagami, and Haas (1978) recently have succeeded in the
purification of the human enzyme. Here again, the use of the pepstatin column and a hemoglobin affinity column along with conven-
tional chromatographic methods, have been used successfully in the
isolation of a small amount of homogeneous human renin with a
specific activity of 830 GU/mg protein.

Our knowledge of renin recently has become very detailed but
confusing. Relatively inactive forms of renin have been found in
man, rabbit, and hog, as well as other species. These can be activated by acidification, incubation at low temperatures, or incubation with various proteolytic enzymes. The activation process may
involve a reduction in molecular weight. In this laboratory (Levine,
Lentz, Kahn, et al., 1978) and in Inagami's laboratory (Inagami,
Murakami, Misono, et al., 1977) it has been shown that conversion of
the partially purified high molecular weight (HMW) material from hog
kidney to 40,000 renin is not accompanied by activation. On the
other hand, Day, Luetscher, and Gonzales (1975) reported HMW renin
from some diseased kidneys which can be activated by acidification
or treatment with trypsin. The activation is not accompanied by
a reduction in molecular weight. A high molecular weight renin from
acidified extracts of hog kidneys has been described which is not
activated nor does its molecular weight change as a result of acidification or treatment with enzymes (Levine, Lentz, Kahn, et al.,
1976). A similar finding from neutral extracts of human kidney has
been reported (Barrett, Eggena, and Sambhi, 1977). The significance
of the inactive or HMW renin in extracts of human kidneys is thus
far unknown. It is also not clear whether the kidney secretes the
HMW renin as such or whether it is an artifact caused by the rupture
of kidney cells.

In human plasma an activable renin has been found in the plasma
in both normal controls and in hypertensive patients (Skinner, Cran,
Gibson, et al., 1975; Derkx, v Gool, Wenting, et al., 1976; Boyd,
1977; Leckie, McConnell, Grant, et al., 1977). In some cases the
renin has a high molecular weight which has been found not to change
in size when activated (Day and Luetscher, 1975). This contrasts
with reports from several laboratories that the activable renin has
a high molecular weight which is reduced to the 40,000 dalton region
upon activation (Boyd, 1977; Leckie, McConnell, and Jordan, 1977).
More recently it has been reported that the inactive renin has a
molecular weight in the 40,000 dalton region both before and after
activation (Shulkes, Gibson, and Skinner, 1978).

It would be of enormous importance if it were found that the inactive renin in human plasma was activated *in vivo* by some as yet unknown mechanism and thus played a role in determining the circulating plasma renin activity (PRA). For this reason a number of laboratories have been searching for such an *in vivo* activating mechanism.

Several investigators (Atlas, Sealey, and Laragh, 1978; Osmond and Loh, 1978) postulate a serine protease as the activating enzyme, based upon inhibition of the activation by diisopropyl fluorophosphate. Factor XII, the initiating component of the blood coagulating cascade, has been implicated (Tatemichi and Osmond, 1978) as has kallikrein, a serine protease, which in turn is activated by Factor XII (Leckie, 1978; Derkx, Tan-Tjiong, and Schalekamp, 1978; Morris and Day, 1978). Recently it has been suggested (Morris, 1978) that pseudorenin or cathepsin D, an acid protease (Dorer, Lentz, Kahn, *et al.*, 1978a) could be involved in the process. The data offered are in all cases sparse, and further investigation is necessary to determine whether and how such *in vivo* activation occurs.

V. ANGIOTENSIN CONVERTING ENZYME

There is still another component of the renin-angiotensin system which we must consider. This is the angiotensin-converting enzyme which converts the inactive decapeptide angiotensin I to the vasoconstrictor octapeptide angiotensin II (Skeggs, Marsh, Kahn, and Shumway, 1954b; Skeggs, Kahn, and Shumway, 1956). The reaction occurs by removal of the C-terminal dipeptide, His-Leu, from angiotensin I (see Figure 1) (Lentz, Skeggs, Woods, *et al.*, 1956). Angiotensin-converting enzyme was first discovered in the mid 1950's. Enzyme activity was shown to require chloride (or another monovalent anion such as bromide, fluoride, or nitrate). The reaction was also inhibited by EDTA, implying that the enzyme was a metallo-protein.

Due to the difficulty of assay, very little was known about the enzyme for many years. More recently, with the availability of synthetic angiotensin I, chemical methods have been developed which are simpler and more precise. In addition, model substrates such as hippuryl-His-Leu (Cushman and Cheung, 1971a) and hippuryl-Gly-Gly (Igic, Erdos, Yeh, *et al.*, 1972) have made possible the routine assay of the enzyme in plasma and tissue extracts as well as in purified enzyme preparations.

Angiotensin-converting enzyme was originally discovered in plasma, and for many years it was assumed that conversion took place in the circulating blood. This seemed an obvious conclusion since the *in vitro* incubation of renin with plasma in the presence of chloride yields exclusively angiotensin II. Furthermore, the intravenous injection of angiotensin I and II have nearly identical

effects on blood pressure. Ng and Vane (1967) showed that angiotensin converting enzyme activity in blood was too low to account for
the rapid conversion of angiotensin I in the intact animal. Their
studies indicated that in dogs the pulmonary circulation was the
most important site for generation of circulating angiotensin II.
Bahkle (1968) showed that angiotensin-converting enzyme activity
was present in a particulate fraction of homogenized dog lung, and
the enzyme has since been demonstrated in extracts of many tissues
(Cushman and Cheung, 1971b; Roth, Weitzman, and Piquilloud, 1969).
Sander and Huggins (1971) carried out subcellular fractionation
studies in which marker enzyme analysis and electron microscopy
suggested that plasma membrane was the site of pulmonary angiotensin-converting enzyme. More recently, the studies of Ryan, Ryan,
Schultz, *et al.* (1975) have demonstrated that the enzyme is localized on the luminal surface of pulmonary endothelial cells. Such
a situation makes the pulmonary vascular bed a unique site for controlling levels of vasoactive peptides entering the arterial circulation.

On the other hand, angiotensin-converting enzyme activity has
been demonstrated in a number of other tissues, and some conversion
must certainly occur in peripheral vascular beds. However, quantitative measurement of the degree of conversion in tissues is difficult and is complicated by the simultaneous degradation of both
angiotensin I and II by tissue angiotensinases. Therefore, the
relative importance of the lung and of the peripheral vascular beds
in the conversion process in different species is not clear.

Angiotensin-converting enzyme has been obtained in purified
form from lung tissue by several groups of workers (Cushman and
Cheung, 1972; Dorer, Kahn, Lentz, *et al.*, 1972; Igic, Erdos, Yeh.
et al., 1972; Lanzillo and Fanburg, 1974; Soffer, Reza, and Caldwell,
1974). The enzyme purified from a particulate fraction of rabbit
lung has been characterized as a glycoprotein containing 26% carbohydrate, a single polypeptide chain, and 1 atom of zinc per molecule of enzyme. The molecular weight is 129,000 (Das and Soffer,
1975). The similarity of the plasma and lung converting enzymes
suggests that pulmonary endothelial cells may be the source of the
plasma enzyme (Das, Hartley, and Soffer, 1977).

In addition to converting angiotensin I to angiotensin II and
hydrolyzing model peptides such as hippuryl-Gly-Gly, angiotensin-
converting enzyme also inactivates bradykinin (see Figure 5). The
hydrolysis of bradykinin proceeds by sequential removal of the di-
peptides Phe-Arg and Ser-Pro from the C-terminal end of the peptide
(Dorer, Kahn, Lentz, *et al.*, 1974; Soffer, Reza, and Caldwell, 1974).
Thus, it appears that the same enzyme which produces the most potent
pressor substance known also inactivates another peptide with potent
vasodepressor effects. Even more striking is the amazing velocity
of these two reactions which may go nearly to completion during a
single passage of blood through the lungs.

VI. INHIBITORS OF THE RENIN-ANGIOTENSIN SYSTEM

The foregoing description of the renin-angiotensin system does
not, in itself, provide us with the all-important answer as to the
degree of responsibility that the renin-angiotensin system bears
for the increase in blood pressure in human and experimental hypertension. It has, however, given us tools which are useful for this
purpose. The most notable of these are the antagonists to angiotensin II, which are effective *in vivo*. The two most widely used
are [Sar[1], Ala[8]] angiotensin II (Saralasin) (Pals, Masucci, Denning,
et al., 1971·) and [Sar[1], Ile[8]] angiotensin II (Khosla, Leese, Maloy,
et al., 1972). The angiotensin-converting enzyme inhibitors that
were originally found in snake venom have already been mentioned.
A number of analogues of these compounds which inhibit the enzyme
have been synthesized by Cushman, Cheung, Sobo, and Ondetti (1977).
The best of these are SQ 20881 and SQ 14225. The latter compound
is effective upon oral administration. Finally, antibodies to
angiotensin I or II may be obtained by immunization of rabbits with
the peptides coupled to larger molecules such as albumin (Vallotton,
1974).

angiotensin I: Asp-Arg-Val-Tyr-Ile-His-Pro-Phe-His-Leu
                                                                ↑

bradykinin: Arg-Pro-Pro-Gly-Phe-Ser-Pro-Phe-Arg
                                                   ↑   ↑

tetradecapeptide
renin
substrate: Asp-Arg-Val-Tyr-Ile-His-Pro-Phe-His-Leu-Leu-Val-Tyr-Ser
                                            ↑   ↑   ↑

Hip-Gly-Gly: Bz-Gly-Gly-Gly
                                                      ↑

*Figure 5. Amino acid sequences of four different substrates for
            angiotensin-converting enzyme. Arrows indicate the
            peptide bonds which are hydrolyzed by the enzyme.*

Both angiotensin antagonists and converting enzyme inhibitors have been used to block the renin-angiotensin system in humans with hypertension. In general, the blood pressure was lowered in those subjects having elevated plasma renin activity (PRA). In one such study using SQ 20881, the diastolic pressure was lowered in 55 out of 65 hypertensive patients. In a third of these the diastolic pressure fell to 90 mm Hg or less. The depressor response occurred in all patients with high renin and in nearly all with normal renin. Those patients having low renin did not respond (Case, Wallace, Keim, et al., 1977).

The effect on the blood pressure produced by blocking the renin-angiotensin system in animals with experimental renal hypertension has been reviewed recently (Skeggs, Dorer, Kahn, et al., 1976). In most studies the blood pressure of acutely hypertensive animals and those with an established form of two-kidney hypertension have been lowered through the use of one or more of the blocking agents. In sharp contrast are the results obtained in animals with chronic one-kidney hypertension. Nearly all investigators who have worked with this form of hypertension have failed to lower the blood pressure even though the renin-angiotensin system was completely blocked. The result of the blockage in both experimental and human hypertension apparently depends upon the PRA. Thus, animals with two-kidney hypertension have elevated PRA and respond to blockade with lowered blood pressure, while those with the one-kidney form have normal or low PRA and do not respond.

One-kidney hypertension in animals resembles low-renin essential hypertension in humans. Both may have low PRA and neither responds to blockage of the renin-angiotensin system. It should be recognized that the persistent form of hypertension produced in dogs by Goldblatt was one-kidney hypertension. The evidence is clear that the hypertension in these animals is sustained by a humoral mechanism which is not the renin-angiotensin system. Recent work in rabbits with chronic one-kidney hypertension suggests that there may be another as yet unknown renal pressor system (Skeggs, Kahn, Levine, et al., 1975, 1976).

The elucidation of the renin-angiotensin system as we now know it represents the work of a large number of investigators over a span of nearly 40 years. During most of this period there was a controversy, frequently acrimonious, as to whether the renin-angiotensin system did, in fact, have anything to do with hypertension. Those of us who were involved in this work and were believers in the system may now take comfort in the fact that the renin-angiotensin system does actually participate in elevating the blood pressure in a good portion of those humans with hypertension.

REFERENCES

Arakawa, K., Nakatani, M., Minohara, A., and Nakamura, M. (1967). Isolation and amino acid composition of human angiotensin I. Biochem. J. 104: 900–906.

Atlas, S. A., Sealey, J. E., and Laragh, J. H. (1978). "Acid"- and "cryo"-activated inactive plasma renin. Similarity of their changes during β-blockage. Evidence that neutral protease(s) participate in both activation procedures. Circ. Res. 43 (suppl. 1): 128–133.

Bahkle, Y. S. (1968). Conversion of angiotensin I to angiotensin II by cell-free extracts of dog lung. Nature 220: 919–921.

Barrett, J. D., Eggena, P., and Sambhi, M. P. (1977). "Big big renin". Enzymatic and partial physical characterization of a new high molecular weight renin from normal human kidney. Circ. Res. 41 (suppl. 2): 7–11.

Biron, P., Koiw, E., Nowaczynski, W., Brouillet, J., and Genest, J. (1961). The effects of intravenous infusions of valine-5 angiotensin II and other pressor agents on urinary electrolytes and corticosteroids, including aldosterone. J. Clin. Invest. 40: 338–347.

Blair-West, J. R., Coghlan, J. P., Denton, D. A., Funder, J. W., Scoggins, B. A., and Wright, R. D. (1971). The effect of the heptapeptide (2–8) and hexapeptide (3–8) fragments of angio- tensin II on aldosterone secretion. J. Clin. Endocrinol. Metab. 32: 575–578.

Boyd, G. W. (1977). An inactive higher-molecular-weight renin in normal subjects and hypertensive patients. Lancet 1: 215–218.

Braun-Menendez, E., Fasciolo, J. C., Leloir, L. F., and Muñoz, J. M. (1940). The substance causing renal hypertension. J. Physiol. 98: 283–298.

Bumpus, F. M., Schwarz, H., and Page, I. H. (1957). Synthesis and pharmacology of the octapeptide angiotensin. Science 125: 886–887.

Bumpus, F. M., Schwarz, H., and Page, I. H. (1956). Partial separa- tion of an oxytocic principal from preparations of angiotonin. Circ. Res. 4: 488–492.

Campbell, W. B., Brooks, S. N., and Pettinger, W. A. (1974). Angio- tensin II and angiotensin III-induced aldosterone release *in vivo* in the rat. Science 184: 994–996.

Case, D. B., Wallace, J. M., Keim, H. J., Weber, M. A., Sealey, J. E., and Laragh, J. H. (1977). Possible role of renin in hypertension as suggested by renin-sodium profiling and inhibi- tion of converting enzyme. New Eng. J. Med. 296: 641–646.

Cushman, D. W. and Cheung, H. S. (1971a). Spectrophotometric assay and properties of the angiotensin-converting enzyme of rabbit lung. Biochem. Pharmacol. 20: 1637–1648.

Cushman, D. W. and Cheung, H. S. (1971b). Concentrations of angio- tensin-converting enzyme in tissues of the rat. Biochim. Biophys. Acta 250: 261–265.

Cushman, D. W. and Cheung, H. S. (1972). Studies *in vitro* of angio-
    tensin-converting enzyme of lung and other tissues. In:
    Hypertension '72 (Genest, J. and Koiw, E., eds.), pp. 532-541,
    Springer-Verlag, New York.
Cushman, D. W., Cheung, H. S., Sabo, E. F., and Ondetti, M. A.
    (1977). Design of potent competitive inhibitors of angiotensin-
    converting enzyme. Carboxyalkanoyl and mercaptoalkanoyl amino
    acids. Biochemistry 16: 5484-5491.
Das, M., Hartley, J. L., and Soffer, R. L. (1977). Serum angiotensin
    converting enzyme. Isolation and relationship to the pulmonary
    enzyme. J. Biol. Chem. 252: 1316-1319.
Das, M. and Soffer, R. L. (1975). Pulmonary angiotensin-converting
    enzyme. Structural and catalytic properties. J. Biol. Chem.
    250: 6762-6768.
Davis, J. O. (1963). Importance of the renin-angiotensin system in
    the control of aldosterone secretion. In: *Hormones and the
    Kidney*. (Williams, P. C., ed.), pp. 325-329, Academic Press,
    New York.
Day, R. P. and Luetscher, J. A. (1975). Biochemical properties of
    big renin extracted from human plasma. J. Clin. Endocrinol.
    Metab. 40: 1085-1093.
Day, R. P., Luetscher, J. A., and Gonzales, C. M. (1975). Occurrence
    of big renin in human plasma, amnionic fluid, and kidney extr-
    acts. J. Clin. Endocrinol. Metab. 40: 1078-1084.
Deodhar, S. D., Haas, E., and Goldblatt, H. (1964). Production of
    antirenin to homologous renin and its effect on experimental
    renal hypertension. J. Exp. Med. 119: 425-432.
Derkx, F. H. M., Tan-Tjionj, H. L., and Schalekamp, M. A. D. H.
    (1978). Endogenous activator of plasma-inactive-renin. Lancet
    2: 217-219.
Derkx, F. H. M., v Gool, J. M. G., Wenting, G. J., Verhoeven, R. P.,
    Man in't Veld, A. J., and Schalekamp, M. A. D. H. (1976).
    Inactive renin in human plasma. Lancet 2: 496-499.
Dorer, F. E., Kahn, J. R., Lentz, K. E., Levine, M., and Skeggs, L. T
    (1972). Purification and properties of angiotensin-converting
    enzyme from hog lung. Circ. Res. 31: 356-366.
Dorer, F. E., Kahn, J. R., Lentz, K. E., Levine, M., and Skeggs, L. T
    (1974). Hydrolysis of bradykinin by angiotensin converting
    enzyme. Circ. Res. 34: 824-827.
Dorer, F. E., Lentz, K. E., Kahn, J. R., Levine, M., and Skeggs, L. T
    (1978a). A comparison of the substrate specificities of
    cathepsin D and pseudorenin. J. Biol. Chem. 253: 3140-3142.
Dorer, F. E., Lentz, K. E., Kahn, J. R., Levine, M., and Skeggs, L. T
    (1978b). Purification of human renin substrate. Anal. Biochem.
    87: 11-18.
Eggena, P., Chu, C. L., Barrett, J. D., and Sambhi, M. P. (1976).
    Purification and partial characterization of human angiotensino-
    gen. Biochim. Biophys. Acta 427: 208-217.

Ferreira, S. H., Bartelt, D. C., and Greene, L. J. (1970). Isolation of bradykinin-potentiating peptides from Bothrops jararaca venom. Biochemistry 9: 2583-2593.

Freeman, R. H. and Rostorfer, H. H. (1972). Hepatic changes in renin substrate biosynthesis and alkaline phosphatase activity in the rat. Am. J. Physiol. 223: 364-370.

Goldblatt, H. (1947). The renal origin of hypertension. Physiol. Rev. 27: 120-165.

Goldblatt, H. (1948). *The Renal Origin of Hypertension.* Charles C. Thomas, Springfield, Ill.

Goldblatt, H., Lynch, J., Hanzal, R. F., and Summerville, W. W. (1934). Studies on experimental hypertension. I. The production of persistent elevation of systolic blood pressure by means of renal ischemia. J. Exp. Med. 59: 347-379.

Goodfriend, T. L. and Peach, M. J. (1975). Angiotensin III: (des-aspartic acid)-angiotensin II. Evidence and speculation for its role as an important agonist in the renin-angiotensin system. Circ. Res. 36-37 (Suppl. 1): 38-48.

Green, A. A. and Bumpus, F. M. (1954). The purification of hog renin substrate. J. Biol. Chem. 210: 281-286.

Haas, E. and Goldblatt, H. (1959). Effects of ganglionic blocking agents, pressor and depressor drugs on renal hypertension. Am. J. Physiol. 197: 1303-1307.

Helmer, O. M. (1957). Differentiation between two forms of angiotonin by means of spirally cut strips of rabbit aorta. Am. J. Physiol. 188: 571-577.

Helmer, O. M. (1958). Studies on renin antibodies. Circulation 17: 648-652.

Hill, R. W., Chester, J. E., and Wisenbaugh, P. E. (1970). The effect of intravenous antirenin injection on chronic experimental and acute renin-induced hypertension in dogs. Lab. Invest. 22: 404-410.

Igic, R., Erdos, E. G., Yeh, H. S. J., Sorrells, K., and Nakajima, T. (1972). Angiotensin I converting enzyme of the lung. Circ. Res. 30-31 (Suppl. 2): 51-61.

Inagami, T. and Murakami, K. (1977). Pure renin. Isolation from hog kidney and characterization. J. Biol. Chem. 252: 2978-2983.

Inagami, T., Murakami, K., Misono, K., Workman, R. J., Cohen, S., and Suketa, Y. (1977). Renin and precursors: Purification, characterization, and studies on active site. In: *Advances in Experimental Medicine and Biology*, Vol. 95, *Acid Proteases. Structure, Function, and Biology.* (Tang, J., ed.), pp. 225-247, Plenum Press, New York.

Kahn, J. R., Skeggs, L. T., Jr., Shumway, N. P., and Wisenbaugh, P. E. (1952). The assay of hypertensin from the arterial blood of normotensive and hypertensive human beings. J. Exp. Med. 95: 523-529.

Khosla, M. C., Leese, R. A., Maloy, W. L., Ferreira, A. T., Smeby, R. R., and Bumpus, F. M. (1972). Synthesis of some analogs of angiotensin II as specific antagonists of the parent hormone. J. Med. Chem. 15: 792–795.

Kremen, S. H. and Wakerlin, G. E. (1955). Renin and antirenin in treatment of long term experimental renal hypertension in the dog. Proc. Soc. Exp. Biol. Med. 90: 99–104.

Lanzillo, J. J. and Fanburg, B. L. (1974). Membrane-bound angiotensin-converting enzyme from rat lung. J. Biol. Chem. 249: 2312–2318.

Laragh, J. H., Angers, M., Kelly, W. G., and Lieberman, S. (1960). Hypotensive agents and pressor substances. J.A.M.A. 174: 234–240.

Leckie, B. (1978). Endogenous activator of plasma-inactive-renin. Lancet 2: 217–218.

Leckie, B. J., McConnell, A., Grant, J., Morton, J. J., Tree, M., and Brown, J. J. (1977). An inactive renin in human plasma. Clin. Chim. Acta 83: 249–257.

Leckie, B. J., McConnell, A., and Jordan, J. (1977). Inactive renin – a renin proenzyme? In: *Advances in Experimental Medicine and Biology*, Vol. 95, *Acid Proteases. Structure, Function, and Biology*. (Tang, J., ed.), pp. 249–269, Plenum Press, New York.

Lentz, K. E., Dorer, F. E., Kahn, J. R., Levine, M., and Skeggs, L. T. (1978). Multiple forms of renin substrate in human plasma. Clin. Chim. Acta 83: 249–257.

Lentz, K. E., Skeggs, L. T., Jr., Woods, K. R., Kahn, J. R., and Shumway, N. P. (1956). The amino acid composition of hypertensin II and its biochemical relationship to hypertensin I. J. Exp. Med. 104: 183–191.

Levine, M., Lentz, K. E., Kahn, J. R., Dorer, F. E., and Skeggs, L. T. (1976). Partial purification of a high molecular weight renin from hog kidney. Circ. Res. 38: (Suppl. 2): 90–94.

Levine, M., Lentz, K. E., Kahn, J. R., Dorer, F. E., and Skeggs, L. T. (1978). Studies on high molecular weight renin from hog kidney. Circ. Res. 42: 368–375.

Morishima, H., Takita, T., Aoyagi, T., Takeuchi, T., and Umezawa, H. (1970). The structure of pepstatin. J. Antibiotics (Tokyo) Ser. A 23: 263–265.

Morris, B. J. (1978). Activation of human inactive ("pro"-) renin by cathepsin D and pepsin. J. Clin. Endocrinol. Metab. 46: 153–157.

Morris, B. J. and Day, R. P. (1978). Activation of inactive renin by kallikrein. Int. Res. Commun. Systems Med. Sci.; Physiology 6: 348.

Ng, K. K. F. and Vane, J. R. (1967). Conversion of angiotensin I to angiotensin II. Nature (Lond) 216: 762–766.

Ng, K. K. F. and Vane, J. R. (1970). Some properties of angiotensin converting enzyme in the lung *in vivo*. Nature (lond.) 226: 1142–1144.

Nasjletti, A. and Masson, G. M. C. (1972). Studies on angiotensinogen formation in a liver perfusion system. Circ. Res. 30-31
(Suppl. 2): 187-198.

Osmond, D. H. and Loh, A. Y. (1978). Protease as endogenous activator of inactive renin. Lancet 1: 102.

Page, I. H. and Helmer, O. M. (1940). A crystalline pressor substance (angiotonin) resulting from the reaction between renin
and renin activator. J. Exp. Med. 71: 29-42.

Page, I. H., McSwain, B., Knapp, G. M., and Andrus, W. D. (1941).
The origin of renin-activator. Am. J. Physiol. 135: 214-222.

Pals, D. T., Masucci, F. D., Denning, G. S., Jr., Sipos, F., and
Fessler, D. C. (1971). Role of the pressor action of angiotensin II in experimental hypertension. Circ. Res. 29: 673-
681.

Peart, W. S., (1956). The isolation of a hypertensin. Biochem. J.
62: 520-527.

Plentl, A. A., Page, I. H., and Davis, W. W. (1973). The nature of
renin activator. J. Biol. Chem. 147: 143-153.

Printz, M. P., Printz, J. M., and Dworschack, R. T. (1977). Human
angiotensinogen. J. Biol. Chem. 252: 1654-1662.

Rittel, W., Iselin, B., Kappeler, H., Riniker, B., and Schwyzer, R.
(1975). Synthese eines hochwirksamen Hypertensin II-amids.
Helv. Chim. Acta 40: 614-624.

Roth, M., Weitzman, A. F., and Piquilloud, Y. (1969). Converting
enzyme content of different tissues of the rat. Experientia
25: 1247.

Ryan, J. W., Ryan, U. S., Schultz, D. R., Whitaker, C., Chung, A.,
and Dorer, F. E. (1975). Subcellular localization of pulmonary
angiotensin-converting enzyme (kininase II). Biochem. J. 146:
497-499.

Sander, G. E. and Huggins, C. G. (1971). Subcellular localization
of angiotensin I converting enzyme in rabbit lung. Nature (New
Biology) 230: 27-29.

Schwarz, H., Bumpus, F. M., and Page, I. H. (1957). Synthesis of a
biologically active octapeptide similar to natural isoleucine
angiotonin octapeptide. J. Am. Chem. Soc. 79: 5697-5703.

Shulkes, A. A., Gibson, R. R., and Skinner, S. L. (1978). The
nature of inactive renin in human plasma and amnionic fluid.
Clin. Sci. Mol. Med. 55: 41-50.

Skeggs, L. T., Dorer, F. E., Kahn, J. R., Lentz, K. E., and Levine,
M. (1976). The biochemistry of the renin-angiotensin system
and its role in hypertension. Am. J. Med. 60: 737-748.

Skeggs, L. T., Jr., Kahn, J. R., Lentz, K., and Shumway, N. P. (1957).
The preparation, purification, and amino acid sequence of a
polypeptide renin substrate. J. Exp. Med. 106: 439-453.

Skeggs, L. T., Kahn, J. R., Levine, M., Dorer, F. E., and Lentz, K.
E. (1975). Chronic one-kidney hypertension in rabbits.
I. Treatment with kidney extracts. Circ. Res. 37: 715-724.

Skeggs, L. T., Kahn, J. R., Levine, M., Dorer, F. E., and Lentz, K.
    E. (1976). Chronic one-kidney hypertension in rabbits. II.
    Evidence for a new factor. Circ. Res. 39: 400-406.
Skeggs, L. T., Kahn, J. R., and Shumway, N. P. (1951). The isolatior
    of hypertensin from the circulating blood of normal dogs with
    experimental renal hypertension by dialysis in an artificial
    kidney. Circulation 3: 384-389.
Skeggs, L. T., Jr., Kahn, J. R., and Shumway, N. P. (1956). The
    preparation and function of the hypertensin-converting enzyme.
    J. Exp. Med. 103: 295-299.
Skeggs, L. T., Jr., Lentz, K. E., Hochstrasser, H., and Kahn, J. R.
    (1963). The purification and partial characterization of
    several forms of hog renin substrate. J. Exp. Med. 118: 73-98.
Skeggs, L. T., Lentz, K. E., Kahn, J. R., and Hochstrasser, H.
    (1967). Studies on the preparation and properties of renin.
    Circ. Res. 20-21 (Suppl. 2): 91-100.
Skeggs, L. T., Lentz, K. E., Kahn, J. R., and Hochstrasser, H.
    (1968). Kinetics of the reaction of renin with nine synthetic
    peptide substrates. J. Exp. Med. 128: 13-34.
Skeggs, L. T., Lentz, K. E., Kahn, J. R., Levine, M., and Dorer, F.]
    (1972). Multiple forms of human kidney renin. In: Hyper-
    tension '72 (Genest, J. and Koiw, E., eds.), pp. 149-160,
    Springer-Verlag, New York.
Skeggs, L. T., Jr., Lentz, K. E., Kahn, J. R., and Shumway, N. P.
    (1958). The synthesis of a tetradecapeptide renin substrate.
    J. Exp. Med. 108: 283-297.
Skeggs, L. T., Jr., Marsh, W. H., Kahn, J. R., and Shumway, N. P.
    (1954a). The purification of hypertensin I. J. Exp. Med.
    100: 363-370.
Skeggs, L. T., Jr., Marsh, W. H., Kahn, J. R., and Shumway, N. P.
    (1954b). The existence of two forms of hypertensin. J. Exp.
    Med. 99: 275-282.
Skeggs, L. T., Jr., Marsh, W. H., Kahn, J. R., and Shumway, N. P.
    (1955). Amino acid composition and electrophoretic properties
    of hypertensin I. J. Exp. Med. 102: 435-440.
Skinner, S. L., Cran, E. J., Gibson, R., Taylor, R., Walters, W. A.
    W., and Catt, K. J. (1975). Angiotensin I and II, active and
    inactive renin, renin substrate, renin activity, and angio-
    tensinase in human liquor amnii and plasma. Am. J. Obstet.
    Gynecol. 121: 626-630.
Soffer, R. L., Reza, R., and Caldwell, P. R. B. (1974). Angioten-
    sin-converting enzyme from rabbit pulmonary particles. Proc.
    Nat. Acad. Sci. U. S. 71: 1720-1724.
Tatemichi, S. R. and Osmond, D. H. (1978). Factor XII in endogenous
    activation of inactive renin. Lancet 1: 1313.
Tewksbury, D. A., Frome, W. L., and Dumas, M. L. (1978). Characteri-
    zation of human angiotensinogen. J. Biol. Chem. 253: 3817-3820
Tewksbury, D. A., Premeau, M. R., and Dumas, M. L. (1976). Isolatio:
    of human angiotensinogen. Biochim. Biophys. Acta 446: 87-95.

Tigerstedt, R. and Bergman, P. G. (1898). Niere und Kreislauf. Scand. Arch. Physiol. 8: 223-271.

Umezawa, H., Aoyagi, T., Morishima, H., Matsuzaki, M., Hamada, M., and Takeuchi, T. (1970). Pepstatin, a new pepsin inhibitor produced by actinomycetes. J. Antibiotics (Tokyo) Ser. A 23: 259-262.

Vallotton, M. B. (1974). Immunogenicity and antigenicity of angiotensin I and II. In: *Handbook of Experimental Pharmacology*, Vol. 37, *Angiotensin*. (Page, I. H. and Bumpus, F. M., eds.), pp. 185-200, Springer-Verlag, New York.

Wakerlin, G. E. (1958). Antibodies to renin as proof of the pathogenesis of sustained renal hypertension. Circulation 17: 653-657.

Wakerlin, G. E., Bird, R. B., Brennan, B. B., Frank, M. H., Kreman, S., Kuperman, I., and Skom, J. H. (1953). Treatment and prophylaxis of experimental renal hypertension with "renin". J. Lab. Clin. Med. 41: 708-728.

Yokosawa, H., Inagami, T., and Haas, E. (1978). Purification of human renin. Biochem. Biophys. Res. Commun. 83: 306-312.

DISCUSSION AFTER DR. SKEGGS' PAPER

Dr. Davis

Thank you very much, Dr. Skeggs. That was the best presentation that I have heard on the history of the development of our knowledge of the renin-angiotensin system. It was delightful to hear about your elegant studies and the many ways that you have contributed to this field. Let me open the discussion by asking a question which is only indirectly related to the renin-angiotensin system, but while we have Dr. Skeggs here we would be remiss if we didn't ask him to say something about other possible humoral substances that are secreted by the kidneys. He is, as you know, one of the leaders in this area and has done extensive work in it, and is very actively engaged in it now. I would like for you to say a word or so about the work you are doing now.

Dr. Skeggs

I didn't go into our recent work because the subject of the conference is the renin-angiotensin system, and I didn't think I should talk about the renin system for fifty minutes and then suddenly say, "I don't think that renin is all that important in hypertension", because, in fact, it is very important. There seems to be no question that the blood pressure of many hypertensives is supported by the renin system. On the other hand, the blood pressure of some hypertensives is not supported by the renin system. This form must resemble one-kidney hypertension in animals, which also is not renin dependent. Let me emphasize that I think that both forms of hypertension have a renal basis. I believe that

Dr. Goldblatt's experiments are still valid. It has to be true
that something comes from the kidney and causes hypertension in
both forms of the disease. That doesn't necessarily mean that
the material coming from the one-kidney hypertensive animal has to
act directly on an arteriole. It could act in a very indirect way.
One could imagine, for example, that the central nervous system is
involved. But there has to be something coming from the kidney
that initiates the hypertensive process.

How can we discover what this substance might be? The best
clue comes from Wakerlin (see Wakerlin *et al.*, 1953), who lowered
the blood pressure of hypertensive dogs by immunization with hog
kidney extracts. It is important to realize that most of the work
of Wakerlin and of Haas and others on this subject was performed
using animals with one-kidney hypertension, and that one-kidney
hypertension is not supported by renin but by some other unknown
substance or system. Consideration of these facts led us to believe
that the blood pressures in Wakerlin's dogs must have been lowered
by antibodies against some unknown agent and not by antibodies
against renin.

We started working with rabbits to produce antibodies against
the hypertensive agent in question. It took us a long time to
achieve success, but we finally were able to obtain extracts from
hog kidneys that would produce antibodies which would lower the
arterial pressure in one-kidney hypertensive rabbits. I have a
slide which summarizes the results of this work (Figure 6). This
is one of our experiments. In this slide, RN,LC means right nephrectomy, left kidney clipped. The arterial pressure measurements
were indirect and were obtained from the central artery of the ear.
The arterial pressures in our hypertensive rabbits generally do not
exceed 110 mm Hg. We started injecting hypertensive rabbits with
an extract obtained from hog kidneys. This particular preparation
contained renin, and therefore an anti-renin titer developed. The
arterial pressure fell in these rabbits, and when we stopped the
immunizations, the arterial pressures went up again. We have performed this experiment using an antigen that did not contain any
renin at all and where no anti-renin titer was produced, and we
obtained the same lowering of arterial pressure. Thus, we are
convinced that our extracts with which we are immunizing and lowering the arterial pressure of hypertensive rabbits do contain an
antigen that is chemically similar to the agent causing one-kidney
hypertension, and we are now working hard to isolate this substance.

Our problems are enormous because the only assay we have is to
test for blood pressure lowering activity in hypertensive rabbits.
As all of you probably know, there is no dose-response relationship
between the amount of antigen given an animal and the antibody
titer that is obtained. I was very optomistic and thought that

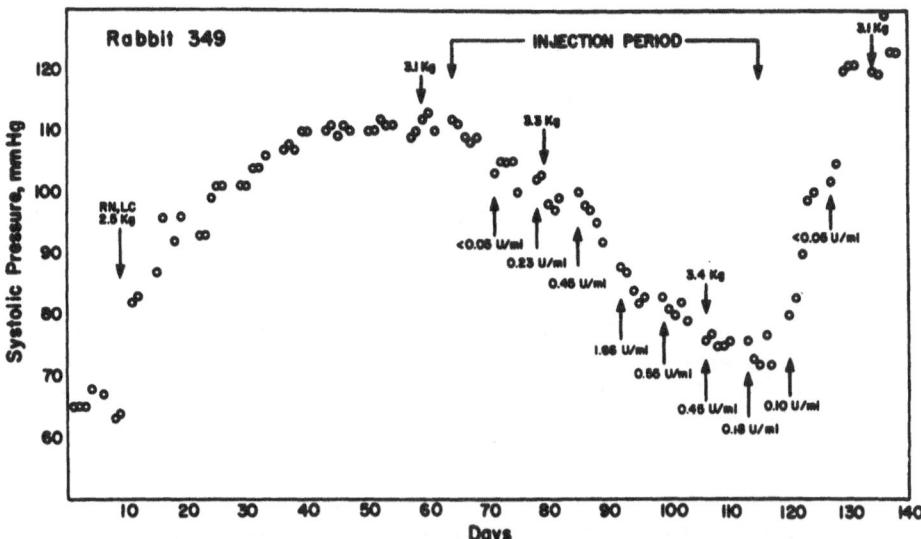

Figure 6. Effect of the injection of a hog kidney cortex prepa-
ration on the blood pressure of a rabbit with one-kidney
hypertension. From Skeggs, L. T. et al. (1975). Circ.
Res. 37: 715-724.

there would be a relationship, but I have to concede now that every-
body who told me there wasn't one was perfectly correct.

In the meantime we have found that we can elevate the blood
pressure of normal rabbits by subcutaneous injection of certain
kidney extracts for a period of 10 to 20 days. A strange thing is
that the arterial pressure usually remains elevated for several days
or weeks after the last injection. The substance that causes this
we call "renopressin". I must say that we have been disappointed
in renopressin, because we have had so little success in purification.
Again, we have the same assay problem: it is totally nonquantitative
as far as we can tell. We give kidney extracts varying in amounts
from 1 to 5 mg per day, and whether or not we get a response doesn't
seem to depend on how much we give.

We have 88 rabbits in our colony, and we are totally dependent
on them for assays, both for renopressin and for the blood pressure
lowering antigen. We're struggling along trying to isolate both
substances. We are up against a very difficult problem. We are
presently trying, by means of immunoelectrophoresis, to identify
that precipitin line on our plates which is the blood pressure
lowering antigen. If we can identify the precipitin line, we can
develop an *in vitro* immunological assay, which we need desperately.

Dr. Goetz

I wonder whether you have any opinions, or if you could tell
us where you think tonin might fit into this system, as far as the
production of angiotensin II?

Dr. Skeggs

I really have no idea. Historically, there have been many
factors brought forth over the years. Prorenin is a case in point.
At the moment this is a very important subject.

Dr. Nishimura

I always become very confused about small renin and big renin.
Do you think prorenin is the same as big renin? It appears they
are both activated similarly by acid, by trypsin, or by cold temperatures. Also, when a peptide is activated during freezing, does that
indicate that its conformation was changed?

Dr. Skeggs

Cold might activate an enzyme, which in turn might act on big
renin to activate it.

Dr. Miller

The hypertensive agent that you have indicated in the slide,
is that a protein?

Dr. Skeggs

I think so, because it serves as an antigen. It could be something else, but usually antigens have fairly high molecular weights.
Usually they are proteins. Also, we used protein methods to isolate it.

Dr. Miller

You have eliminated the possibility of a lipid, then?

Dr. Skeggs

Not entirely, no. A lipid can serve as an antigen, and therefore it could be a lipid.

Dr. Miller

We spent about three years trying to isolate a lipid which was
not a prostaglandin, from the kidney, and finally gave up. The
purer we got it, the less activity it had.

Dr. Skeggs

Was that with Dr. Muirhead, or along his line of work?

Dr. Miller

That type of thing, yes, although apparently ours was slightly
different from his. We don't think it was the same substance he

has been studying. However, I was wondering if your substance
might be in that same class. Another thing I was wondering, I don't
know whether you are familiar with our work on the so-called "sustained pressor principle" which we reported some years ago.

Dr. Skeggs
I have read that paper many times.

Dr. Miller
When that material is injected, it does not give the sustained
pressor response in an intact animal, but does so only in the nephrectomized animal. I was wondering if the material you're talking
about could be assayed better in nephrectomized animals?

Dr. Skeggs
I have speculated the same thing myself.

Dr. Peach
Dr. Skeggs, I would like to ask about the location of the angio
tensin converting-enzyme. You showed a micrograph from Dr. Ryan's
work on the location of the enzyme. As I recall their work in looking at different vascular beds, don't you think that converting enzyme is an endothelial enzyme and will be located in any vascular
bed, since vessels contain endothelial cells? Does this influence
your thinking from the standpoint of Dr. Vane's slide that you
showed?

Dr. Skeggs
I think this is quite possible. But the question really is,
which is the predominant pathway? We are still in the position of
guessing, because there doesn't seem to be any way to do a truly
physiological experiment. One can't get a meaningful result by
using enormous doses of angiotensin. The real question is, what
happens when tiny amounts of angiotensin I circulate? Where is
it converted?

Dr. Cushman
Have you ruled out the possibility that the small amount of
converting enzyme which might be present in the kidney could be
antigenic, and that your studies with the antibodies could actually
be antibody production to converting enzyme?

Dr. Skeggs
No, we really don't have any way to rule that out, except that
I don't believe you will lower the blood pressure of these rabbits
with a converting enzyme inhibitor.

COMPARATIVE ENDOCRINOLOGY OF RENIN AND ANGIOTENSIN[1]

Hiroko Nishimura

Department of Physiology and Biophysics
University of Tennessee Center for Health Sciences
Memphis, TN 38163

OUTLINE

I. Introduction

II. Evolution of the juxtaglomerular apparatus and renal renin
    A. Juxtaglomerular apparatus in primitive vertebrates
    B. Occurrence of renal renin activity
    C. Extrarenal renin

III. Biochemistry of the renin-angiotensin system
    A. Renin-substrate and renin reaction
    B. Angiotensin
    C. Angiotensin converting enzyme
    D. Angiotensinases

IV. Vasopressor action of angiotensin and angiotensin receptors
    A. Vasopressor action of exogenously administered angiotensin
    B. Angiotensin receptors in blood vessels

V. The role of hemodynamic factors in control of renin release
    A. Effect of hemorrhage
    B. Effect of vasodilatory drugs
    C. Effect of blood volume

---

[1]Unpublished research from the author's laboratory described in the text is supported by a research grant from the National Science Foundation, PCM 75-20645, and by research grant AM 17824 from the National Institute of Arthritis, Metabolism, and Digestive Diseases. H. Nishimura is an Established Investigator, American Heart Assn.

I. INTRODUCTION

The renin-angiotensin system evolved during early evolution of
bony fishes and is found in a variety of teleosts and tetrapods.
However, the morphological appearance of the juxtaglomerular (JG)
apparatus, the biochemical properties of renin and angiotensin, the
characteristics of the angiotensin receptors, and presumably the
physiological functions and roles of the renin-angiotensin system
differ in primitive vertebrates from those in mammals. Because of
difficulties in obtaining taxonomically appropriate species and
problems in establishing appropriate laboratory conditions for these
species, plus the necessity of using unique surgical and analytical
techniques, the number of investigators involved in this field is
limited. Thus, the information available to date on the comparative
aspects of the renin-angiotensin system is not large. Sokabe and
Ogawa (1974) reviewed the literature extensively and summarized the
comparative studies of the JG apparatus. The present article will
review primarily the recent advancements in the biochemical and
physiological aspects of the renin-angiotensin system in nonmammalian
vertebrates. Based on currently available information, this article
also will speculate on the evolutionary trend of the role of this
hormonal system and will examine the phylogenetical relationship
between the adrenergic nervous system and the renin-angiotensin system. The phylogeny of the renal effects of angiotensin (Sokabe,
1974) and the role of the renin-angiotensin system in hydromineral
regulation (Taylor, 1977) were reviewed previously. Details of the
literature on the physiological aspect has been published elsewhere
(Nishimura, 1978).

Comparative studies provide unique approaches which may unravel the chemical and functional evolution of the renin-angiotensin system and which may answer questions such as: What were the original functions of this system in primitive animals, and how did the functions change during adaptation of living creatures to diverse environments, from marine to the freshwater environment, and from aquatic to terrestrial life? The renin-angiotensin system exerts multiple actions and functions in man and other mammals. Some of these functions may have been more important in primitive animals, although a similar function remains in man as a relic of the primitive system, since man is the result of a long history of natural selection of physiological processes (C. Ladd Prosser). By providing a perspective in the "developmental process" of the renin-angiotensin system, comparative approaches will aid in understanding and dissecting out the underlying mechanisms operating in mammals.

II. EVOLUTION OF THE JUXTAGLOMERULAR APPARATUS AND RENAL RENIN

A. Juxtaglomerular Apparatus in Primitive Vertebrates

The JG apparatus of the mammalian kidney is composed of the afferent (JG cells) and efferent arterioles, the convoluted distal tubule (macula densa), and the extracellular mesangium (Barajas and Latta, 1967). The JG cells in mammals possess a rich sympathetic innervation (Barajas, 1964). The JG apparatus in nonmammalian vertebrates is incomplete. Primitive bony fishes, teleosts, lungfishes, amphibians, and reptiles have granulated epitheloid cells, resembling mammalian JG cells, in the media of small arteries and arterioles of the kidney (Sokabe, Ogawa, Oguri, and Nishimura, 1969; Nishimura, Ogawa, and Sawyer, 1973). Krishnamurthy and Bern (1969) identified six types of distribution of JG cells in teleosts in relation to arteries, arterioles, and glomeruli, and five different types of granules have been identified microscopically in teleost JG cells (Bulger and Trump, 1969). Kidneys from the aglomerular teleosts also possess granulated cells (Oguri, Ogawa, and Sokabe, 1972).

Granulated cells have not been found in the more primitive vertebrates, the cyclostomes and elasmobranchs (Nishimura, Oguri, Ogawa, et al., 1970). Holocephalians, a cartilagenous fish differing from elasmobranchs, do possess granulated cells, although the appearance and distribution pattern of the granules differ slightly from those seen in teleost fishes (Nishimura, Ogawa, and Sawyer, 1973; Oguri, 1978). It has been shown that holocephalians resemble teleosts in some endocrinological aspects, although morphologically they resemble elasmobranchs.

In the majority of the species examined, the distal tubules do not attach to the vascular pole of their parent glomerulus (Sokabe, Ogawa, Oguri, and Nishimura, 1969; Nishimura, Ogawa, and Sawyer,

1973). Thus, they lack a macula densa and an extraglomerular mesangium. In elasmobranchs, holocephalians, and presumably in some amphibians (Edwards, 1940; Capelli, Wesson, and Aponte, 1970), distal tubules return to their own glomeruli and attach to the afferent arterioles, but no cells which resemble mammalian macula densa cells are present (Sokabe, Ogawa, Oguri, and Nishimura, 1969). The available literature does not agree as to the presence of a macula densa in amphibians. Avian kidneys, however, possess macula densa cells which show some characteristics of a mammalian macula densa (Ogawa and Sokabe, 1971). Therefore, the JG apparatus in birds represents a transitional form between the primitive type and mammalian type of JG apparatus.

B. Occurrence of Renal Renin Activity

The presence or absence of renal renin activity has been determined in various species of nonmammalian vertebrates. This is done by incubating extracts of their kidneys with homologous plasma under adequate inhibition of angiotensinases and then testing the vasopressor activity of the product in the anesthetized rat (Sokabe and Ogawa, 1974). Vasopressor substances were produced in this manner from kidneys of primitive bony fishes, teleosts, lungfishes, amphibians, reptiles, and birds (Sokabe, Ogawa, Oguri, and Nishimura, 1969; Nishimura, Ogawa, and Sawyer, 1973). The vasopressor substance is biologically similar to that obtained using mammalian kidneys. However, the pressor activity of the product from holocephalians was low (Nishimura, Ogawa, and Sawyer, 1973) and no vasopressor substance was formed by incubating the kidney and plasma from several species of cyclostomes and elasmobranchs (Nishimura, Oguri, Ogawa, *et al.*, 1970).

The amount of renal renin activity is in accord with the occurrence of granulated cells except in some holosteans and chondrosteans in which granules do not take up stain. This suggests that the histochemical properties of renin granules may differ in these fishes. Also, in teleost fish the intensity of the stainable granules does not necessarily agree with that of the biochemically determined renin activity (Oguri and Sokabe, 1968).

Figure 1 summarizes the occurrence of the JG apparatus and renin among vertebrates. Renal renin activity and JG cells probably evolved during early development of bony fishes, whereas macula densa cells evolved in a more recent stage of phylogeny. Therefore, the vascular component of the JG apparatus evolved phylogenetically earlier than the tubular component. This is important when we consider the function of the renin-angiotensin system in nonmammalian vertebrates.

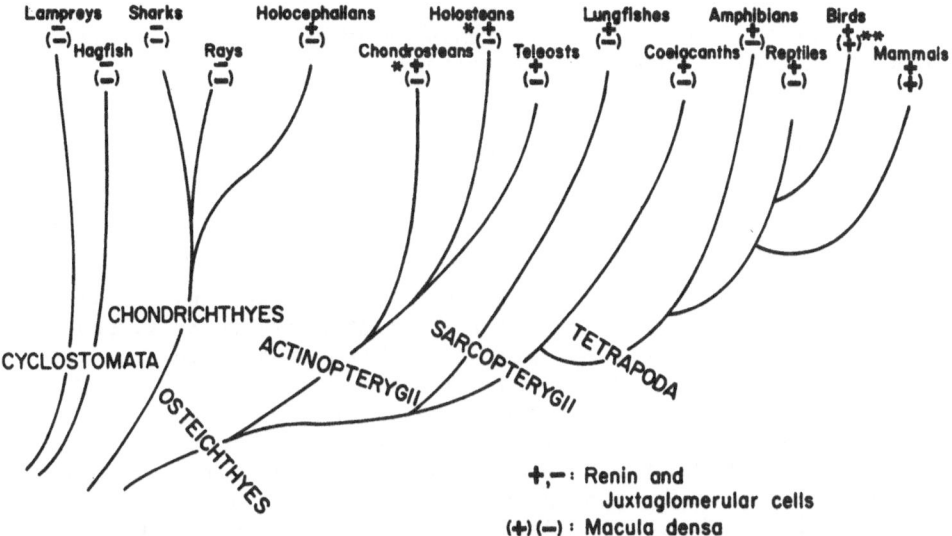

Figure 1. A diagram of the vertebrate phylogenetic tree and the presence and absence of the renin-angiotensin system among various classes of the vertebrates. Studies from several groups are summarized. *Renin activity was noted, but granules were not stained or showed different properties by Bowie's method. **A primitive form of macula densa.

C.   Extrarenal Renin

Saline extracts of the corpuscles of Stannius (CS) from the European eel (Chester-Jones, Henderson, Chan, *et al.*, 1966), carp, goldfish, and aglomerular Japanese goosefish (Sokabe, Nishimura, Ogawa, and Oguri, 1970) formed an angiotensin-like substance when incubated with homologous plasma. The CS had granules which were stained by periodic acid-Schiff and Bowie's method, but the granules were coarse and their appearance differed slightly from that of JG granules in the kidney (Sokabe, Nishimura, Ogawa, and Oguri, 1970). The CS contain a calcium-decreasing substance named hypocalcin (Pang, Pang, and Sawyer, 1974). An angiotensin-like substance produced in CS homogenate from the carp by incubating with carp plasma decreased plasma calcium levels of intact eels (Ogawa, 1977). It remains to be determined whether the CS angiotensin or renin is chemically the same substance as "hypocalcin".

The presence or absence of renin activity in the brain has not been determined in nonmammalian vertebrates.

III. BIOCHEMISTRY OF THE RENIN-ANGIOTENSIN SYSTEM

A. Renin-Substrate and Renin Reaction

Plasma from nonmammalian vertebrates contains renin-substrate (angiotensinogen). The angiotensin-forming activity of kidney extracts added to heterologous plasma has been studied in a variety of species (Schaffenburg, Haas, and Goldblatt, 1960; Grill, Granger, and Thurau, 1972; Nolly and Fasciolo, 1972). The reaction of renin on renin-substrate shows relatively strong species specificity. Angiotensinogen levels in the plasma appear to be higher in taxonomically more-advanced animals than in lower vertebrates (Nolly and Fasciolo, 1972; Nishimura, Ogawa, and Sawyer, 1973). The optimum pH for the reaction of plasma renin on renin-substrate in the aglomerular toadfish was 6.2 to 6.5 (Nishimura, Crofton, Norton, and Share, 1977), but the generation of angiotensin from plasma and kidney extracts in nonmammalian vertebrates usually is better at pH 7.4 (Mizogami, Oguri, Sokabe, and Nishimura, 1968) than at an acidic pH, presumably because angiotensinases are inhibited more completely at a neutral pH (Nishimura and Sokabe, 1968). Incubation of renin with substrate at 20° C is suitable for cold-blooded animals (Mizogami, Oguri, Sokabe, and Nishimura, 1968; Nishimura, Ogawa, and Sawyer, 1973).

Kidney extracts from the eel, toadfish, fowl, and rat produce angiotensin from the synthetic [Asp^1, Ile^5, His^9] tetradecapeptide substrate (human TDP substrate) and from [Asp^1, Val^5, Ser^9] TDP (fowl TDP substrate[2]) (Mugaas, Khosla, and Nishimura, unpublished). Angiotensin formation at pH 7.4 is higher with human TDP than with fowl TDP in all species examined; however, there is a possibility that the enzyme which hydrolyzes TDP is pseudorenin.

B. Angiotensin

The amino acid sequence of angiotensin I (AI) from three nonmammalian species, a fowl (white Leghorn, *Gallus gallus*) (Nakayama, Nakajima, and Sokabe, 1973), a snake (*Elaphe climocophora*) (Nakayama, Nakajima, and Sokabe, 1977), and a fish (Japanese goosefish, *Lophius litulon*) (Hayashi, Nakayama, Nakajima, and Sokabe, 1978) have been determined (Figure 2). It appears that the variation

---

[2]Synthesized by Dr. M. C. Khosla, Cleveland Clinic Foundation.

Equine, Hog, Human, Rat, Dog

$$\underline{Asp}^1 - Arg^2 - Val^3 - Tyr^4 - \underline{Ile}^5 - His^6 - Pro^7 - Phe^8 - \underline{His}^9 - Leu^{10}$$

Bovine

$$\underline{Asp}^1 - Arg^2 - Val^3 - Tyr^4 - \underline{Val}^5 - His^6 - Pro^7 - Phe^8 - \underline{His}^9 - Leu^{10}$$

Fowl

$$\underline{Asp}^1 - Arg^2 - Val^3 - Tyr^4 - \underline{Val}^5 - His^6 - Pro^7 - Phe^8 - \underline{Ser}^9 - Leu^{10}$$

Japanese goosefish
Lophius litulon

$$\underline{Asn}^1 - Arg^2 - Val^3 - Tyr^4 - \underline{Val}^5 - His^6 - Pro^7 - Phe^8 - \underline{His}^9 - Leu^{10}$$

Snake
Elaphe climocophora

$$\underline{Asp}^1 - Arg^2 - Val^3 - Tyr^4 - \underline{Val}^5 - His^6 - Pro^7 - Phe^8 - \underline{Tyr}^9 - Leu^{10}$$
$$(X - \underline{Asx})$$

*Figure 2. Amino acid sequence of currently known native angio-
tensin I in vertebrates. Changes of the structure of
angiotensin seem to have occurred at the 1st, 5th, and
9th amino acids during vertebrate evolution.*

of the amino acid of the decapeptide AI occurred in positions 1, 5, and 9 during phylogeny of the vertebrates. It is of interest to note that [Asn^1, Val^5] angiotensin II (AII-amide), which has been synthesized and used for clinical and experimental studies, is the native angiotensin for the goosefish.

Three angiotensin-like substances were identified in the incubation product from snake kidney and plasma: 1) [Asp^1, Val^5] AII (so-called bovine AII), 2) nona- and 3) decapeptide with tyrosine at position 9. However, the N-terminal of both the nona- and decapeptides contained an unidentified substance (Nakayama, Nakajima, and Sokabe, 1977).

Nakajima, Nakayama, and Sokabe (1971) attempted to characterize angiotensin-like substances in selected species of teleost fishes,

amphibians, reptiles, birds, and other mammals by fractionating them
with SE-Sephadex column chromatography. Products derived from
teleost fishes were eluted with pH and ionic strength gradients in
two peaks, neither of which exactly coincided with those of known
mammalian angiotensins I or II.

Partially purified angiotensins (angiotensin I preparation)
from an aglomerular teleost, the toadfish (*Opsanus tau*), the African
lungfish (*Protopterus aethiopicus*), and the rainbow trout (*Salmo
gairdneri*) were bound by a human angiotensin I antibody (Nishimura,
Crofton, Norton, and Share, 1977, and unpublished), suggesting that
a part, or all, of the angiotensin molecule of these animals is
similar to that of human AI. Angiotensin from the American eel,
the channel catfish, and the South American lungfish, as well as
synthetic fowl AI, were not bound by human AI antibody. Plasma
renin activity (determined by the rate of angiotensin I generation)
and plasma angiotensinogen levels (determined by the maximal amount
of angiotensin formed after incubation of the plasma with an excess
of renal renin), measured in toadfish by radioimmunoassay using
human AI antibody, correlated well with the values obtained when
measured by the rat pressor bioassay.

C. Angiotensin Converting Enzyme

Dorsal aortic pressure in eels was increased during the administration of [Asp^1, Val^5]AII, [Asp^1, Val^5, Ser^9]AI (fowl AI), and by
a partially purified preparation of natural eel AI (Nishimura,
Norton, and Bumpus, 1978). Pretreatment of eels with a converting
enzyme inhibitor, SQ 20,881 (Squibb) which has been shown to inhibit
angiotensin converting enzyme in mammals, inhibited the pressor responses to eel and fowl AI, but not those to AII. This suggests that
a converting enzyme-like substance may exist in eels.

Opdyke and Holcombe (1976) found that the vasopressor effect of
[Asp^1, Ile^5, His^9]AI in the spiny dogfish, *Squalus acanthias*, was
inhibited by SQ 20,881. This finding is particularly interesting
since neither renin nor JG cells have been found in elasmobranchs
(Nishimura, Oguri, Ogawa, *et al.*, 1970). Thus, the evolution of
converting enzyme may precede the evolution of renin. It is also
possible that the enzyme which was blocked by SQ 20,881 was brady-
kininase in elasmobranchs. Converting enzyme activity also has
been shown in the fowl (Sokabe and Watanabe, 1977).

D. Angiotensinases

Angiotensinase activities have been shown in the plasma and

kidney from a variety of nonmammalian species including the cyclostomes and elasmobranchs, which do not possess renin (Nishimura and
Sokabe, 1968). As in mammals, plasma from the lamprey, a cyclo-
stome, contains an angiotensinase which is active at neutral pH.
Kidney extracts contain at least two angiotensinases; one of these
is active at pH 7.4 and the other at pH 5.0. Angiotensinases in
plasma and kidneys of nonmammalian vertebrates are inhibited by
acid- or alkaline treatment, EDTA, diisopropyl fluorophosphate
(DFP), phenylmethylsulfonylfluoride (PMSF: Sigma), adsorption of
angiotensin onto Dowex-resin, or a combination of these treatments
(Mizogami, Oguri, Sokabe, and Nishimura, 1968; Nishimura and Sokabe,
1968; Nishimura, Crofton, Norton, and Share, 1977). Thus, it is
unlikely that angiotensinases are specific enzymes which are
involved only in inactivation of angiotensin II.

IV. VASOPRESSOR ACTION OF ANGIOTENSIN AND ANGIOTENSIN RECEPTORS

A. Vasopressor Action of Exogenously Administered Angiotensin

Exogenous administration of a homologous kidney extract,
natural homologous angiotensin (product of the incubation of kidney
extract with homologous plasma), or synthetic angiotensins I or II
produced vasopressor actions in an elasmobranch (Opdyke and Holcombe,
1976), teleost fishes (Chester-Jones, Henderson, Chan, *et al.*, 1966;
Nishimura and Sawyer, 1976), lungfishes (Sawyer, 1970; Sawyer,
Blair-West, Simpson, and Sawyer, 1976), amphibians (Johnston, Davis,
Wright, and Howards, 1967; Taylor and Davis, 1971; Grill, Granger,
and Thurau, 1972), reptiles (Nothstine, Davis, and DeRoos, 1971),
and birds (Taylor, Davis, Breitenbach, and Hartroft, 1970; Chan and
Holmes, 1971; Moore, 1978). Thus, vasopressor action appears to be
a phylogenetically old function of angiotensin (see Table 1).

Injection of homologous kidney extract produced a prolonged
pressor effect (Johnston, Davis, Wright, and Howards, 1967), whereas
injections of angiotensins showed rapid onset and shorter vasopressor
responses. No study has been reported on the pressor effect of
angiotensin or renin in cyclostomes. The pressor activity of
$[Asp^1, Val^5, Ser^9]AI$ (the native fowl AI) is approximately half
of that of $[Asp^1, Val^5]AII$ (the native fowl AII) in the anesthetized
chicken (Sumner, Mugaas, and Nishimura, unpublished). In the
conscious chicken, however, the response to $[Asn^1, Val^5]AII$ is
biphasic--an initial depressor response followed by a pressor
response (Moore, Strong, and Buckley, 1978). The depressor response
was inhibited during tachyphylaxis to vasopressin, suggesting that
AII induces a release of posterior pituitary hormone.

Table 1. VASOPRESSOR ACTION OF ANGIOTENSIN

| | | Vasopressor Response | | |
Class	Renin-Angiotensin System	Angiotensin	Blockade by α-adrenergic blocking drugs	References
Elasmobranchs	–	↑	100%	Opdyke and Holcombe, 1976
Teleosts	+	↑	30-40%	Nishimura, Norton and Bumpus, 1978
Lungfishes	+	↑	-----	
Amphibians	+	↑	-----	
Reptiles	+	↑	50%	J. E. Zehr, personal communication
Birds	+	↑	100%	Harvey, Copen, Ekelson et al., 1954, Moore, 1978

References listed in this table are those for "blockade of angiotensin's pressor action by α-adrenergic blocking drugs."

B. Angiotensin Receptors in Blood Vessels

Since the renin-angiotensin system evolved in primitive bony fishes, and since selected animals from all classes from elasmobranchs to mammals respond to angiotensin or renin by increases in blood pressure, we presume that the angiotensin receptor also evolved in the early stage of vertebrate phylogeny. However, angiotensin receptors in primitive vertebrates appear to have different properties from those in mammals. In mammals, angiotensin analogues in which the aromatic structure of phenylalanine in position 8 of the peptide was replaced by aliphatic residues (leucine, valine, isoleucine) have been shown to act as specific antagonists at various angiotensin receptor sites (Regoli, Park, and Rioux, 1974; Turker, Page, and Bumpus, 1974; Peach, 1977). However, [Sar[1], Ile[8]]AII and [Sar[1], Thr[8]]AII (10 µg/kg per min) did not inhibit the vasopressor action of either [Asn[1], Val[5]]AII or natural eel angiotensin in eels (Nishimura, Norton, and Bumpus, 1978). On the other hand, angiotensin analogues which have an aromatic-group amino acid in position 8 appears to be important in determining the affinity of angiotensin for receptors, as well as in evoking intrinsic action through the secondary mechanism in the receptor (Bumpus, 1977). In eels, the aromatic group in position 8 may be necessary both for inducing pressor action and for binding to the receptors on the vascular smooth muscle cells.

Furthermore, in some species of primitive vertebrates a part or perhaps even all of the pressor action of AII appears to be due to a release of catecholamines (Table 1). In the unanesthetized spiny dogfish shark, *Squalus acanthias*, in which neither renin nor JG cells have been detected, the pressor response to [Asn[1], Val[5]]AII was entirely inhibited by the alpha adrenergic blocking drug, phentolamine (Opdyke and Holcombe, 1976). This interesting observation raises two questions: 1) Did angiotensin receptors evolve prior to the emergence of renin and angiotensin? 2) Is the vasopressor action of angiotensin entirely indirect, possibly being mediated by catecholamines?

Possible interaction between angiotensin and the sympathoadrenal system has been observed in several nonmammalian species. In unanesthetized eels the vasopressor response to [Asn[1], Val[5]]AII was reduced by 30-40% by the administration of phentolamine or phenoxybenzamine, and was reduced by 70% following depletion of catecholamines by reserpine (Nishimura, Norton, and Bumpus, 1978). In the unanesthetized turtle (J. E. Zehr, personal communication) approximately 50% of the vasopressor action induced by [Asn[1], Val[5]] AII was inhibited by phentolamine; the remainder of the pressor action was abolished by the simultaneous application of the mammalian AII antagonist, [Sar[1], Ile[8]]AII. Angiotonin, an earlier, cruder preparation of AII, either produced pressor or depressor effects or caused no response in the anesthetized chicken (Harvey, Copen, Eskelson, *et al*., 1954); this pressor action of angiotonin was entirely blocked by phentolamine. Vasopressor responses to [Asn¹, Val⁵]AII and to norepinephrine were equally inhibited by phentolamine in the anesthetized chicken (Moore, 1978).

In vitro studies also indicate that angiotensin may not exert a direct action on vascular smooth muscle in some species. Somlyo, Somlyo, and Woo (1967) observed that isolated vascular strips of pulmonary and sciatic arteries from domestic chickens showed no contractile responses to [Asn¹, Val⁵]AII (10 µg/ml). Isolated spirally-cut fowl aortas failed to contract in response to AI, AII, or AIII at concentrations up to 5 x 10⁻⁵ g/ml (Moore, 1978). No changes in vascular resistance occurred in the isolated, perfused dogfish gut preparation after application of [Asp¹, Ile⁵, His⁹]AI or [Asn¹, Val⁵] AII (Opdyke and Holcombe, 1978), whereas epinephrine caused a marked increase in flow resistance. Indeed, also in mammals a considerable portion of the pressor action of angiotensin may be ascribed to catecholamine release from the adrenal medulla and to a complex interaction between the angiotensin molecule and the sympathoadrenal system (Muñoz-Ramírez, Khosla, Bumpus, and Khairallah, 1975).

It has been shown that in mammals the presence of the [Phe⁸] residue of angiotensin is an absolute requirement for stimulation of catecholamine release (Peach, 1977). Also, there is some evidence to suggest that the NH_2-terminal amino acid may be important for the stimulation of catecholamine release. Removal of the aspartic acid in position 1 or its replacement by sarcosine almost totally abolished the secretory activity of [Ala⁸]AII and [Ile⁸]AII in the isolated cat adrenal medulla (Peach and Ober, 1974; Peach and Ackerly, 1976; Bumpus and Khosla, 1977). [Asn¹]AII appears to be more potent in stimulating catecholamine release than is [Asp¹]AII (P. Khairallah, personal communication).

Preliminary results from our laboratory also indicate that [Asn¹, Val⁵]AII and [Asn¹, Ile⁵]AII exert more potent vasopressor actions in unanesthetized eels than do [Asp¹, Ile⁵]AII or [Asp¹, Val⁵]AII. These AII analogues, as well as norepinephrine, increased the heart rate in eels, and their vasopressor actions were considerably inhibited by phentolamine. [Sar¹, Ile⁵]AII had less pressor action and did not increase the heart rate in eels (Nishimura, Madey, and Khairallah, unpublished). It is of interest to note that the amino acids in positions 1, 5, and 9 have changed during the evolution of vertebrates. Stimulation of catecholamine release may be one of the phylogenetically older functions of angiotensin, and the change in this function of angiotensin with evolution may be related to a structural change in position 1. Recent studies in mammals also show that [Val⁵]AII and [Ile⁵]AII have different pressor potencies (Watanabe, Sokabe, Honda, *et al*., 1977; Khosla, Bumpus, Hayashi, *et al*., 1977).

V. THE ROLE OF HEMODYNAMIC FACTORS IN CONTROL OF RENIN RELEASE

A. Effect of Hemorrhage

Since the kidneys from primitive vertebrates lack a macula densa, the possible baroreceptor function in JG cells may be important in the regulation of renin release in these animals. The toadfish, an aglomerular teleost, provides an ideal model to determine whether a baroreceptor exists in primitive vertebrates for controlling renin release. In addition, plasma renin activity (PRA) can be measured by radioimmunoassay in the toadfish under various experimental conditions. Graded hemorrhages (Figure 3) or a single massive bleeding (50-60% of the estimated blood volume) from unanesthetized toadfish kept in 50% seawater caused immediate and significant decreases in mean aortic pressure and stepwise increases in PRA (Nishimura, Lunde, and Zucker, 1979). These results indicated that the toadfish responds to decreases in blood pressure and/or blood volume by increases in renin release, in spite of the absence of a macula densa; these findings suggest that primitive vertebrates have a functional renal baroreceptor mechanism for controlling renin release.

Blaine, Davis, and Witty (1970) developed a nonfiltering kidney model in the dog, in which the macula densa was made nonfunctional by permanently ligating the ureters and clamping the renal arteries for 2 hours; hemorrhage increased the renin release from these dogs with denervated, nonfiltering kidneys. Our studies in the toadfish support their conclusion from studies in the nonfiltering dog kidney, that a change in sodium delivery to the macula densa is not essential for renin release during hemorrhage. A difference in studying renin release in the toadfish as compared to the nonfiltering dog model is that in the toadfish the macula densa is absent morphologically, and the excretory function of the kidney remains intact.

Chan and Holmes (1971) found that acute hemorrhage increased PRA in intact and in hypophysectomized pigeons in proportion to the amount of blood withdrawn. Hypophysectomized pigeons had low blood pressures and high PRA values as compared to the intact pigeons.

B. Effect of Vasodilatory Drugs

The intraarterial injection of papaverine (10 mg/kg) in the toadfish increased PRA (5-20 fold) with a concomitant decrease in blood pressure. Neither PRA nor blood pressure were altered after minoxidil (Nishimura, Lunde, and Zucker, 1979). Both papaverine and minoxidil have been shown to increase PRA in man and other mammals. These results imply that renin is released in the toad-

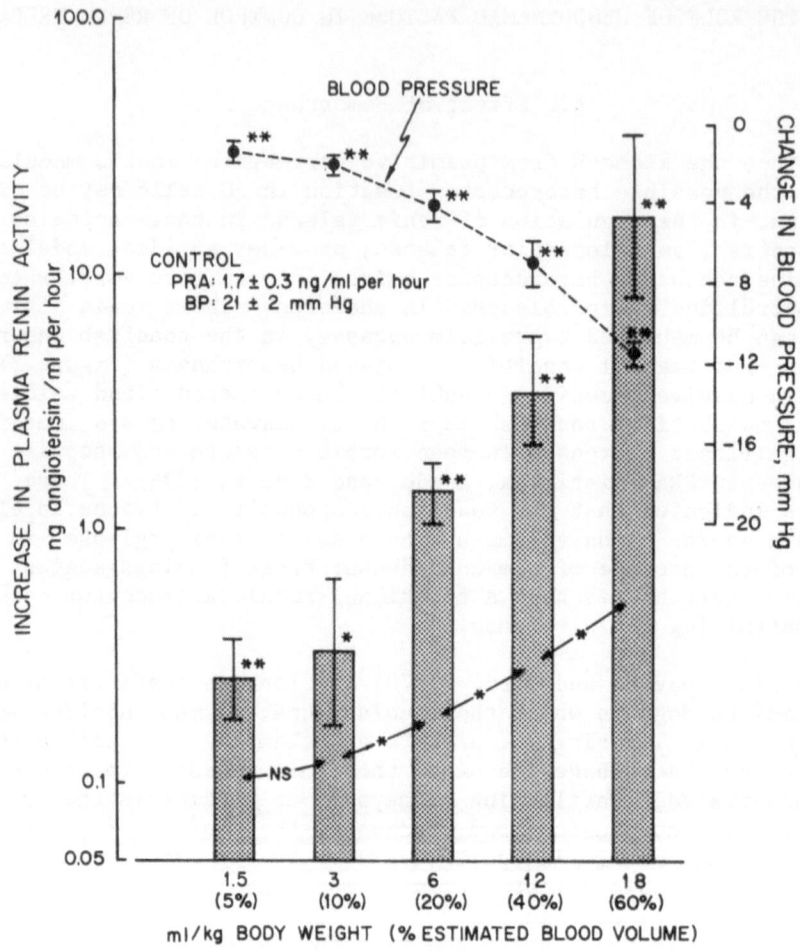

Figure 3.   *Increase of plasma renin activity (PRA) and decrease of blood pressure after graded hemorrhage (n = 7) in the unanesthetized aglomerular toadfish adapted to 50% seawater. The statistical significance of the differences between prehemorrhage levels of PRA and the levels after 1.5, 3, 6, 12, and 18 ml/kg (total blood loss) of bleeding, and the difference in PRA between two adjacent hemorrhages were determined by a paired "t" test using logs of data (transformed). The figure was drawn after the means were transformed. Decreases in blood pressure after cumulative hemorrhage from prehemorrhage level were analyzed with a paired "t" test (nontransformed). From Nishimura, Lunde, and Zucker (1979), Am. J. Physiol. 237: H105-H111.*

fish, most likely in response to a reduction in blood pressure.

These hemorrhage and hypotensive drug studies in toadfish raise two questions: 1) Did the reduction in renal perfusion pressure, due to decreased dorsal aortic pressure, stimulate a possible baro-receptor in the granulated cells, or did hypotension or hypovolemia affect the activity of granulated cells reflexly by signals trans-mitted by the renal nerves? 2) Does increased PRA reflect increased release of renin, or does it reflect both increased release and decreased clearance of renin?

Regarding the first question, it is not possible to measure or regulate renal perfusion pressure directly in the toadfish, since the renal arteries are small branches of the brachial arteries, and renal blood flow is supplied primarily by the segmental and the caudal vein through the renal portal system. Also, the teleost kidney is innervated segmentally, and thus it is difficult to dener-vate. It has been shown in some teleost fishes that adrenergic nerves innervate blood vessels in the kidney (Gannon, 1972), but the morphological relationship between granulated cells and adrenergic nerve endings has not been studied. Regarding the second question, it is most likely that increased PRA after hemorrhage or hypotension in the toadfish largely reflects renin release. The rate of renin clearance has not been determined in fishes, but it is presumably lower than in mammals. Although decreased renal and hepatic renin clearances due to hypotension and hypovolemia may contribute par-tially to the increased PRA, this contribution should be relatively minor. A more than 20-fold increase in PRA within one hour is far beyond the increase which can be accounted for by decreased renin clearance. It is ideal, however, to determine renin secretion rate instead of PRA.

C. Effect of Blood Volume

It has been shown in mammals that cardiopulmonary receptors are involved in renin release. An increase in left atrial pressure, which reflects a change of blood volume, reflexly reduces the rate of renin secretion via vagal afferent and renal sympathetic efferent pathways (Zehr, Hasbargen, and Kurz, 1976). Isosmotic volume expan-sion in the Australian lungfish, *Neoceratodus forsteri*, produced by injecting an isosmotic saline solution, decreased PRA and increased the mean dorsal aortic pressure by 2 mm Hg (Blair-West, Coghlan, Denton, *et al*., 1977). The receptor which detects the change in blood volume, and the pathway through which the stimulus is trans-mitted are not known.

VI.   THE ROLE OF THE ADRENERGIC NERVOUS SYSTEM IN CONTROL OF RENIN
RELEASE

There is no clear evidence that sympathetic vasomotor tone
exists in elasmobranchs (Opdyke, McGreehan, Messing, and Opdyke,
1972). Vascular resistance is likely to be regulated by circulating
catecholamines and other vasoactive substances, suggesting that
humoral control of vascular beds preceded neural control phylogenetically. However, it is not known whether the renin-angiotensin
system has a role in the control of cardiovascular function in
primitive vertebrates either by working directly on the cardiovascular system or by interacting with the adrenergic nervous system.

It appears that the large arteries of teleosts are supplied both
by "constrictor adrenergic" and by "constrictor cholinergic" nerves
(Kirby and Burnstock, 1969; Holmgren and Nilsson, 1974). Cholinergic
vasoconstrictor nerves appear to be both of sympathetic and parasympathetic origin. Adrenergic receptors (Wood, 1976) and adrenergic
innervation in the blood vessels are present but are rudimentary in
fishes (Burnstock, 1969). Adrenergic innervation increased, whereas
cholinergic innervation diminished in the evolution of the vertebrates. The innervation of the vertebrate heart by inhibitory vagal
cholinergic fibers and by excitatory sympathetic adrenergic fibers
was established phylogenetically early in teleost fishes and was
retained virtually unchanged through evolution to mammals (Gannon
and Burnstock, 1969; Gannon, 1971).

In mammals, beta adrenergic receptors, which are presumably
located in the JG cells, appear to mediate renin release (Johnson,
Davis, Gotshall, *et al.*, 1976). Intrarenal infusion of isoproterenol,
norepinephrine, or electrical stimulation of renal nerves caused
renin release in the dog, which was blocked by beta adrenergic
blocking drugs (for review, see Davis and Freeman, 1976).

Isoproterenol (1 µg/kg) caused transient hypotension with a
concomitant increase in PRA and heart rate in the aglomerular toadfish (Nishimura, Lunde, and Zucker, 1978, and unpublished); propranolol (1 mg/kg per hr), a beta adrenergic blocking drug, abolished
both the vasodepressor and PRA responses to isoproterenol. The
increase in PRA after isoproterenol in the toadfish raises two
questions: 1) Does isoproterenol stimulate a release of renin from
the granulated cells? 2) Is the increase in response to isoproterenol due simply to a reduction in blood pressure? Infusion of a
low dose of isoproterenol (1 ng/kg per min) in the toadfish did not
decrease blood pressure, but PRA still showed a slight transient
increase. However, we still cannot exclude the possibility that
isoproterenol acted on the renal vasculature and altered renal hemodynamics without changing the systemic pressure, which then stimu-

lated the vascular receptors in the granulated cells. It will be
necessary to determine whether isoproterenol has a direct action on
the granulated cells by using *in vitro* kidney slices.

Norepinephrine (1 µg/kg), on the other hand, increased blood
pressure and heart rate remarkably but did not alter PRA (Nishimura
and Madey, unpublished). Phentolamine, an alpha adrenergic blocking
drug, caused a transient decrease in blood pressure, presumably due
to a nonspecific vasodilatory effect of this drug, and resulted in
increases in PRA and heart rate.

Another way to determine whether the neural component is
involved in renin release in primitive animals is to denervate the
kidney pharmacologically. Preliminary results from our laboratory
indicate that neither propranolol nor pentolinium tartrate
(Ansolysen) abolished the increase in PRA after papaverine. The
effects of neuron blocking drugs or catecholamine depleters have
not yet been studied. The participation of the adrenergic nerves
in the control of renin release may have evolved in a later stage
in vertebrate phylogeny.

VII. RELATIONSHIP AMONG THE RENIN-ANGIOTENSIN SYSTEM, SODIUM BALANCE, AND MINERALOCORTICOIDS

A. Stimulation of Steroid Secretion by Angiotensin

The effect of angiotensin or kidney extract (renin) on mineralocorticoid secretion has been studied in various nonmammalian vertebrates by Davis and coworkers. Intravenous administration of the
homologous kidney extract increased aldosterone (Johnston, Davis,
Wright, and Howards, 1967), or aldosterone and corticosterone
(Taylor, Davis, and Braverman, 1972) secretion rates in the hypophysectomized, anesthetized frog and also in the pithed frog
(Johnston, Davis, Wright, and Howards, 1967). Corticosterone
secretion increased in the anesthetized, dexamethasone-treated
turtle, *Pseudemys sueanniensis*, after infusion of homologous kidney
extract, but no increase in steroid secretion occurred in the croco-
dile, *Caiman sclerops* (Nothstine, Davis, and DeRoos, 1971). Homologous kidney extract failed to increase aldosterone or corticosterone secretion in intact or hypophysectomized chickens (Taylor,
Davis, Breitenbach, and Hartroft, 1970). In these experiments,
however, arterial blood pressure, and often postcaval plasma flow
also, increased after infusion of kidney extracts (see Table 2).

It is difficult to determine the effect of renin or angiotensin on steroid secretion in bony fishes since the adrenal
(interrenal) tissues of teleosts are not comprised of a single

Table 2.   STIMULATION OF ADRENOCORTICOID SECRETION BY ANGIOTENSIN OR RENIN

Species	Experimental Conditions	Injected Substance	Steroid Secretion	References
TELEOSTS				
European eel (Anguilla anguilla)	Intact or hypophysectomized	Homologous kidney extract, [Asn^1, Val^5] angiotensin II	Cortisol (plasma)	Henderson, Jotisankasa, Mosley, and Oguri, 1976
AMPHIBIANS				
Frog (Rana catesbeiana)	Hypophysectomized	Homologous kidney extract	Aldosterone, or aldosterone and corticosterone	Johnston, Davis, Wright, and Howards, 1967; Taylor, Davis, and Braverman, 1972
Frog (Rana catesbeiana)	Hypophysectomized	Natural carp angiotensin[a]	Aldosterone and corticosterone	Taylor and Davis, 1971
REPTILES				
Turtle (Pseudemys sueanniensis)	Dexamethasone-treated	Homologous kidney extract	Corticosterone	Nothstine, Davis, and DeRoos, 1971
Crocodile (Caimen sclerops)	Dexamethasone-treated	Homologous kidney extract	No increase	Nothstine, Davis, and DeRoos, 1971
BIRDS				
Cockerel (Gallus gallus)	Hypophysectomized	Homologous kidney extract	No increase	Taylor, Davis, Breitenbach, and Hartroft, 1970

[a] Product from incubation of carp plasma and kidney. Experiments were performed in anesthetized animals except in the eel.

structure. Aldosterone has been demonstrated in a few species of bony fishes (Chavin and Singley, 1972; Idler, Sangalang, and Truscott, 1972), but it is unlikely that aldosterone has any physiological role. The major mineralocorticoid in teleost fishes is cortisol, but cortisone and corticosterone also have been demonstrated. Synthetic angiotensin II (amide) or eel kidney extract increased the cortisol level in the arterial blood in intact and hypophysectomized eels (Henderson, Jotisankasa, Mosley, and Oguri, 1976). However, since test materials were injected into the systemic circulation in these experiments and thus produced increases in blood pressure, the possibility cannot be excluded that the increased steroid secretion may have been due to increased blood flow to the interrenal cells. Injection of natural carp angiotensin (the product from the incubation of carp kidney extract with homologous plasma) into the hypophysectomized, anesthetized frog increased aldosterone and corticosterone secretion (Taylor and Davis, 1971). On the other hand, carp kidney extract or synthetic angiotensin II (amide) increased the blood pressure of the frog but had no effect on steroid secretion.

B. Renin Activity in Sodium-Depleted and Sodium-Loaded Animals

Since the renin-angiotensin system is important in the regulation of sodium balance, and sodium depletion usually is a potent stimulus for renin release in man and other mammals, evidence for a homologous function has been sought in primitive animals, particularly in fishes. Osmoregulation in teleost fishes differs depending on their external media (Hickman and Trump, 1969). Teleost fishes in fresh water are always exposed to the danger of excessive water intake along the osmotic gradient; thus, the primary role of the kidney of fresh water teleosts is to excrete excess water as dilute urine and to reabsorb the electrolytes. Marine fishes, on the other hand, are exposed to a salt load and dehydration; they drink seawater and absorb both minerals and water through the gut to compensate for their osmotic water loss. Thus, their kidneys have an important function in conserving water and excreting divalent ions, such as magnesium, sulfate, and phosphate; sodium and chloride ions are extruded from the gills.

Euryhaline teleosts, such as eels or salmon, can survive both in seawater and in fresh water and can maintain their internal osmolality relatively constant in spite of the large concentration gradients between them and either of these two media. When euryhaline fish are introduced from seawater to fresh water, glomerular filtration rate and urine flow increase immediately (primary adjustment). Renal tubules appear to become less permeable to water within a few days (secondary adjustment), resulting in a larger volume of urine (Hickman and Trump, 1969).

It will be of interest to determine whether the renin-angiotensin system participates in osmoregulation in fishes by influencing
renal function or epithelial transport through the gills or the gut.
However, there is no clear indication that the renin-angiotensin
system helps to conserve sodium in teleosts in hyposmotic media.
Plasma renin activity either did not change or decreased when the
euryhaline fish *Tilapia mossambica* (Malvin and Vander, 1967), the
eel, or the toadfish (Nishimura, Sawyer, and Nigrelli, 1976;
Henderson, Jotisankasa, Mosely, and Oguri, 1976) were transferred
from seawater to hyposmotic media, despite decreases in plasma sodium
concentration. The JG cells of the euryhaline fish *Cymatogaster
aggregata* showed involutional changes after the animals were transferred from brackish to hyposmotic media (Lagios, 1968). There were
no differences in PRA between toads acclimated to saline and those
acclimated to distilled water (Garland and Henderson, 1975). Glomerular filtration rates and the secretion rates of adrenocorticosteroids
were much higher in toads in distilled water than in toads in saline
(Garland and Henderson, 1975).

On the contrary, PRA (Sokabe, Oide, Ogawa, and Utida, 1973;
Henderson, Jotisankasa, Mosely, and Oguri, 1976) and cortisol levels
(Ball, Chester-Jones, Forster, *et al.*, 1971; Hirano, 1969) increased
in eels loaded with sodium by being adapted to seawater. Also, the
JG cells increased in number and size in a euryhaline, *Tilapia mossambica*, after it was transferred from fresh water to seawater
(Krishnamurthy and Bern, 1973). This apparent paradox may be understandable if we consider that angiotensin may stimulate the secretion
of cortisol (a mineralocorticoid) in teleosts. Cortisol in teleosts
has an important function in seawater osmoregulation by promoting
the extrusion of sodium across the gill (Maetz, 1969) and by increasing water absorption in the gut (Hirano and Utida, 1971).

Available reports on the relation of external salinity to renal
renin content, however, do not agree with those of PRA. The renin
content of the kidneys decreased when Japanese eels *(Anguilla japonica)* or *Tilapia mossambica* were adapted from fresh water to seawater
over 3 weeks (Sokabe, Mizogami, and Sato, 1968). Kidney renin activity was higher in freshwater stanohaline teleosts or euryhaline
fishes adapted to hyposmotic media than in marine species (Mizogami,
Oguri, Sokabe, and Nishimura, 1968; Capelli, Wesson, and Aponte,
1970). Nolly and Fasciolo (1972), however, did not find any significant differences in renal renin activity among five species of teleosts, despite differences in external salinity (seawater or fresh
water). In toads, decreases in plasma sodium concentration, produced
by peritoneal dialysis, furosemide administration, or by placing them
in distilled water, did not result in significant changes in renal
renin content (Nolly and Fasciolo, 1971). It should be pointed out
that decreases or increases in PRA, which presumably reflect the
changes in renin release and/or renin metabolism, may not necessarily

be associated with measurable changes in renal renin. It is also
necessary to note that the plasma renin activities in available
reports were all determined by measuring the angiotensin I generation rates using the rat pressor bioassay, and by using group com-
parisons. A change in PRA should be determined with respect to
changes in external salinity in a given animal with a more sensitive renin assay method.

    In more advanced vertebrates, the renin response to sodium
depletion resembles that seen in mammals. Renal renin activity
and granularity of JG cells increased in the sodium-depleted fowl
(Taylor, Davis, Breitenbach, and Hartroft, 1970). Both PRA and
renal renin increased in a monotreme, *Tachyglossus aculeatus*,
depleted of Na by daily injections of furosemide (Reid, 1971). The
sodium-conserving function of the renin-angiotensin system may have
evolved in a relatively recent stage of vertebrate phylogeny.

    The effects of sodium depletion and sodium loading on the
renin-angiotensin system in several animal species are given in
Tables 3 and 4.

VIII.   DIPSOGENIC ACTION OF ANGIOTENSIN

    Systemic and intracranial injection of angiotensin II (amide)
stimulates drinking behavior in a variety of mammalian and nonmammalian vertebrates (Table 5). It has been suggested that the
renin-angiotensin system may participate in normal thirst mechanisms in mammals (Fitzsimons, 1972). Eels which were adapted to
seawater and drank seawater to compensate for their osmotic water
loss showed a dipsogenic response to exogenously administered
angiotensin in lower doses than did eels in fresh water (Hirano,
Takei, and Kobayashi, 1978). This dipsogenic effect of angiotensin was observed in eels with hypothalamic lesions and in
"decerebrated" eels, whereas vagotomy abolished the effect.
"Decerebrated" eels from fresh water began to drink when they were
transferred to seawater. These findings suggest that angiotensin
may act on the drinking or swallowing center(s) in the rhomb-
encephalon or on receptors outside the central nervous system in
this fish (Hirano, Takei, and Kobayashi, 1978). It has been shown
that drinking in the eel is regulated at a level lower than the
diencephalon and that the vagus nerve is involved in the regulation
of water intake (Hirano, Satou, and Utida, 1972).

    Large doses of angiotensin failed to induce drinking in the
frog. However, the frogs started to drink water when they were
immersed in 50% seawater (Hirano, Takei, and Kobayashi, 1978).
Intraperitoneal injection of angiotensin II (amide) into the
turtle, lizard, snake (Kobayashi, Uemura, Wada, and Takei, 1979),

Table 3. *ACTIVITIES OF THE RENIN-ANGIOTENSIN SYSTEM IN SODIUM-*
DEPLETED ANIMALS

Species	Na Depletion	Activity	References
PLASMA RENIN ACTIVITY			
TELEOSTS			
Tilapia (*Tilapia mossambica*)	SW to FW	No change	Malvin and Vander, 1967
American eel (*Anguilla rostrata*)	SW to FW	Decreased	Nishimura, Sawyer, and Nigrelli, 1976
Aglomerular toadfish (*Opsanus tau*)	50% SW to 5% SW	No change	Nishimura, Sawyer, and Nigrelli, 1976
European eel (*Anguilla anguilla*)	SW to FW	Decreased	Henderson, Jotisankasa, Mosely, and Oguri, 1976
AMPHIBIANS			
Toad (*Bufo marinus*)	Distilled water	No change	Garland and Henderson, 1975
JUXTAGLOMERULAR CELLS			
TELEOSTS			
(*Cymatogaster aggregata*)	68% SW to hyposmotic media	Involutional change	Lagios, 1968
BIRDS			
Cockerel (*Gallus gallus*)	Low Na diet plus diuretics	Increased granularity	Taylor, Davis, Breitenbach, and Hartroft, 1970

SW: Seawater.   FW: Fresh water

Table 4. *ACTIVITIES OF THE RENIN-ANGIOTENSIN SYSTEM IN SODIUM-LOADED ANIMALS*

Species	Na load	Activity	References
PLASMA RENIN ACTIVITY			
TELEOSTS			
Japanese eel (*Anguilla japonica*)	FW to SW	Transiently increased	Sokabe, Oide, Ogawa, and Utida, 1973
European eel (*Anguilla anguilla*)	FW to SW	Increased	Henderson, Jotisankasa, Mosely, and Oguri, 1976
AMPHIBIANS			
Toad (*Bufo marinus*)	Hyper-osmotic saline	No change	Garland and Henderson, 1975
JUXTAGLOMERULAR CELLS			
TELEOSTS			
Tilapia (*Tilapia mossambica*)	FW to SW	Increase in number and size	Krishnamurthy and Bern, 1973

SW: Seawater. *FW: Fresh water*

Table 5. STIMULATION OF DRINKING BY ANGIOTENSIN

Species	Conditions	Treatment	Route	Dose	Response	References
TELEOSTS						
Japanese eel (Anguilla japonica)	FW	[Asn[1],Val[5]]AII; natural eel angiotensin[a]	i.a.	50 ng/100g BW[b]	Induced drinking	Hirano, Takei, and Kobayashi, 1978
Japanese eel (Anguilla japonica)	SW	[Asn[1],Val[5]]AII	i.a.	5 ng/100g BW[b]	Induced drinking	Hirano, Takei, and Kobayashi, 1978
Japanese eel (Anguilla japonica)	FW	"decerebration"[c] plus[Asn[1],Val[5]]AII	i.a.	1–10 µg/fish	Induced drinking	Hirano, Takei, and Kobayashi, 1978
AMPHIBIANS						
Japanese frog (Rana brevipoda)	FW	[Asn[1],Val[5]]AII	i.v.	5–2500 µg/100 g. BW	No response	Hirano, Takei, and Kobayashi, 1978
Japanese frog (Rana brevipoda)	FW	Dehydration[d]		————	No response	Hirano, Takei, and Kobayashi, 1978
REPTILES						
Common iguana (Iguana iguana)		[Asn[1],Val[5]]AII	i.p.	2×10^{-8} mole/100 g BW[e]	Induced drinking	Fitzsimons and Kaufman, 1977
Turtle, lizard, snake		[Asn[1],Val[5]]AII	i.p.	1–30 µg/100 g BW	Induced drinking	Kobayashi, Uemura, Wada, and Takei, 1979

Table 5. STIMULATION OF DRINKING BY ANGIOTENSIN (*Continued*)

Species	Treatment	Route	Dose	Response	References
BIRDS					
White-crowned sparrow (*Zonotrichia leucophrys gambelii*)	$[Asn^1,Val^5]AII$	i.v.	50 µg/animal[b]	Induced drinking	Wada, Kobayashi, and Farner, 1975
White-crowned sparrow (*Zonotrichia leucophrys gambelii*)	$[Asn^1,Val^5]AII$	anterior hypothalamus	500 ng/animal[b]	Induced drinking	Wada, Kobayashi, and Farner, 1975
White leghorn cocks (*Gallus domesticus*)	$[Asn^1,Val^5]AII$	i.v.	300 µg/animal[b]	Induced drinking	Snapir, Robinzon, and Godschalk, 1976
White leghorn cocks (*Gallus domesticus*)	$[Asn^1,Val^5]AII$	anterior diencephalon	2.5 µg/animal[b]	Induced drinking	Snapir, Robinzon, and Godschalk, 1976
White leghorn chicken (*Gallus domesticus*)	$[Asn^1,Val^5]AII$	i.m.	100 µg/animal[b]	Induced drinking	Schwab and Johnson, 1977
White leghorn chicken (*Gallus domesticus*)	$[Asn^1,Val^5]AII$	i.c.	75 ng/animal[b]	Induced drinking	Schwab and Johnson, 1977
Japanese quail (*Coturnix coturnix japonica*)	$[Asn^1,Val^5]AII$	i.v.	5 µg/animal[b]	Induced drinking	Takei, 1977a,b
Japanese quail (*Coturnix coturnix japonica*)	$[Asn^1,Val^5]AII$	preoptic area, or subfornical organ	1-5 ng/100 g BW[b]	Induced drinking	Takei, 1977a,b

Table 5. STIMULATION OF DRINKING BY ANGIOTENSIN (Continued)

Species	Treatment	Route	Dose	Response	References
BIRDS (Continued)					
Pigeon (*Columba livia*)	[Asn^1,Val^5]AII; [Asn^1,Ile^5]AII	i.p.	5 x 10^{-9} mole/animal^b	Induced drinking	Evered and Fitzsimons, 1976
Pigeon (*Columba livia*)	[Asn^1,Val^5]AII; [Asn^1,Ile^5]AII	i.c.	10^{-12} mole/animal^b	Induced drinking	Evered and Fitzsimons, 1976

FW: fresh water   i.a.: intraarterial   i.v.: intravenous   i.p.: intraperitoneal
SW: seawater   i.c.: intracranial   i.m.: intramuscular
BW: body weight

[a] Activity of partially purified natural eel angiotensin was expressed in terms of nanograms of [Asn^1,Val^5]AII (Hypertensin, CIBA) with equivalent vasopressor activity in the rat.

[b] Minimum effective dose.

[c] Prosencephalon, mesencephalon and diencephalon were removed.

[d] Cellular dehydration was induced by infusing 10% NaCl solution (i.v.).

[e] Maximum response to dose induced.

or into the iguana (Fitzsimons and Kaufman, 1977) induced drinking. Reptiles which live in arid regions and those under hibernation failed to respond or responded only to very high doses (500-1000 μg/100 gm body weight) of angiotensin (Kobayashi, Uemura, Wada, and Takei, 1979).

Intracranial injection of angiotensin II (amide) stimulated drinking in birds (Table 5). Sensitive sites to angiotensin are the medial preoptic area and subfornical organ in the Japanese quail (Takei, 1977 a, b) and the minimum effective dose was 5 ng per 100 gm body weight, which is comparable to the minimum effective dose in the rat. [Asn^1, Val^5]AII or [Asn^1, Ile^5]AII injected intraperitoneally, intravenously, or into the forebrain stimulated drinking in the pigeon (Evered and Fitzsimons, 1976) and the doses of both intracranially and intraperitoneally administered angiotensin which caused drinking in the pigeon were smaller than in the rat. Pigeons also responded to intracranial injection of hog renin, tetradecapeptide renin substrate, and angiotensin I (Evered and Fitzsimons, 1976). Intracranial injection of a higher dose of angiotensin was necessary to induce drinking in the sparrow (Wada, Kobayashi, and Farner, 1975) and the fowl (Snapir, Robinzon, and Godschalk, 1976; Schwob and Johnson, 1977). Birds which depend on food for most of their ingested water and thus drink little water in their natural state were insensitive to angiotensin (Kobayashi, Uemura, Wada, and Takei, 1977, 1978). Electrical destruction of the subfornical organ of the quail attenuated water intake induced by angiotensin injected into the preoptic area (Takei, 1977a). When the fluorescent fibers connecting the medial preoptic area and the subfornical organ were cut, injection of angiotensin into the preoptic area did not induce drinking. Thus, it appears that the information generated by angiotensin at the preoptic area is transmitted to the subfornical organ through neural pathways (Takei, 1977a).

Assuming from the structures of angiotensin I, determined in the fowl, the snake, and the Japanese goosefish (Fig. 2), [Asp^1, Val^5]AII, [Asn^1, Val^5]AII, and perhaps angiotensins whith other chemical structures as well, are present as native angiotensin among nonmammalian vertebrates. The angiotensin used for inducing the dipsogenic effect in most of the literature is [Asn^1, Val^5]AII. Therefore, variability of sensitivity to this angiotensin among species may be partially because it may not be their native angiotensin.

IX. THE RENIN-ANGIOTENSIN SYSTEM AND RENAL FUNCTION

A. Renal Action of Exogenous Angiotensin

The kidneys of most nonmammalian vertebrates receive two blood supplies: the renal arterial system which supplies the glomerulus, and the renal portal system which carries blood to the renal tubules. The efferent arterioles from the glomeruli anastomose with the capillary network of afferent veins of the renal portal system; thus, peritubular blood is mixed with arterial and venous (renal portal) blood. In primitive animals, therefore, the effects of drugs and hormones on renal tubular function can be determined independent of the influences of glomerular hemodynamics.

The effects of angiotensin on renal function have been determined in various vertebrates (Table 6). It appears that angiotensin acts both on the glomerulus and on the tubules in some species, and that the effect depends on the dose of angiotensin. Pressor doses of angiotensin cause diuresis and natriuresis in eels, lungfishes, and toads. It appears that the diuresis due to angiotensin is largely a consequence of an increase in glomerular filtration rate (GFR) due to increased dorsal aortic pressure. Natriuresis presumably reflects "glomerular-tubular imbalance", i.e., the renal tubules fail to reabsorb sodium proportionately to the increased sodium load. In the rainbow trout, three groups of nephrons (filtering, nonfiltering but with perfused glomeruli, and nonperfused) were observed by dissection of the nephrons after ferrocyanide injection (Henderson, Brown, Oliver, and Haywood, 1978). Infusion of angiotensin II (amide) reduced total GFR and urine flow in rainbow trout both in seawater and in fresh water. Single nephron GFR, however, did not change in fresh water trout, while it was reduced markedly in seawater trout, suggesting that in fresh water trout angiotensin may produce a redistribution of the nephron types mentioned above (Brown, Oliver, and Henderson, 1978; Henderson, Brown, Oliver, and Haywood, 1978). However, norepinephrine was used in these preparations to maintain a normal rate of urine production, and thus it is possible that the three differing types of nephrons and the effect of angiotensin on single nephron GFR may have been partially due to the effects of norepinephrine, or due to the additive effects of norepinephrine and angiotensin.

If the diuresis observed in some bony fishes is ascribed to the increased GFR secondary to the elevated aortic pressure produced by angiotensin, then this diuresis should be minimal in the aglomerular fish. Infusions of large doses of angiotensin into the aglomerular toadfish produced no significant diuresis or natriuresis (Zucker and Nishimura, 1977). Churchill and Churchill (1976), however, found a mild diuresis and natriuresis during angiotensin infusion in the American goosefish, *Lophius americanus*. This diuresis and natriuresis may have been the consequence of increased renal blood flow rather than a direct effect of angiotensin on the sodium transport mechanisms in the renal tubules.

Pang, Galli-Gallardo, and Sawyer (1977) perfused the renal arterial system and the renal portal system individually under constant pressure (*in situ* preparation) in toads and reported that angiotensin injected into the renal portal system caused anti-

Table 6. RENAL EFFECTS OF EXOGENOUS ANGIOTENSIN

Species	Glomerular Action		Tubular Action		References
	Nonpressor Dose	Pressor Dose	Nonpressor Dose	Pressor Dose	
TELEOSTS					
American eel (*Anguilla rostrata*)	No effect	Diuresis and natriuresis	------	------	Nishimura and Sawyer, 1976
Aglomerular goosefish (*Lophius americanus*)	------	------	------	Diuresis and natriuresis	Churchill and Churchill, 1976
Aglomerular toadfish (*Opsanus tau*)	------	------	No effect	No effect	Zucker and Nishimura, 1977
Rainbow trout[a] (*Salmo gairdneri*)	------	Antidiuresis	------	------	Henderson, Brown, Oliver, and Haywood, 1978
DIPNOANS					
African lungfish (*Protopterus aethiopicus*)	------	Mild diuresis and natriuresis	------	------	Sawyer, 1970
Australian lungfish (*Neoceratodus forsteri*)	------	Moderate diuresis and natriuresis	------	------	Sawyer, Blair-West, Simpson, and Sawyer, 1976

Table 6. RENAL EFFECTS OF EXOGENOUS ANGIOTENSIN (Continued)

Species	Glomerular Action		Tubular Action		References
	Nonpressor Dose	Pressor Dose	Nonpressor Dose	Pressor Dose	
AMPHIBIANS					
Chilean toads[b] (Calyptocephalela caudiverbeia)	Antidiuresis and antinatriuresis	Diuresis and natriuresis	Antidiuresis and antnatriuresis	Antidiuresis and antinatriuresis	Pang, Galli-Gallardo, and Sawyer, 1977
Toad[c] (Bufo paracnemis)	----	----	----	Antidiuresis and antinatriuresis	Coviello, 1969
Toad (Xenopus laevis)	----	No change in GFR	----	Diuresis and natriuresis	Henderson and Edwards, 1969
BIRDS					
Chicken (Gallus domesticus)	----	----	----	Diuresis and natriuresis	Langford and Fallis, 1966

[a] Single nephron GFR was determined.

[b] *In situ* perfusion of renal portal system

[c] Isolated perfused kidney

diuresis and antinatriuresis, regardless of the dose. However,
Henderson and Edwards (1969) reported that angiotensin II (amide)
increased the urine flow and urinary sodium excretion without
changes in GFR in *Xenopus laevis* which were maintained in distilled
water and had a high GFR. It has been shown that angiotensin II
increases the permeability of the urinary bladder to water in
Bufo paracnemis (Coviello, 1969).

In birds, the angiotensin effect resembles that seen in mammals.
Angiotensin II (amide) infused into the leg vein of the chicken and
which eventually drains into the renal portal system, caused diuresis
and natriuresis in spite of decreases in GFR (Langford and Fallis,
1966).

B. Possible Role of the Renin-Angiotensin System in Renal Function

The structure of the nephron in primitive vertebrates is incomplete. The kidneys of teleost fishes (freshwater stenohaline and
euryhaline), amphibians and reptiles possess proximal and distal
tubules and collecting tubules and ducts, but they lack a loop of
Henle. Marine teleosts lost the distal tubule and in some species
even the glomerulus and a part of the proximal tubule. Thus,
primitive vertebrates cannot concentrate urine hyperosmotic to the
plasma. Also renal autoregulation in teleosts kidneys is poor and
the GFR is readily affected by the dorsal aortic pressure.

Sokabe (1974) proposed the hypothesis that the renin-angiotensin
system regulated GFR by constricting the efferent arteriole in
amphibians. GFR and PRA increased in the frog infused with isotonic
saline or glucose, whereas PRA was low in dehydrated frogs (Sokabe,
Nishimura, Kawabe *et al.,* 1972). However, this relationship between
GFR and PRA was not observed in teleost fishes.

The structure of the nephron of birds is unique. It is a
transitional form from the primitive type to a highly integrated
mammalian type of nephron. Birds possess two basic types of
nephrons (Shoemaker, 1972); short reptilian type cortical nephrons
and long juxtamedullary nephrons which possess a loop of Henle.
The bird kidneys have the ability to produce hyperosmotic urine, and
the presence of a countercurrent multiplier system has been
suggested (Poulson, 1965). Relatively small, but convincing, osmotic
and ionic differences between medullary and cortical tissues were
noted in dehydrated and salt-loaded chickens and turkeys
(Skadhauge and Schmidt-Nielsen, 1967). In birds, urine flow appears
to be controlled by both filtration rate and tubular water reabsorption and the ability to handle loaded salt varies depending on
species. The osmolalities (mOsm/liter) of urine after salt loading
range from 400 in the chicken, which has a poor ability to excrete
salt load (Dantzler, 1966), to 2000 in the salt marsh sparrow

(Poulson and Bartholomew, 1962). Furthermore, bird kidneys possess
a primitive form of macula densa. It would be of interest to study
whether a functional relationship exists among JG cells, glomerular
hemodynamics, and macula densa cells which detect electrolyte changes
in tubular urine, and to study whether the renin-angiotensin system
participates in the urine concentrating mechanisms in birds.

X.   EVOLUTIONARY SPECULATION

Based on currently available information (Figures 4 and 5),
I would pose several questions:

1. Does the renin-angiotensin system play a role in the control of
    blood pressure or blood volume?

Hemorrhage and acute hypotension are potent stimuli for renin
release in teleosts, birds, and mammals. A possible baroreceptor
function for the control of renin release appears to exist in
primitive vertebrates. When we consider this fact, together with
the anatomical evidence that evolution of the JG cells precedes
that of the macula densa, and the fact that a vasopressor action
of angiotensin has been demonstrated throughout the vertebrate
phylogenetic scale, it may be reasonable to speculate that the
renin-angiotensin system evolved in close relation to blood pressure homeostasis. A reduction in systemic blood pressure decreases the renal perfusion pressure, which then acts as a stimulus
to renal arterial baroreceptors and produces increased renin
release; the angiotensin thus formed helps to restore blood pressure levels either by directly contracting the vascular smooth
muscle cells or by releasing catecholamines. The increased renin
release then will be attenuated by a negative feedback mechanism.

It has been shown in several species of birds, including the
domestic fowl, the turkey, pigeon, and canary, that both systolic
and diastolic blood pressures are high (Sturkie, 1976; Jones and
Johansen, 1972) and atherosclerotic lesions are often observed in
the aorta and other major arteries (Roberts and Straus, 1965; Wagner,
Clarkson, Feldner, and Pritchard, 1973). Systolic pressure in the
adult unanesthetized male chicken measured by a direct method is
approximately 190 mm Hg, and the diastolic pressure is about 150 mm
Hg. Blood pressure tends to increase with age in some species and
shows some heritability (Sturkie, 1970). Treatment of the hypertensive turkeys with l- or dl-propranolol lowers the blood pressure
and heart rate and decreases the mortality due to rupture of the
aorta induced by β-aminopropionitrile (Simpson, Boucek, and Noble,
1976). However, the etiology of this elevated blood pressure in
birds is not known. A recent report indicates that the hypertensive
turkeys have low PRA and normal plasma aldosterone levels (Pagnan,
Pessina, Thiene, and Dal Palu, 1978). In a later stage (48 weeks)

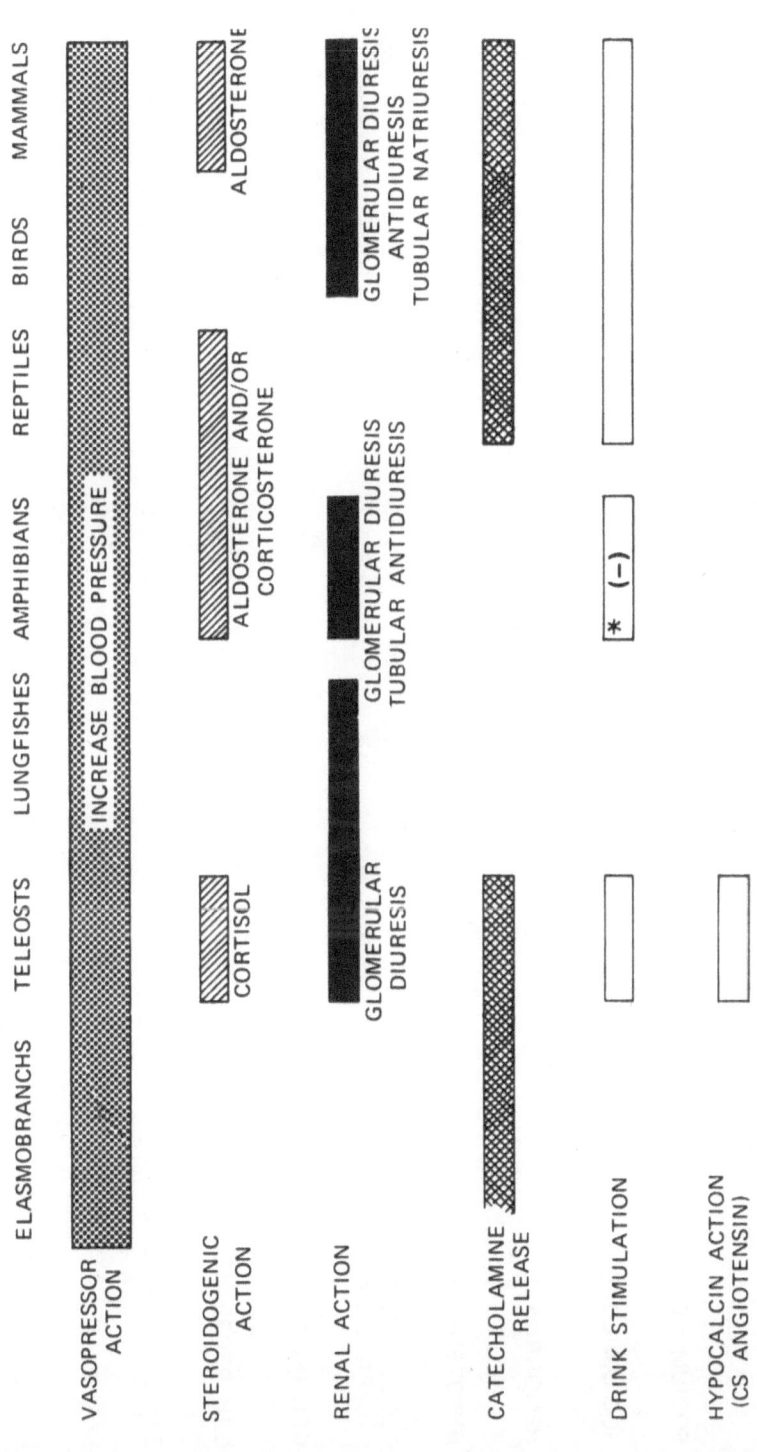

Figure 4. Current summary of the actions of exogenous angiotensin in various classes of vertebrates. *No drink stimulation occurred in frogs. Reproduced from Nishimura (1978). Jpn. Heart J. 19: 806-822.

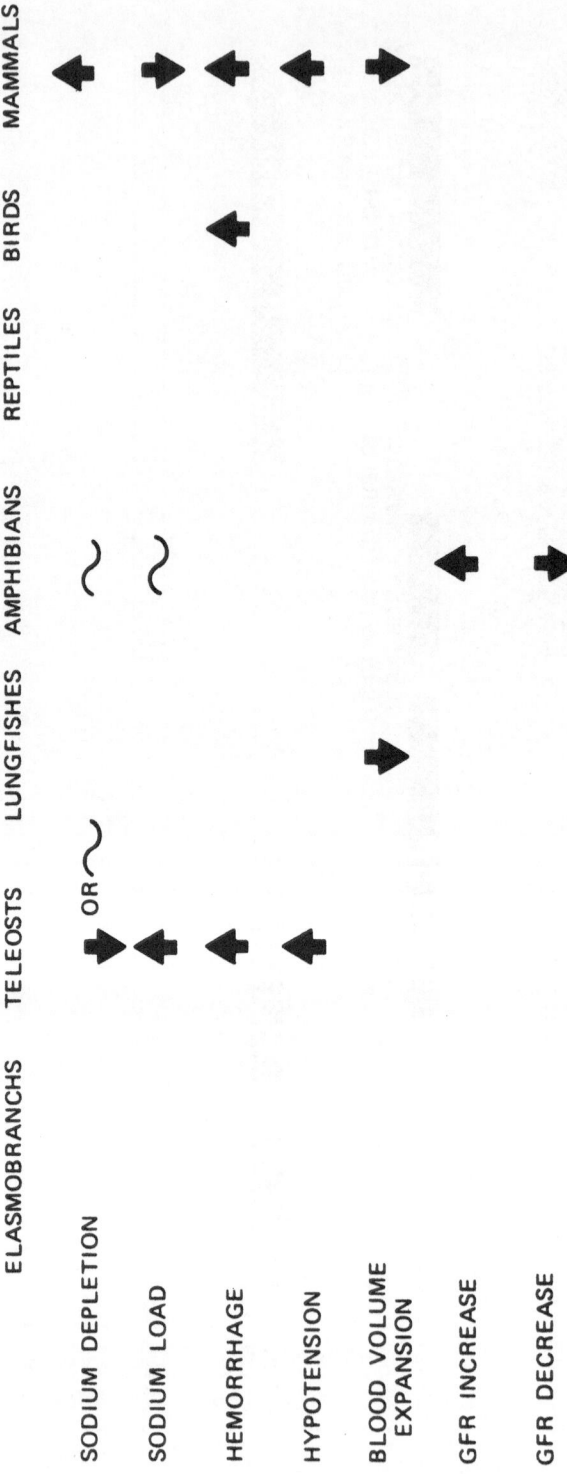

Figure 5. Factors influencing plasma renin activity determined in various classes of vertebrates. ↑ increase, ↓ decrease, ~ no change. Reproduced from Nishimura (1978). Jpn. Heart J. 19: 806-822.

when the kidney and the heart exhibit nephroangiosclerosis and cardiac hypertrophy, aldosterone levels are increased with hyperkalemia, whereas PRA values remain low. It will be of interest to determine the relationship among the adrenergic nervous system, the renin-angiotensin system, and hydromineral balance with respect to high blood pressure in birds.

2. Does the adrenergic nervous system interact with the renin-angiotensin system?

Hypotension may increase sympathetic discharge to granulated cells and stimulate renin release in primitive vertebrates. There is some evidence to suggest the possible presence of baroreceptors in the circulatory system of teleost fishes (Randall and Stevens, 1967). Adrenergic nerves have been demonstrated in the renal blood vessels of some teleosts, but this system generally is rudimentary in fishes. Adrenergic innervation increases in more advanced vertebrates. In the aglomerular teleosts, isoproterenol increases PRA with concomitant decreases in blood pressure; this renin response can be ascribed either to a direct stimulation of granulated cells by this beta adrenergic drug, or to a reduction in blood pressure. Furthermore, increases in PRA after acute hypotension induced by a vasodilatory drug were not diminished by a beta adrenergic drug or by a ganglionic blocking drug in the toadfish. It will be of interest to determine the innervation of theJG cells in nonmammalian vertebrates.

It appears that a considerable portion of the pressor action of angiotensin results from the release of catecholamines, and this phenomenon can be demonstrated throughout the vertebrates. In elasmobranchs and birds the alpha adrenergic blocking drugs almost completely abolish the vasopressor action of angiotensin. This fact is of particular interest when we consider that the amino acid in position 1 appears to be important for stimulating catecholamine release, in addition to that in position 8, and that changes in the chemical structure at position 1 occurred during vertebrate evolution. Kidneys of primitive animals contain abundant chromaffin cells. Thus, angiotensin may participate physiologically in the regulation of catecholamine release (Opdyke and Holcombe, 1976).

3. Does the renin-angiotensin-mineralocorticoid axis exist in non-mammalian vertebrates?

Exogenous administration of angiotensin or homologous renin increased the mineralocorticoid secretion in frogs and reptiles, and possibly in teleosts. It remains to be determined whether endogenous levels of renin correlate with those of mineralocorticoids under various physiological and pathological conditions before we can conclude that the renin-angiotensin system participates in the control of mineralocorticoid secretion in nonmammalian vertebrates.

Sodium depletion does not stimulate the renin-angiotensin system in teleosts and amphibians. On the other hand, PRA increases in teleosts during seawater adaptation. This paradox may be understandable if the renin-angiotensin system regulates the secretion of cortisol, which is an important mineralocorticoid in seawater teleosts. Another explanation for increased PRA during seawater adaptation of teleosts would be that angiotensin stimulates drinking in fishes. The sodium-conserving function of the renin-angiotensin system may have evolved in a more recent stage of vertebrate phylogeny.

4. Does the renin-angiotensin system regulate renal function by its systemic or intrarenal action?

Glomerular filtration rate is important for determining urine flow in primitive vertebrates (Hickman and Trump, 1969; Schmidt-Nielsen and Forster, 1954). The kidneys in teleost fishes appear to have poor autoregulation, and the GFR is readily influenced by changes in dorsal aortic pressure, although blood pressure is not the sole factor for controlling GFR. Administration of pressor doses of angiotensin causes glomerular diuresis and natriuresis in teleosts, lungfishes, and amphibians. Angiotensin may participate in the control of GFR through its influence on blood pressure in these animals. In addition, the renin-angiotensin system may control GFR by producing contraction of the afferent or efferent arteriole. It appears that angiotensin also has a tubular action in amphibians, but the mechanism by which angiotensin affects the transport of water or electrolytes across renal tubules is not known.

Birds possess an intermediate type of kidney which is similar to the kidneys both of mammals and of primitive vertebrates. The bird kidney has the ability to produce urine hyperosmotic to plasma, achieved by tubular water reabsorption as in mammalian kidneys, although GFR also perticipates in the regulation of urine flow (Shoemaker, 1972). As in mammals, angiotensin causes tubular natriuresis. On the other hand, birds have a renal portal system, and a majority of their nephrons are the short, reptilian-type. It will be interesting to determine if the renin-angiotensin system has a role in the regulation of GFR or renal sodium handling in birds.

In mammals, the macula densa senses some changes in composition or flow of the renal tubular fluid, which then influences GFR in the same nephron through a feedback mechanism. Thurau, Dahlheim, Gruner, *et al.* (1972) and Thurau (1974) demonstrated that retrograde perfusion

of the macula densa with a hypertonic sodium chloride solution increased the renin activity in a single JG apparatus. They proposed
that angiotensin, generated locally in the JG area, regulates GFR
by constricting the afferent arteriole. Does this functional inter-
relationship among the JG cells, glomerular hemodynamics and renal
tubules exist in primitive vertebrates? Or, is this feedback system
inoperative since they lack a macula densa? In birds, sodium
depletion appears to stimulate the renin-angiotensin system. Does
this indicate that a functional relationship between JG cells and
Na or Cl transport at the macula densa site evolved in birds?

Distribution of the JG cells appears to have changed along the
phylogenetic advancement of the vertebrate. Granulated cells are
distributed diffusely along the small renal arteries and arterioles
in fishes and tend to be localized near the glomeruli in more
advanced animals (Sokabe and Ogawa, 1974). If we are allowed to
speculate, this distribution pattern of granulated cells appears to
suggest that some shift occurred in the function of the renin-
angiotensin system, probably from a systemic endocrine action to a
local regulator of glomerular circulation.

XI. SUMMARY AND CONCLUSION

1. Renal renin and the juxtaglomerular (JG) cells presumably
evolved in primitive bony fishes and have been found in a variety
of teleost fishes and tetrapods. Neither renin nor the JG cells
have been found in the elasmobranchs or cyclostomes, whereas both
have been shown in holocephalians. Bony fishes, lungfishes,
amphibians and reptiles lack a macula densa. Birds have a primitive
form of macula densa cells. Only mammals have all the components
of the JG apparatus.

2. Primitive vertebrates possess renin substrate, renin,
angiotensin-converting enzyme (or a like substance), angiotensins I
and II, and angiotensinases. It appears that the chemical
structure of angiotensin changed in the amino acids at positions 1,
5 and 9 during vertebrate evolution.

3. Properties of angiotensin receptors in the blood vessels
differ in fishes from those of mammals.

4. A vasopressor action of angiotensin has been demonstrated
in selected species of all vertebrate classes from elasmobranchs
to mammals. A considerable portion of its pressor effect appears
to be an indirect action, presumably due to the stimulation of
catecholamine release.

5. Hemorrhage and acute hypotension increase plasma renin
activity (PRA) in the aglomerular toadfish, which lacks a macula

densa and glomerulus. Decreases in renal perfusion pressure may
cause renin release by stimulating a possible baroreceptor function
of the granulated cells.

6. It is not known whether adrenergic nerves innervate JG
cells in primitive animals. Isoproterenol increases PRA with concomitant decreases in blood pressure, and propranolol blocks both
effects. Norepinephrine increases blood pre-sure but does not alter
PRA. It remains to be determined, however, whether isoproterenol
has a direct action on the granulated cells.

7. Exogenously administered renin (kidney extract) or angiotensin stimulates mineralocorticoid secretion in amphibians, reptiles,
and possibly teleosts. However, sodium depletion does not stimulate
the renin-angiotensin system in teleosts and amphibians, whereas
sodium loading causes transient increases in PRA in teleosts. In
birds, sodium depletion increases renal renin activity and granularity of the JG cells.

8. Systemic or intracranial injection of angiotensin II stimulates drinking in birds, reptiles, and teleosts, but not in anuran
amphibians. Reptiles which live in arid regions and those under
hibernation fail or require higher doses to elicit a dipsogenic
effect of angiotensin.

9. Angiotensin causes glomerular "pressure diuresis" in
teleosts and lungfishes. Angiotensin appears to exert both glomerular and tubular actions in some amphibians. Tubular natriuresis has
been observed in birds. The renin-angiotensin system may participate
in the regulation of GFR through the control of blood pressure in
teleosts, and by constricting efferent arterioles in amphibians.

10. Evolutionary trends and perspectives with respect to
possible functions and role of the renin-angiotensin system in nonmammalian vertebrates were discussed.

REFERENCES

Ball, J. N., Chester-Jones, I., Forster, M. E., Hargreaves, G.,
    Hawkins, E. F., and Milne, K. P. (1971). Measurement of
    plasma cortisol levels in the eel, *Anguilla anguilla*, in
    relation to osmotic adjustments. J. Endocrinol. 50: 75-96.
Barajas, L. (1964). The innervation of the juxtaglomerular
    apparatus. An electron microscopic study of the innervation
    of the glomerular arterioles. Lab. Invest. 13: 916-929.
Barajas, L. and Latta, H. (1967). Structure of the juxtaglomerular
    apparatus. Circ. Res. 20-21 (Suppl. 2): 15-28.

Blaine, E. H., Davis, J. O., and Witty, R. T. (1970). Renin release after hemorrhage and after suprarenal aortic constriction in dogs without sodium delivery to the macula densa. Circ. Res. 27: 1081-1089.

Blair-West, J. R., Coghlan, J. P., Denton, D. A., Gibson, A. P., Oddie, C. J., Sawyer, W. H., and Scoggins, B. A. (1977). Plasma renin activity and blood corticosteroids in the Australian lungfish, *Neoceratodus forsteri*. J. Endocrinol. 74: 137-142.

Brown, J. A., Oliver, J. A., and Henderson, I. W. (1978). Angiotensin and glomerular perfusion patterns in trout. In: *Comparative Endocrinology* (Gaillard, P. J. and Boer, H. H., eds.), pp. 236, Elsevier/North Holland Biomedical Press, Amsterdam.

Bulger, R. E. and Trump, B. F. (1969). Ultrastructure of granulated arteriolar cells (juxtaglomerular cells) in kidney of a fresh and a salt water teleost. Am. J. Anat. 124: 77-88.

Bumpus, F. M. (1977). Mechanisms and sites of action of newer angiotensin agonists and antagonists in terms of activity and receptor. Fed. Proc. 36: 2128-2132.

Bumpus, F. M. and Khosla, M. C. (1977). Pathogenic factors involved in renovascular hypertension. State of the art. Mayo Clin. Proc. 52: 417-423.

Burnstock, G. (1969). Evolution of the autonomic innervation of visceral and cardiovascular systems in vertebrates. Pharmacol. Rev. 21: 247-324.

Capelli, J. P., Wesson, L. G., Jr., and Aponte, G. E. (1970). A phylogenetic study of the renin-angiotensin system. Am. J. Physiol. 218: 1171-1178.

Chan, M. Y. and Holmes, W. H. (1971). Studies on a "renin-angiotensin" system in the normal and hypophysectomized pigeon (*Columba livia*). Gen. Comp. Endocrinol. 16: 304-311.

Chavin, W. and Singley, J. A. (1972). Adrenocorticoids of the goldfish, *Carassius auratus*. Comp. Biochem. Physiol. 42B: 547-562.

Chester-Jones, I., Henderson, I. W., Chan, D. K. O., Rankin, J. C., Mosely, W., Brown, J. J., Lever, A. F., Robertson, J. I. S., and Tree, M. (1966). Pressor activity in extracts of the corpuscles of Stannius from the European eel (*Anguilla anguilla* L.). J. Endocrinol. 34: 393-408.

Churchill, P. C. and Churchill, M. C. (1976). Renal effects of angiotensin II in *Lophius americanus*. Bull. Mt. Desert Island Biol. Lab. 16: 5-8.

Coviello, A. (1969). Tubular effects of angiotensin II on the toad kidney. Acta Physiol. Lat. Am. 19: 73-82.

Dantzler, W. H. (1966). Renal response of chickens to infusion of hyperosmotic sodium chloride solution. Am. J. Physiol. 210: 640-646.

Davis, J. O. and Freeman, R. H. (1976). Mechanisms regulating
    renin release. Physiol. Rev. 56: 1-56.
Edwards, J. G. (1940). The vascular pole of the glomerulus in the
    kidney of vertebrates. Anat. Rec. 76: 381-389.
Evered, M. D. and Fitzsimons, J. T. (1976). Drinking induced by
    angiotensin in the pigeon (*Columba livia*). J. Physiol. 263:
    193P-194P.
Fitzsimons, J. T. (1972). Thirst. Physiol. Rev. 52: 468-561.
Fitzsimons, J. T. and Kaufman, S. (1977). Cellular and extracellu-
    lar dehydration, and angiotensin as stimuli to drinking in the
    common iguana, *Iguana iguana*. J. Physiol. 265: 443-463.
Gannon, B. J. (1971). A study of the dual innervation of the teleost
    heart by a field stimulation technique. Comp. Gen. Pharmacol.
    2: 175-183.
Gannon, B. J. (1972). Comparative and developmental studies of
    autonomic nerves in visceral and cardiovascular systems. Ph.D.
    Thesis, Dept. of Zoology, University of Melbourne, Melbourne,
    Australia.
Gannon, B. J. and Burnstock, G. (1969). Excitatory adrenergic inner-
    vation of the fish heart. Comp. Biochem. Physiol. 29: 765-773.
Garland, H. O. and Henderson, I. W. (1975). Influence of environ-
    mental salinity on renal and adrenocortical function in the
    toad, *Bufo marinus*. Gen. Comp. Endocrinol. 27: 136-143.
Grill, G. Granger, P. and Thurau, K. (1972). The renin angiotensin
    system of amphibians. I. Determination of the renin content
    of amphibian kidneys. Pflügers Arch.; Eur. J. Physiol. 331:
    1-12.
Harvey, S. C., Copen, E. G., Ekelson, D. W., Graff, S. R., Poulsen,
    L. D., and Rasmussen, D. L. (1954). Autonomic pharmacology of
    the chicken with adrenergic blockade. J. Pharmacol. Exp. Ther.
    112: 8-22.
Hayashi, T., Nakayama, T., Nakajima, T., and Sokabe, H. (1978).
    Comparative studies on angiotensins. V. Structure of angio-
    tensin formed by the kidney of Japanese goosefish and its
    identification by dansyl method. Chem. Pharm. Bull. 26: 215-
    219.
Henderson, I. W., Brown, J. A., Oliver, J. A., and Haywood, G. P.
    (1978). Hormones and single nephron function in fishes. In:
    Comparative Endocrinology (Gaillard, P. J. and Boer, H. H.,
    eds.), pp. 217-222, Elsevier/North Holland Biomedical Press,
    Amsterdam.
Henderson, I. W. and Edwards, B. R. (1969). Effect of angiotensin-
    II-amide on renal function in the clawed toad, *Xenopus laevis*
    Daudin. J. Endocrinol. 44: iii-iv.
Henderson, I. W., Jotinsankasa, V., Mosely, W., and Oguri, M. (1976).
    Endocrine and environmental influences upon plasma cortisol
    concentrations and plasma renin activity of the eel, *Anguilla
    anguilla* L. J. Endocrinol. 70: 81-95.

Hickman, C. P. and Trump, B. F. (1969). The kidney. In: *Fish Physiology* (Hoar, W. S. and Randall, eds.), Vol. 1, pp. 91–239, Academic Press, New York.

Hirano, T. (1969). Effects of hypophysectomy and salinity changes on plasma cortisol concentration in the Japanese eel, *Anguilla japonica*. Endocrinol. Jpn. 16: 557–560.

Hirano, T., Satou, M., and Utida, S. (1972). Central nervous system control of osmoregulation in the eel (*Anguilla japonica*). Comp. Biochem. Physiol. 43A: 537–547.

Hirano, T., Takei, Y., and Kobayashi, H. (1978). Angiotensin and drinking in the eel and the frog. In: Alfred Benzon Symposium XI (1977), *Osmotic and Volume Regulation* (Jorgensen, C. B. and Skadhauge, E., eds.), pp. 123–134, Munksgaard, Copenhagen.

Hirano, T. and Utida, S. (1971). Plasma cortisol concentration and the rate of intestinal water absorption in the eel, *Anguilla japonica*. Endocrinol. Jpn. 18: 47–52.

Holmgren, S. and Nilsson, S. (1974). Drug effects on isolated artery strips from two teleosts, *Gadus morhua* and *Salmo gairdneri*. Acta Physiol. Scand. 90: 431–437.

Idler, D. R., Sangalang, G. B., and Truscott, B. (1972). Corticosteroids in the South American lungfish. Gen. Comp. Endocrinol. Suppl. 3: 238–244.

Johnson, J. A., Davis, J. O., Gotshall, R. W., Lohmeier, T. E., Davis, J. L., Braverman, B., and Tempel, G. E. (1976). Evidence for an intrarenal beta receptor in control of renin release. Am. J. Physiol. 230: 410–418.

Johnston, C. I., Davis, J. O., Wright, F. S., and Howards, S. S. (1967). Effects of renin and ACTH on adrenal steroid secretion in the American bullfrog. Am. J. Physiol. 213: 393–399.

Jones, D. R. and Johansen, K. (1972). The blood vascular system of birds. In: *Avian Biology* (Farner, D. S. and King, J. R., eds.), Vol. II, pp. 157–285, Academic Press, New York.

Khosla, M. C., Bumpus, F. M., Hayashi, Y., Nakajima, T., Watanabe, T. X., and Sokabe, H. (1977). Synthesis and specific pressor activity of [1-Aspartic acid, 5-valine, 9-serine] angiotensin I ("fowl angiotensin I"). J. Med. Chem. 20: 315–316.

Kirby, S. and Burnstock, G. (1969). Comparative pharmacological studies of isolated spiral strips of large arteries from lower vertebrates. Comp. Biochem. Physiol. 28: 307–319.

Kobayashi, H., Uemura, H., Wada, M., and Takei, Y. (1979). Ecological adaptation of angiotensin-induced thirst mechanism in tetrapods. Gen. Comp. Endocrinol. 38: 93–104.

Krishnamurthy, V. G. and Bern, H. A. (1969). Correlative and histologic study of the corpuscles of Stannius and the juxtaglomerular cells of teleost fishes. Gen. Comp. Endocrinol. 13: 313–335.

Krishnamurthy, V. G. and Bern, H. A. (1973). Juxtaglomerular cell changes in the euryhaline freshwater fish, *Tilapia mossambica*, during adaptation to sea water. Acta Zool. 54: 9–14.

Lagios, M. D. (1968). Granular epithelioid cell involution in the
    renal arteries of a euryhaline fish, *Cymatogaster*, adapted
    to hypotonic salinities. Gen. Comp. Endocrinol. 11: 248-250.
Langford, H. G. and Fallis, N. (1966). Diuretic effect of angio-
    tensin in the chicken. Proc. Soc. Exp. Biol. Med. 123: 317-
    321.
Maetz, J. (1969). Observations on the role of the pituitary-intra-
    renal axis in the ion regulation of the eel and other teleosts.
    Gen. Comp. Endocrinol. Suppl. 2: 299-316.
Malvin, R. L. and Vander, A. J. (1967). Plasma renin activity in
    marine teleosts and Cetacea. Am. J. Physiol. 213: 1582-1584.
Mizogami, S., Oguri, M., Sokabe, H., and Nishimura, H. (1968).
    Presence of renin in the glomerular and aglomerular kidney of
    marine teleosts. Am. J. Physiol. 215: 991-994.
Moore, A. F. (1978). Vascular actions of angiotensin II (AII) in
    the fowl (*Gallus domesticus*). Fed. Proc. 37: 387 (abstract).
Moore, A. F., Strong, J. H., and Buckley, J. P. (1978). Angioten-
    sin (AII) and chicken blood pressure. 7th International Cong-
    ress of Pharmacology, Paris, p. 57 (abstract).
Muñoz-Ramirez, H., Khosla, M. C., Bumpus, F. M., and Khairallah, P.
    A. (1975). Influence of the adrenal gland on the pressor
    effect and antagonist potency of angiotensin II analogs. Eur.
    J. Pharmacol. 31: 122-135.
Nakajima, T., Nakayama, T., and Sokabe, H. (1971). Examination of
    angiotensin-like substances from renal and extrarenal sources
    in mammalian and nonmammalian species. Gen. Comp. Endocrinol.
    17: 458-466.
Nakayama, T., Nakajima, T., and Sokabe, H. (1973). Comparative
    studies on angiotensins. III. Structure of fowl angiotensin
    and its identification by DNA-method. Chem. Pharm. Bull. 21:
    2085-2087.
Nakayama, T., Nakajima, T., and Sokabe, H. (1977). Comparative
    studies on angiotensins. IV. Structure of snake (*Elaphe
    climocophora*) angiotensin. Chem. Pharm. Bull. 25: 3255-3260.
Nishimura, H. (1978). Physiological evolution of the renin-
    angiotensin system. Jpn. Heart J. 19: 806-822.
Nishimura, H., Crofton, J. T., Norton, V. M., and Share, L. (1977).
    Angiotensin generation in teleost fish determined by radio-
    immunoassay and bioassay. Gen. Comp. Endocrinol. 32: 236-247.
Nishimura, H., Lunde, L. G., and Zucker, A. (1978). Renin response
    to hypotension and adrenergic drugs in the aglomerular toadfish.
    Fed. Proc. 37: 294 (abstract).
Nishimura, H., Lunde, L. G., and Zucker, A. (1979). Renin response
    to hemorrhage in the aglomerulat toadfish, *Opsanus tau*. Am. J.
    Physiol. 237: H105-H111.
Nishimura, H., Norton, V. M., and Bumpus, F. M. (1978). Lack of
    specific inhibition on angiotensin II in eels by angiotensin
    antagonists. Am. J. Physiol. 235: H95-H103.

Nishimura, H., Ogawa, M., and Sawyer, W. H. (1973). Renin-angiotensin system in primitive bony fishes and a holocephalin. Am. J. Physiol. 224: 950-956.

Nishimura, H., Oguri, M., Ogawa, M., Sokabe, H., and Imai, M. (1970). Absence of renin in kidneys of elasmobranchs and cyclostomes. Am. J. Physiol. 218: 911-915.

Nishimura, H. and Sawyer, W. H. (1976). Vasopressor, diuretic, and natriuretic responses to angiotensins by the American eel, *Anguilla rostrata*. Gen. Comp. Endocrinol. 29: 337-348.

Nishimura, H., Sawyer, W. H., and Nigrelli, R. F. (1976). Renin, cortisol and plasma volume in marine teleost fishes adapted to dilute media. J. Endocrinol. 70: 47-59.

Nishimura, H. and Sokabe, H. (1968). The role of angiotensinases in the renin-angiotensin system. *Proceedings of the Symposium on Chemical Physiology and Pathology* 8: 116-120.

Nolly, H. and Fasciolo, J. C. (1971). Renin-angiotensin system and sodium homeostasis in *Bufo arenarum*. Comp. Biochem. Physiol. 39A: 833-841.

Nolly, H. L. and Fasciolo, J. C. (1972). The renin-angiotensin system through the phylogenetic scale. Comp. Biochem. Physiol. 41A: 249-254.

Nothstine, S. A., Davis, J. O., and DeRoos, R. M. (1971). Kidney extracts and ACTH on adrenal steroid secretion in a turtle and a crocodilian. Am. J. Physiol. 221: 726-732.

Ogawa, M. (1977). Effects of homologous angiotensins on plasma calcium in Japanese eel. In: *Japan-U.S. Cooperative Science Program, Seminar: Comparative Studies of the Renin-Angiotensin System*, Tochigi, Japan, November, 1977 (abstract).

Ogawa, M. and Sokabe, H. (1971). The macula densa site of avian kidneys. Zeit. Zellforsch. Mikroskop. Anat. 120: 29-36.

Oguri, M. (1978). Presence of juxtaglomerular cells in the holocephalian kidney. Gen. Comp. Endocrinol. 36: 170-173.

Oguri, M., Ogawa, M., and Sokabe, H. (1972). Juxtaglomerular cells in aglomerular teleosts. Bull. Jpn. Soc. Sci. Fish. 38: 195-200.

Oguri, M. and Sokabe, H. (1968). Juxtaglomerular cells in the teleost kidneys. Bull. Jpn. Soc. Sci. Fish. 34: 882-888.

Opdyke, D. F. and Holcombe, R. (1976). Response to angiotensins I and II and to AI-converting enzyme inhibitor in a shark. Am. J. Physiol. 231: 1750-1753.

Opdyke, D. F. and Holcombe, R. F. (1978). Effect of angiotensins and epinephrine on vascular resistance of isolated dogfish gut. Am. J. Physiol. 234: R196-R200.

Opdyke, D. F., McGreehan, J. R., Messing, S., and Opdyke, N. E. (1972). Cardiovascular responses to spinal cord stimulation and autonomically active drugs in *Squalus acanthias*. Comp. Biochem. Physiol. 42A: 611-620.

Pagnan, A., Pessina, A. C., Thiene, G., and Dal Palu, C. (1978).
     The natural history of hypertension in turkeys. Fifth Scien-
     tific Meeting of the International Society of Hypertension,
     Paris, June 12-14. (abstract).
Pang, P. K. T., Gali-Gallardo, S. M., and Sawyer, W. H. (1977).
     Renal and vascular responses of some amphibians to vasoactive
     substances. In: *Japan-U.S. Coopertaive Science Program,
     Seminar: Comparative Studies of the Renin-Angiotensin System.*
     Tochigi, Japan, November, 1977 (abstract).
Pang, P. K. T., Pang, R. K., and Sawyer, W. H. (1974). Environ-
     mental calcium and the sensitivity of killifish (*Fundulus
     heteroclitus*) in bioassays for the hypocalcemic response to
     Stannius corpuscles from killifish and cod (*Gadus morhua*).
     Endocrinology 94: 548-555.
Peach, M. J. (1977). Renin angiotensin system: Biochemistry and
     mechanisms of action. Physiol Rev. 57: 313-370.
Peach, M. J. and Ackerly, J. A. (1976). Angiotensin antagonists
     and the adrenal cortex and medulla. Fed. Proc. 35: 2502-2507.
Peach, M. J. and Ober, M. (1974). Inhibition of angiotensin-induced
     adrenal catecholamine release by 8-substituted analogs of
     angiotensin II. J. Pharmacol. Exp. Ther. 190: 49-58.
Poulsen, T. L. (1965). Countercurrent multipliers in avian kidneys.
     Science 148: 389-391.
Poulsen, T. L. and Bartholemew, G. A. (1962). Salt balance in the
     savannah sparrow. Physiol. Zool. 35: 109-119.
Randall, D. J. and Stevens, E. D. (1967). The role of adrenergic
     receptors in cardiovascular changes associated with exercise
     in salmon. Comp. Biochem. Physiol. 21: 415-424.
Regoli, D. Park, W. K., and Rioux, F. (1974). Pharmacology of
     angiotensin. Pharmacol. Rev. 26: 69-123.
Reid, I. A. (1971). Renin secretion in a monotreme (*Tachyglossus
     aculeatus*). Comp. Biochem. Physiol. 40A: 249-255.
Roberts, J. C., Jr., and Straus, R. (eds.), (1965). *Comparative
     Atherosclerosis.* Hoeber, New York.
Sawyer, W. H. (1970). Vasopressor, diuretic, and natriuretic res-
     ponses by lungfish to arginine vasotocin. Am. J. Physiol. 218:
     1789-1794.
Sawyer, W. H., Blair-West, J. R., Simpson, P. A., and Sawyer, M. K.
     (1976). Renal responses of Australian lungfish to vasotocin,
     angiotensin II and NaCl infusion. Am. J. Physiol. 231: 593-602.
Schaffenburg, C. A., Haas, E., and Goldblatt, H. (1960). Concen-
     tration of renin in kidneys and angiotensinogen in serum of
     various species. Am. J. Physiol. 199: 788-792.
Schmidt-Nielsen, B. and Forster, R. P. (1954). The effect of dehyd-
     ration and low temperature on renal function in the bullfrog.
     J. Cell. Comp. Physiol. 44: 233-246.
Schwob, J. E. and Johnson, A. K. (1977). Angiotensin-induced dipso-
     genesis in domestic fowl (*Gallus gallus*). J. Comp. Physiol.
     Psych. 91: 182-188.

Shoemaker, V. H. (1972). Osmoregulation and excretion in birds. In: *Avian Biology* (Farner, D. S. and King, J. R., eds.), Vol. II, pp. 527-574. Academic Press, New York.

Simpson, C. F., Boucek, R. J., and Noble, N. S. (1976). Influence of *d*-, *l*-, and *dl*-propranolol, and practolol on β-aminopropio-nitrile-induced aortic ruptures of turkeys. Toxicol. Appl. Pharmacol. 38: 169-175.

Skadhauge, E. and Schmidt-Nielsen, B. (1967). Renal medullary electrolyte and urea gradient in chickens and turkeys. Am. J. Physiol. 212: 1313-1318.

Snapir, N., Robinzon, B., and Godschalk, M. (1976). The drinking response of the chicken to peripheral and central administration of angiotensin II. Pharmacol. Biochem. Behav. 5: 5-10.

Sokabe, H. (1974). Phylogeny of the renal effects of angiotensin. Kidney Int. 6: 263-271.

Sokabe, H., Mizogami, S., and Sato, A. (1968). Role of renin in adaptation to sea water in euryhaline fishes. Jpn. J. Pharmacol. 18: 332-343.

Sokabe, H., Nishimura, H., Kawabe, K., Tenmoku, S., and Arai, T. (1972). Plasma renin activity in varying hydrated states in the bullfrog. Am. J. Physiol. 222: 142-146.

Sokabe, H., Nishimura, H., Ogawa, M. and Oguri, M. (1970). Determination of renin in the corpuscles of Stannius of the teleost. Gen. Comp. Endocrinol. 14: 510-516.

Sokabe, H. and Ogawa, M. (1974). Comparative studies of the juxta-glomerular apparatus. Int. Rev. Cytol. 37: 271-327.

Sokabe, H., Ogawa, M., Oguri, M., and Nishimura, H. (1969). Evolution of the juxtaglomerular apparatus in the vertebrate kidneys. Tex. Rep. Biol. Med. 27: 867-885.

Sokabe, H., Oide, H., Ogawa, M., and Utida, S. (1973). Plasma renin activity in Japanese eels (*Anguilla japonica*) adapted to sea-water or in dehydration. Gen. Comp. Endocrinol. 21: 160-167.

Sokabe, H. and Watanabe, T. X. (1977). Evolution of the chemical structure of angiotensins and their physiological roles. Gunma Symposium Endocrinol. 14: 83-97.

Somlyo, A. P., Somlyo, A. V., and Woo, C. (1967). Neurohypophyseal peptide interaction with magnesium in avian vascular smooth muscle. J. Physiol. 192: 657-668.

Sturkie, P. D. (1970). Seven generations of selection for high and low blood pressure in chickens. Poultry Sci. 49: 953.

Sturkie, P. D. (1976). Heart and circulation: anatomy, hemodynamics, blood pressure, blood flow, and body fluids. In: *Avian Physiology* (Sturkie, P. D., ed.), pp. 76-101. Springer-Verlag, New York.

Takei, Y. (1977a). The role of the subfornical organ in drinking induced by angiotensin in the Japanese quail, *Coturnix coturnix japonica*. Cell. Tiss. Res. 185: 175-181.

Takei, Y. (1977b). Angiotensin and water intake in the Japanese quail (*Coturnix coturnix japonica*). Gen. Comp. Endocrinol. 31: 364-372.

Taylor, A. A. (1977). Comparative physiology of the renin-angiotensin system. Fed. Proc. 36: 1776–1780.

Taylor, A. A. and Davis, J. O. (1971). Effects of carp kidney extracts and angiotensin II on adrenal steroid secretion. Am. J. Physiol. 221: 652–657.

Taylor, A. A., Davis, J. O., and Braverman, B. (1972). Deoxycorticosterone secretion in the bullfrog: Effects of ACTH, hypophysectomy, and renin. Am. J. Physiol. 223: 858–863.

Taylor, A. A., Davis, J. O., Breitenbach, R. P., and Hartroft, P. M. (1970). Adrenal steroid secretion and a renal-pressor system in the chicken (*Gallus domesticus*). Gen. Comp. Endocrinol. 14: 321–333.

Thurau, K. (1974). Intrarenal action of angiotensin. In: *Handbook of Experimental Pharmacology: Angiotensin* (Page, I. H. and Bumpus, F. M., eds.), Vol. 37, pp. 475–489. Springer-Verlag, Heidelberg.

Thurau, K. W. C., Dahlheim, H., Gruner, A., Mason, J., and Granger, P. (1972). Activation of renin in the single juxtaglomerular apparatus by sodium chloride in the tubular fluid at the macula densa. Circ. Res. 30–31 (Suppl. 2): 182–186.

Turker, R. K., Page, I. H., and Bumpus, F. M. (1974). Antagonists of angiotensin II. In: *Handbook of Experimental Pharmacology: Angiotensin* (Page, I. H. and Bumpus, F. M., eds.), Vol. 37, pp. 162–169. Springer-Verlag, Heidelberg.

Wada, M., Kobayashi, H., and Farner, D. S. (1975). Induction of drinking in the white-crowned sparrow, *Zonotrichia leucophrys gambelii*, by intracranial injection of angiotensin II. Gen. Comp. Endocrinol. 26: 192–197.

Wagner, W. D., Clarkson, T. B., Feldner, M. A., and Prichard, R. W. (1973). The development of pigeon strains with selected atherosclerotic characteristics. Exp. Mol. Pathol. 19: 304–319.

Watanabe, T. X., Sokabe, H., Honda, I., Sakakibara, S., Nakayama, T., and Nakajima, T. (1977). Specific pressor activity and stability of synthetic angiotensins. Jpn. J. Pharmacol. 27: 137–144.

Wood, C. M. (1976). Pharmacological properties of the adrenergic receptors regulating systemic vascular resistance in the rainbow trout. J. Comp. Physiol. 107: 211–228.

Zehr, J. E., Hasbargen, J. A., and Kurz, K. D. (1976). Reflex suppression of renin secretion during distention of cardiopulmonary receptors in dogs. Circ. Res. 38: 232–239.

Zucker, A. and Nishimura, H. (1977). The renal response of the aglomerular toadfish to vasoactive hormones. Am. Zool. 17: 858.

DISCUSSION AFTER DR. NISHIMURA'S PAPER

Dr. Zehr
    I might add a bit of information to one of your slides having
to do with reptiles. I had a student who was looking at the action
of angiotensin on vascular beds in turtles. It turns out, in agreement with what you said, that when we administered angiotensin II
to these turtles we got very nice pressor responses. If we infused
[Sar[1], Ile[8]] angiotensin II, the pressor response was reduced by
about 50 percent, but when we combined this with an alpha adrenergic
blocker, the response was completely gone. So it looks like reptiles
release substantial amounts of catecholamines in response to angiotensin.

Dr. Nishimura
    Thank you. That is a very interesting observation. We also
did a preliminary study on a chicken to determine how it responded
to angiotensin. The angiotensin II antagonist, [Sar[1], Thr[8]] angiotensin II, at a dose of 10 µg/kg per minute reduced the pressor response to [Asn[1], Val[5]] angiotensin II by about one half. I haven't
tried alpha adrenergic blockers yet, but I will. However, in the
fish I couldn't see any blockade of the pressor effect of angiotensin II by using a mammalian angiotensin II antagonist, so perhaps
between the bony fishes and the reptiles the properties of angiotensin receptors may have changed.

Dr. Davis
    I would like to ask you a little more about the appearance of
the macula densa phylogenetically. As I recall, when Hartroft was
working with us she found what looked like a macula densa in the
frog. Since I know you are very familiar with the literature, what
species of amphibia have been studied and the presence of a macula
densa been excluded?

Dr. Nishimura
    Dr. Ogawa examined juxtaglomerular cells and macula densa in
*Triturus pyrrhogaster, Rana catesbeiana, Rana japonica, Rana nigro-
maculata,* and *Bufo vulgaris.* Although he found that in some species
the renal distal tubule returns to the JG cells, he couldn't find
the characteristic macula densa cells, so he concluded that macula
densa cells are absent in amphibia. However, Edwards reported that
a macula densa exists in frogs, and Capelli observed a primitive
form of macula densa in *Rana pipiens.* So there certainly is controversy among investigators.

Dr. Freeman
    Dr. Nishimura, you didn't say anything about the effects of
angiotensin on other organs involved in sodium excretion. I am
thinking particularly about the nasal glands of some birds. Could

you comment on this? What kind of work has been done along those
lines?

Dr. Nishimura

I don't think there have been any studies done on the effects
of angiotensin on the nasal glands, or if there have been, they
probably didn't report it because there was no effect. The major
regulator of sodium excretion by nasal glands appears to be a
mineralocorticoid - corticosterone or cortisol. We did a little
study on whether angiotensin acts on the fish gills, because gills
are important for sodium regulation in the aquatic environment.
In the freshwater eel I couldn't see any effect of angiotensin on
either sodium or water flux.

As I mentioned in my talk, there is no clear evidence to suggest that the renin-angiotensin system is stimulated in teleosts
and amphibians in hyposmotic media, possibly to help in conserving
sodium. In birds, however, Taylor demonstrated that the renal renin
content and granularity is increased in the sodium depleted cockerel.
At present, I am hypothesizing that the relationship between the
renin-angiotensin system and blood pressure homeostasis evolved
first, and that the role of this hormonal system in the regulation
of sodium balance evolved in a more recent stage of vertebrate
phylogeny, possibly in relation to the development of the macula
densa.

Dr. Peach

Don't you have evidence that several of the 8-substituted
analogues of angiotensin II are actually full agonists in some of
the teleosts? I bring this up because in some of the work we've
done it is fairly clear that some of the 8-substituted analogues
are full agonists for the release of catecholamines from certain
structures. If you find the right one, it becomes a partial agonist.
Studies done in Dr. Munday's lab. at Southampton have clearly shown
that all of the 8-substituted analogues they have studied so far are
very active in stimulating water transport from the gut. They have
seen no blockade by a wide variety of these analogues. They also
have found that the [des-Phe^8] angiotensin II homologue has a remarkable activity on gut water transport. The angiotensin-induced water
transport in the gut is blocked by alpha adrenergic blockade or by
depletion of catecholamines (Mariscotti, *et al.*, 1977). Do you have
evidence of agonist responses to any of the 8-substituted analogues?

Dr. Nishimura

We studied only the pressor action of angiotensins in teleosts.
We examined both agonist and antagonist effects of [Sar^1, Ile^8] angiotensin II, [Sar^1, Thr^8] angiotensin II, and [Tal^8] angiotensin II
(8-thienylalanine angiotensin II). [Sar^1, Thr^8] angiotensin II
showed no pressor activity itself, but [Sar^1, Ile^8] angiotensin II and
[Tal^8] angiotensin II showed considerable agonistic action.

Dr. Peach
    You haven't tried alpha blockade with those?

Dr. Nishimura
    Yes, I did. I did for [Tal[8]]angiotensin II. In eels the pressor responses to this angiotensin decreased after phentolamine.
Also, after treatment with reserpine the pressor responses to [Tal[8]]
angiotensin II became lower.

Dr. Davis
    I want to say, Dr. Nishimura, that this is the most complete,
most sophisticated presentation I have seen on this subject. We
are really indebted to you for it. Thank you very much.

DISCUSSION REFERENCES

Capelli, J. P., Wesson, L. G., Jr., and Aponte, G. E. (1970).
    A phylogenetic study of the renin-angiotensin system. Am. J.
    Physiol. 218: 1171-1178.
Edwards, J. G. (1940). The vascular pole of the glomerulus in the
    kidney. Anat. Rec. 76: 381-389.
Levens, N. R., Munday, K. A. and Poat, J. A. (1976). Effect of
    (Sar[1], Leu[8])-angiotensin on rat jejunal fluid transport in vivo.
    J. Endocrinol. 68: 7P-8P.
Mariscotti, S. P., Levens, N. R., and Munday, K. A. (1977). Importance of 8-phenylalanine for the biological activity of the
    angiotensin molecule. J. Endocrinol. 72: 2P.
Sokabe, H., Ogawa, M., Oguri, M., and Nishimura, H. (1969).
    Evolution of the juxtaglomerular apparatus in the vertebrate
    kidneys. Tex. Rep. Biol. Med. 27: 867-885.
Taylor, A. A., Davis, J. O., Breitenbach, R. P., and Hartroft, P. M.
    (1970). Adrenal steroid secretion and a renal-pressor system
    in the chicken (*Gallus domesticus*).

THE ACTIONS OF ANGIOTENSIN II IN THE CHICKEN

Alan Moore[1]

Department of Pharmacology
Institute for Cardiovascular Studies
University of Houston
Houston, TX 77004

The actions of angiotensin II and its analogues have been studied in several nonmammalian species, most extensively in eels (Nishimura, Norton, and Bumpus, 1978). The dorsal aorta of the eel and the aorta of the boa constrictor, when cut spirally and suspended in an organ bath, showed dose-dependent contractions in response to both angiotensin II and norepinephrine (Moore and Khairallah, unpublished observations). The isolated ventral aorta of the eels, however, showed no response. Although Taylor, Davis, Breitenbach, and Hartroft (1970) described a pressor response to angiotensin II in the hypophysectomized, anesthetized fowl, no studies have been performed *in vitro*. We found that although the isolated, spirally-cut chicken aorta responded to both norepinephrine and serotonin in a dose-dependent manner, it did not respond to either angiotensin II or its agonist analogues (Moore, 1978; Moore, Strong, and Buckley, 1979).

The chicken rectum, unlike intestinal smooth muscle from other species, also does not respond to angiotensin II (Ng, 1968). Therefore, rather than systematically working through all of the blood vessels in the chicken, we used the whole animal as a conscious preparation for blood pressure recording, with the conscious rabbit as a comparison. We found that norepinephrine in both species gave a pressor response, and in the conscious rabbit a pressor response also occurred with angiotensin II. However, in the conscious chicken the administration of angiotensin II resulted in a biphasic response; an initial clear depressor response, followed by a smaller pressor response (Figure 1).

[1]Present address: Norwich-Eaton Pharmaceuticals, P. O. Box 191, Norwich, NY 13815

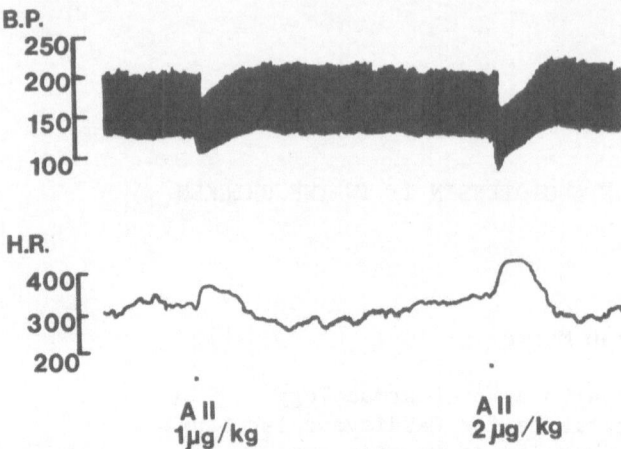

Figure 1. Response of the conscious chicken to angiotensin II (AII). Blood pressure (BP) and heart rate (HR) responses are shown to two concentrations of AII. At the higher con- contration of AII the biphasic nature of the response is, more apparent.

Many possibilities for the mechanisms of this depressor response were explored, including the use of a combination of α- and β-adreno-receptor blockade, atropine, hexamethonium, histamine$_1$ and histamine$_2$ receptor blockade, indomethacin pretreatment, and the use of various routes of injection (jugular, brachial, and femoral veins). However, none of these compounds caused any significant variation in the angio-tensin II depressor response (Moore, Strong, and Buckley, 1979). Finally, it was realized that as vasopressin is depressor in chickens rather than pressor as in mammals (British Pharmacopoeia, 1968), it was possible that release of the closely-related equivalent avian hormone, vasotocin, by angiotensin II could be responsible for the depressor effect.

As no specific vasopressin antagonists were available, the next experimental approach we used was to induce tachyphylaxis to vaso-pressin. In the conscious chicken made nonresponsive to vasopressin, the administration of angiotensin II gave a purely pressor response rather than a depressor response (Figure 2). We have shown subse-quently that this pressor response is totally sympathetically mediated (Moore, Strong, and Buckley, 1979). Therefore, it is suggested that in the chicken all of the observed blood pressure

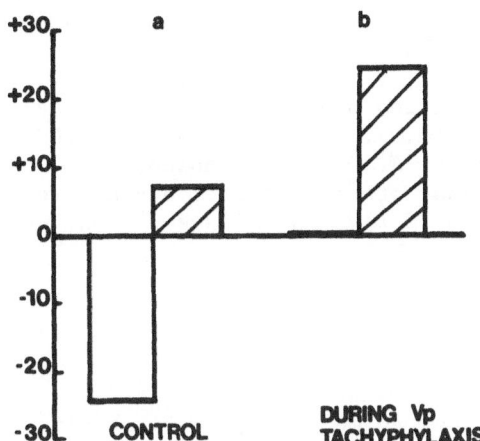

Figure 2.   *The depressor (open columns) and pressor (diagonally
striped columns) response to angiotensin II in the
conscious chicken are shown (a) as control animals, and
(b) after induction of tachyphylaxis to vasopressin
(Vp). Changes in blood pressure are expressed as
percent change from control pressure (N = 5).*

responses to angiotensin II are indirect;   i.e., the depressor
effect is mediated by a release of vasotocin and the pressor effect
by sympathetic activation. We feel that the possible contribution
of indirect mechanisms to the observed response to angiotensin II
in nonmammalian species should be examined carefully in each case.

REFERENCES

British Pharmacopoeia (1968). p. 1341. Pharmaceutical Press,
     London.
Moore, A. F. (1978). Vascular action of angiotensin II (AII) in the
     fowl (*Gallus domesticus*). Fed. Proc. 37: 387 (abstract).

Moore, A. F., Strong, J. H., and Buckley, J. P. (1979). Cardio-
    vascular actions of angiotensin in the fowl (*Gallus domesticus*).
    I. Analysis of response. Eur. J. Pharmacol. (in press).
Ng, K. K. F. (1968). Cited in: Khairallah, P. A. (1971).
    Pharmacology of Angiotensin. In: *Kidney Hormones*. (Fisher,
    J. W., ed.), Academic Press, New York.
Nishimura, H., Norton, V. M., and Bumpus, F. M. (1978). Lack of
    specific inhibition of angiotensin II in eels by angiotensin
    antagonists. Am. J. Physiol. 235: H95-H103.
Taylor, A. A., Davis, J. O., Breitenbach, R. P., and Hartroft, P. M.
    (1970). Adrenal steroid secretion and a renal pressor system
    in the chicken (*Gallus domesticus*). Gen. Comp. Endocrinol.
    14: 321-333.

DISCUSSION AFTER DR. MOORE'S PAPER

Dr. Nishimura
    It was not clear to me from your first slide, do the aortic
strips not show any response to angiotensin?

Dr. Moore
    Yes, that's right.

Dr. Nishimura
    Dr. Khairallah, of the Cleveland Clinic, is studying angiotensin
responses in eels in collaboration with my laboratory by using intact
animals and isolated dorsal aortic strips. The dorsal aorta showed
a good response to norepinephrine but a relatively small response to
angiotensin, even when a high dose was given.

Dr. Moore
    Actually, I started these experiments with Phil Khairallah in
Cleveland, and found the same thing. Evidently the ventral aorta
doesn't respond to angiotensin II whereas the dorsal aorta does, but
it does give a good response. You have to watch out for tachyphylaxis in these. One way we found recently of avoiding tachyphylaxis
was to increase the sodium in the medium by 20 percent. It is rather
an artificial way, but it does give you good dose-response curves.

    One other thing we found. I was discussing our work recently
with Dr. Sokabe, and he pointed out that fowl angiotensin has valine
in position 5, and we were using isoleucine-5 angiotensin II. We
have since gone back and redone it, so it appears, in our animals
anyway, that there is no angiotensin pressor receptor on vascular
smooth muscle in the fowl.

Dr. Goetz
    This may be a jump in your logic, but are you saying that the
conscious chicken releases vasopressin or oxytocin in response to

angiotensin, and in the anesthetized chicken the angiotensin activates the catecholamine system or the sympathetic nervous system?

Dr. Moore
  Yes.

Dr. Goetz
  You are speculating I take it. What does the anesthetic do to change the picture?

Dr. Moore
  I think that the anesthetic mostly inhibits the release of vasopressin by angiotensin. In fact, Dr. Buckley, with whom I now work, has proposed before that in anesthetized animals you are less likely to get release of vasopressin by angiotensin. Obviously, as you say, I am guessing right now. I don't know, because we haven't measured it. That is purely a working hypothesis. It seems to explain what we see, but we haven't tested it yet.

Dr. Peach
  Do birds get vascular hypertension?

Dr. Moore
  Actually, birds are very hypertensive.

Dr. Peach
  No, I mean if you mess around with their kidneys?

Dr. Moore
  I don't know.

Dr. Peach
  With brain lesions in birds, for example, hypertension is very easy to produce, but what about renal hypertension?

Dr. Moore
  I don't know, to be quite honest with you.

Dr. Nishimura
  People at the Mayo Clinic attempted to produce renal hypertension in the pigeon by constricting the renal artery. The birds became uremic and died. Also, Dr. W. D. Wagner of Bowman Gray School of Medicine has pigeons that are genetically susceptible to atherosclerosis. Currently he is in the process of producing genetically hypertensive pigeons. He also has tried to induce salt hypertension in the pigeon, but this attempt was not quite successful. The pigeons just could not tolerate salt loading, and their blood pressure decreased and they died.

Dr. Moore
      I plan to start looking at hypertensive turkeys before Thanks-
giving, myself!

STRUCTURE OF THE JUXTAGLOMERULAR APPARATUS[1]

L. Barajas and J. Müller

Department of Pathology
University of California at Los Angeles
School of Medicine, Harbor–UCLA Medical Center
Torrance, CA 90509

OUTLINE

  I. Introduction

 II. Definition of the juxtaglomerular apparatus

III. Structure of the juxtaglomerular cell

 IV. Structure of the macula densa

  V. Relationship between components of the juxtaglomerular apparatus
  A. Serial section light microscopy
  B. Serial section electron microscopy
  C. Analysis of serial sections
     1. The limits of the juxtaglomerular apparatus
     2. Surfaces of contact
     3. Three dimensional reconstructions
     4. Cellular composition

 VI. Structural-functional correlations

VII. Innervation of the juxtaglomerular apparatus
  A. The juxtaglomerular nerves by catecholamine fluorescent histochemistry
  B. The juxtaglomerular nerves by localization of acetyl-cholinesterase
  C. The juxtaglomerular nerves by electron microscopy
  D. The juxtaglomerular nerves by serial section electron microscopy
  E. Nerves in a juxtaglomerular cell tumor

VIII. Summary

---

[1]Supported by PHS Grant R01 HL 18340 from the National Heart & Lung Institute

I.   INTRODUCTION

The demonstration by Edelman and Hartroft (1961) that fluores-
cent-labeled antibodies to partially purified renin were selectively
localized in the granulated cells of the juxtaglomerular apparatus
provided convincing evidence, after a long period of search, of the
anatomical site of renin in the kidney and gave credence to the
earlier hypothesis of Goormaghtigh (1939, 1945). Prior to the
fluorescent antibody studies, however, there was a considerable body
of evidence implicating the granular cells as the source of renin.
The isolation and microdissection of glomeruli by Cook and Pickering
(1959) showed that most of the renin was present in the hilar region,
where the granular cells were located. Studies which found a positive correlation between the renin content of the kidney and the
degree of juxtaglomerular granularity further supported the view
that the granular cells were the source of renin (Hartroft, 1968).
More recently, Cook (1971) has carried out microextractions of renin
directly from juxtaglomerular cells, and Faarup (1967, 1968) has
succeeded in analyzing the distribution of renin in the different
parts of the vascular pole·by using microdissection techniques.

II.   DEFINITION OF THE JUXTAGLOMERULAR APPARATUS

We use the term juxtaglomerular apparatus (complex) to mean the
anatomical unit situated at the hilus of the glomerulus, made up of
a tubular and a vascular component. The vascular component consists
of the afferent and the efferent arteriole and an ill-defined region
containing both granular and agranular cells situated between the
arterioles, which has received many names in the literature: Polkissen (Zimmermann, 1933), lacis (Oberling and Hatt, 1960), and
juxtaglomerular body (Goormaghtigh, 1939). Because of its continuity with the glomerular mesangium, it has been called the extraglomerular mesangial region (Barajas, 1970). The tubular component
consists of a portion of the distal tubule that runs toward the
glomerulus and comes in contact with the vascular component. In this
region of contact the nuclei of the tubular cells appear accumulated,
and for this reason it was called the "macula densa" (Zimmermann,
1933). Cells which contain renin granules are called juxtaglomerular
cells; they may be found in all parts of the vascular component.

The above definition of the juxtaglomerular apparatus is based
on studies of the mammalian kidney. For information concerning the
comparative biology of the juxtaglomerular apparatus, the excellent
reviews of Sokabe (1974) and Sokabe and Ogawa (1974) may be consulted

III.   STRUCTURE OF THE JUXTAGLOMERULAR CELL

The vascular component of the juxtaglomerular apparatus is
the site of a unique cell type: a smooth muscle cell with endocrine morphologic and functional features.   The presence of secretory granules indicates its endocrine nature, although many of the
ultrastructural characteristics of its smooth muscle origin are
retained (attachment bodies, myofibrils, etc.).

By far the most useful stain for the light microscopic study
of renin granules is the Bowie method as modified by Hartroft (1968).
It has been applied successfully to assess the granularity of the
juxtaglomerular apparatus in experimental animals (Figure 1) and in
man, and has also been used to demonstrate the presence of renin
granules in mature, embryonic, and fetal kidneys in a variety of
vertebrate species.

Early electron microscopic studies showed that the juxtaglomerular cells of the rat (Oberling and Hatt, 1960; Hartroft and Newmark,
1961) and the mouse (Bohle, 1959) contain large, often multilobulated, membrane-bound granules which were found to be larger and
more irregular than those previously seen in most endocrine cells
(Figure 2).   The observations of some investigators suggested that
the juxtaglomerular granules originated in the Golgi apparatus
(Barajas and Latta, 1963; Chandra, Hubbard, Skelton, *et al.*, 1965).
Later, in studies of human, monkey, and rat kidneys, a different
type of granule, which was called a protogranule, was observed
(Barajas and Latta, 1965; Barajas, 1966; Biava and West, 1966).
They seemed to be more numerous in juxtaglomerular cells of kidneys
with increased renin production, such as those with constricted
renal arteries.   The smallest protogranules appeared in the cisternae
of the Golgi apparatus and had crystalline shape and substructure
(Figure 3).   Near the Golgi region, sacs were seen to include several
protogranules and, invariably, some small vesicles.   Conglomerates
of protogranules retaining their individual crystalline patterns
could be observed in the cytoplasm of the juxtaglomerular cell
(Figure 4).   The large granules, although usually amorphous, occa-
sionally displayed areas with crystalline substructure.   Based on
these observations it was proposed that the large amorphous granules developed from the protogranules observed in the Golgi cisternae.   According to this scheme, the sacs containing protogranules
and the conglomerates represent intermediate granular forms (Figure
5) (Barajas, 1966).   Observations made on juxtaglomerular cell tumors
also are consistent with this scheme (MacCallum, Conn, and Baker,
1973; Barajas, Bennett, Connor, and Lindstrom, 1977).

By contrast with the large, often multilobulated granules, the
small protogranules were similar in their morphology to other endocrine granules.   For example, in monkey and in man their rhomboidal
shape and the clear halo that separated them from their surrounding

membrane gave the protogranules considerable resemblance to beta-cell granules of the pancreas of some species (Barajas, 1966).

The fate of the granules and their relation to renin secretion remains an open question. It has been proposed that secretion might occur via release of the secretory product from granules into the cytoplasm (Lee, Hurley, and Hopper, 1966). The discharge would be mediated by changes in permeability of the granular membrane. This hypothesis is based on the observation of paler granules with intact limiting membrane, but no exocytosis, after the injection of agents to induce granule release.

More recent investigations carried out in other endocrine cells such as the beta cells of the pancreas, the adrenal medulla, as well as anterior and posterior pituitary support the view that the final step in the release of the hormone is by exocytosis (emiocytosis) (Lacy, 1975). In this process the membrane enveloping the granules fuses with the plasma membrane. This is followed by opening of the sac at the site of fusion and release of the granule contents into the interstitial space. In the juxtaglomerular cell the evidence for exocytosis is inconclusive. However, some investigators have observed areas of increased density in the interstitium, adjacent to the granular cells, in adrenalectomized rats (Peters, 1976) and in *Tupaia belangeri* after renal nerve stimulation (Taugner, Forssmann, Billich, *et al.*, 1978). This finding, as well as observations made by freeze-fracturing experiments, have been interpreted as suggestive of exocytosis (Taugner, Forssman, Billich, *et al.*, 1978).

In addition to the granular cells, the vascular component of the juxtaglomerular apparatus includes cells without renin granules. In the extraglomerular mesangium these agranular cells predominate (Barajas, 1971). In that location, their cytoplasm shows not only an absence of renin granules but also a relative scarcity of other cytoplasmic organelles. A few fibrillar bundles and attachment bodies provide evidence for their smooth muscle cell origin. In the wall of the arterioles, especially the afferent, typical vascular smooth muscle cells intermingle with juxtaglomerular granular cells. These smooth muscle cells are indistinguishable from those found in arterioles throughout the body. It should be added that serial section electron microscopy shows that a smooth muscle or agranular cell which in a given section may reveal no granules in its cytoplasm, might show them in sections at different levels. Therefore, in the juxtaglomerular apparatus, labeling a cell as agranular, based on random sections, should be done with caution.

In the juxtaglomerular apparatus of man, lipofuscin-like granules may be abundant in the granular juxtaglomerular cells (Biava and West, 1965; Barajas and Latta, 1967). In our experience these granules do not stain with the Bowie stain (Barajas, Sampson, and Latta, 1965; Barajas and Latta, 1967). We repeatedly have been able

to demonstrate them in great numbers with the electron microscope
in the juxtaglomerular apparatus from kidneys in which light microscopy shows no Bowie positive granules in the juxtaglomerular apparatus. These lipofuscin granules, therefore, most likely do not
interfere with the quantitative evaluation of granularity using the
Bowie stain.

IV. STRUCTURE OF THE MACULA DENSA

Besides the characteristic accumulation of nuclei, other morphologic changes occur in the distal tubule at the site of contact with
the vascular component. The most intriguing one is that the Golgi
apparatus appears in the basal, rather than the apical part of the
cell, close to the vascular component (McManus, 1943). When observed
with the electron microscope (Figure 6), the macula densa also shows
differences from other segments of the distal tubule in the size,
shape, and distribution of the mitochondria and in the extent of the
lateral interdigitations of the tubular cells. In the macula densa
the mitochondria are predominantly ovoid in shape and are scattered
throughout the cytoplasm. They are only rarely found inside the
lateral cytoplasmic interdigitations, which are only slightly developed in the macula densa. By contrast, in other segments of the
distal tubule the prevalent finding is elongated mitochondrial pro-
files perpendicular to the base of the cell which are enclosed by
invaginations of the plasma membrane.

V. RELATIONSHIPS BETWEEN COMPONENTS OF THE JUXTAGLOMERULAR APPARATUS

Goormaghtigh (1939) hypothesized in the late thirties, before
good evidence was available about the site of renin, that the macula
densa might act as a sensor to control the function of the adjacent
granular (juxtaglomerular) cells. With the juxtaglomerular cells
established as a source of renin, the old observation that at the
hilus of every glomerulus a part of the distal tubule (macula densa)
comes in contact with the vascular component, acquired a new and
potentially important significance in the understanding of regulation
of renin secretion. To establish the anatomical basis for a possible
participation of the distal tubule in the control of renin secretion,
a detailed investigation was undertaken in the rat of the tubulo-
vascular relationships at the hilus of the glomerulus.

A. Serial Section Light Microscopy

Serial semi-thin sections were prepared about 1 μ in thickness,
of plastic-embedded tissue. The sections were cut with glass knives
on a Porter-Blum MT1 Ultramicrotome and were stained with toluidine
blue. From the light microscopic photographs of the semi-thin

sections, freehand clay reconstructions of several juxtaglomerular apparatuses were made (Figure 7) (Barajas and Latta, 1963a, 1963b). These reconstructions in the rat showed a long and constant assoc- iation between the distal tubule and the efferent arteriole (Barajas and Latta, 1963a, 1963b; Faarup, 1964) and little contact of the distal tubule with the afferent arteriole. These observations were of interest from two standpoints: first, they showed the need to revise the widely-held notion that the juxtaglomerular apparatus included only contact between the distal tubule and the afferent arteriole; second, they revealed the surprising fact that most of the granular cells, which are located in the afferent arteriole, are not in contact with the distal tubule. The technique of cutting semi-thin serial sections of plastic-embedded material has the addi- tional advantage that it can be combined with ultra-thin sectioning for electron microscopy. It permitted, therefore, ultrastructural confirmation of the contact of the distal tubule with the efferent arteriole (Barajas and Latta, 1963b).

Recently Christensen, Meyer, and Bohle (1975) have reported that in man there is a more extensive association of the distal tubule with the afferent arteriole than with the efferent arteriole. Their studies, however, were carried out in tissues fixed by immer- sion, a method of fixation which results in closure of the tubular lumen and requires cutting of the unfixed tissue into small blocks. This procedure is likely to produce compression of the tissues and possibly increase contact between structures. Their studies, there- fore, are not comparable to those previously reported in rat kidneys fixed by dripping of osmium tetraoxide or perfusion with glutaralde- hyde. Both of these methods of fixation maintain the lumen of the tubules open and permit cutting the blocks after fixation of the tissues. Furthermore, the lack of ultrastructural confirmation of their findings is in contrast with the studies in the rat where, as has been mentioned above and will be discussed later, extensive electron microscopic studies have confirmed the light microscopic observations.

B. Serial Section Electron Microscopy

Electron microscopic observations by Oberling and Hatt (1960), Hartroft and Newmark (1961), Latta and Maunsbach (1962), Barajas and Latta (1963a) and others have established that the distal tubule is in intimate contact with the vascular component. This special type of contact is formed by projections of tubule cells into the tubulovascular space and fusion of the basement membranes of the two structures with formation of a network (Figure 6). A relation- ship of this kind suggests that the macula densa of the distal tubule and the vascular pole (arterioles and extraglomerular mesan- gial region) of the glomerulus form a single functional unit.

In the early sixties, Vander and Miller (1964) provided experimental evidence by the use of diuretics, suggesting that an increase in the sodium load in the distal tubule could decrease renin secretion. About the same time, Thurau (1964) and Guyton, Langston, and Navar (1964) independently proposed the juxtaglomerular apparatus as the site of a tubulo-arteriolar feedback mechanism controlling glomerular filtration rate. In the last 15 years much work from many laboratories has been carried out to elucidate the role of the distal tubule in the control of renin secretion and the function of the juxtaglomerular apparatus in the feedback control of single nephron filtration rate. Both of these topics have been recently reviewed (Davis and Freeman, 1976; Wright and Briggs, 1979). Interpretation of the results of Vander and Miller (1964) as well as the hypothesis that assigned the juxtaglomerular apparatus a role as feedback controller of single nephron filtration rate, relied heavily on the presence in the juxtaglomerular apparatus of a close association between the macula densa and the granular cells of the afferent arteriole. Thurau (1964) considered it a key fact supporting his hypothesis which included mediation of the renin-angiotensin system in the function of the feedback mechanism. In view of the results obtained by serial section light microscopy mentioned above, which showed very little contact between the afferent arteriole and the macula densa, it appeared pertinent to investigate at the cellular level the anatomical relationship between the distal tubule and vascular pole by means of the serial section electron microscopy technique. This method, although time consuming, provides the resolution necessary to analyze and quantify the type and number of cells in contact with the tubule, as well as the anatomical characteristics of the contact involved.

The methods used have been discussed in detail elsewhere (Barajas, 1970). Briefly, rat kidneys were used that had been fixed either by perfusion with 1% glutaraldehyde followed by osmium tetroxide or by dripping and immersion in osmium tetroxide. The tissue was embedded in Vestopal and large semi-thin sections were cut and stained with toluidine blue. Serial semi-thin sections of renal cortex which included many glomeruli were cut and examined by light microscopy. When the appearance of the juxtaglomerular apparatus in one of the glomeruli was thought to be imminent, then serial thin sections of that glomerulus were started. Series of 500 sections were cut and mounted on Formvar-coated, single-hole grids. A montage of electron micrographs was required for each section.

C. Analysis of Serial Sections

1. The limits of the juxtaglomerular apparatus. An analysis of the juxtaglomerular apparatus at the cellular level required a more precise definition of its boundaries than was customarily

employed. The vascular component was defined as: 1) those portions of the afferent and efferent arterioles from the point where the granular cells distal to the glomerulus first make their appearance, up to the glomerular hilus, and 2) the extraglomerular mesangial and arteriolar areas in contact with the distal tubule. The tubular component included the macula densa and was defined as that part of the distal tubule in contact with the vascular components.

　　2. Surfaces of contact. The initial measurements were of the surfaces of contact between the distal tubule and the vascular components. A good estimate of the true thickness of the sections was obtained by measuring the diameters of the spherical lysosomes in the proximal convoluted tubule and counting the number of sections required to go through an entire one. The average section thickness was found to be about 850 Å. The line of contact was measured in the electron micrographs by rolling a map measurer over it; the approximate area of the surface of contact was then easily obtained by multiplying this one-dimensional measurement by the section thickness. In all, the surfaces of contact of four juxtaglomerular apparatuses were measured. These measurements confirmed our light microscopic observations of prolonged contact between the efferent arteriole and the distal tubule. The distance between the vascular and tubular components in the regions of contact was 1000-2000 Å. Another central feature which emerged from this study was an appreciation of the extent and nature of the specialized contact between the distal tubule and the extraglomerular mesangium. It was in this area that cellular cytoplasmic projections of one component into the other was seen, with fusion and continuity of their basement membranes (Figure 6). This was in contrast to the arteriolar-tubular contact which, on the whole, consisted simply of apposition of the basement membranes. The occurrence of two distinct types of contact, and the fact that granular cells were involved in both types, indicated the possibility that this arrangement might have physiological significance, a point to be discussed later.

　　3. Three dimensional reconstructions. The relationships between tubular and vascular components of the juxtaglomerular apparatus are best studied and illustrated in three-dimensional models. Graphic models were obtained by outlining onto transparent plastic sheets the different components of the juxtaglomerular apparatus from the montages of electron micrographs. The two-dimensional representations were then superimposed and were offset a constant amount to give a three-dimensional effect (Figure 8a). Models of the tubular and vascular component were produced either separate or mounted together, and the area of tubulovascular contact was represented separately. More details of the methods used and illustrations of the models are given elsewhere (Barajas, 1970). A solid model was built using essentially the same procedures as for the graphic ones except that instead of outlining the juxtaglomerular

apparatus from montages onto plastic sheets, outline tracings were cut out of urethane foam sheets, using a modified Bruning drafting machine fitted with a soldering iron with a gold-plated tip. The resulting models corroborated the graphic ones and permitted us to see regions of the juxtaglomerular apparatus not visible in the graphic representations (Figure 8b).

  4. Cellular composition. Each cell of the vascular component was characterized according to position (afferent arteriole, extraglomerular mesangium, efferent arteriole) and granularity, and its nucleus was located and numbered on the montages (Barajas, 1971). The cells were then traced through the series of montages and their contact, if any, with the macula densa was noted. The previous observation that the majority of the granular cells are not in contact with the distal tubule was confirmed and quantified. In addition, serial sections showed that the extraglomerular mesangium, the region of the vascular component most consistently and extensively in contact with the macula densa, is extremely poor in granular cells. This observation has been corroborated recently by Latta and Johnston (1978) who found also an increase in the number of agranular cells in the extraglomerular mesangial region of rats with unilateral renovascular hypertension.

                VI. STRUCTURAL-FUNCTIONAL CORRELATIONS

  Physiological studies indicate that changes in sodium or chloride load at the distal tubule (macula densa hypothesis) or changes in the volume and stretch of the afferent arteriole (stretch receptor hypothesis) are involved in control of renin secretion. Davis and Freeman (1976) have recently reviewed the experimental evidence supporting both theories and other mechanisms controlling renin release. Taking into account the wealth of morphological data derived from the serial section studies, an interpretation was suggested for the mechanism of control of renin secretion (Barajas, 1971). The type of contact in which projections from the bases of the cells of the distal tubule penetrate the vascular component with fusion and network formation of the basement membranes was considered to be permanent and to represent the site at which the distal tubule is anchored to the vascular component. The type of contact involving a simple adjacency of basement membranes was interpreted as reversible. Variations in the extent of contact could, of course, be due to the different responses of individual nephrons to the preparatory technique; however, the fact that most of the granular cells are located where contact, if any, would be reversible, could indicate that variations in contact might occur under physiological conditions. A model in which variations in contact between the elements of the juxtaglomerular apparatus are responsible for the control of renin secretion may unify the supporting evidence for both hypotheses (Figure 9).

Many proponents of the macula densa hypothesis interpret their data as indicating that lowered sodium or chloride transport through the distal tubule increases renin secretion (Davis and Freeman, 1976). A smaller sodium or chloride load in the distal tubule would probably be accompanied by a decrease in the tubular volume and, therefore, decreased contact with granular cells. This mechanism also fits the stretch receptor hypothesis which is based on the fact that lowering the blood volume passing through the afferent arteriole increases renin secretion, and vice versa. On this basis, less contact would lead to an increase, while more contact would produce a decrease in renin secretion. On the other hand, the results of micropuncture experiments suggest that an increase in tubular fluid sodium concentration or more likely an increase in the reabsorptive transport of chloride are requirements to elicit the feedback response (Wright and Briggs, 1979). If it is assumed that the renin-angiotensin system is involved in the vasoconstriction of the afferent arteriole, a point that is uncertain at present, then it appears that high sodium or chloride levels in the macula densa would lead to an increase in renin secretion. From the anatomical standpoint, however, regardless of the mechanisms involved, the structure of the juxtaglomerular apparatus suggests that changes in the extent of contact between the tubular and vascular components are quite possible; these changes in contact are likely to alter whatever influence the distal tubule exerts on the granular cells, and might be physiologically significant. Following this line of reasoning, permanent contact can be viewed as more than just an anchoring device for the distal tubule, but also as providing a permanent site for functional exchange between the cells of the extraglomerular mesangial region and the macula densa.

In addition, it should be noted that there are granular cells in both arterioles so far removed from the distal tubule that any contact with it seems unlikely. In the efferent arteriole, these granular cells are on occasion seen to be in contact with the proximal tubule. Although this contact may very well be a fixation artifact, it opens the possibility of the existence of reversible contact between some of these cells and the proximal tubule, and suggests that physiological changes in the proximal tubule might modify renin secretion.

VII.   INNERVATION OF THE JUXTAGLOMERULAR APPARATUS

Light microscopists described a rich innervation of the renal cortex using silver impregnation and other staining methods (De Muylder, 1952). Although there was agreement among these early workers on the existence of an innervation of the glomerular arterioles, important questions regarding the nature and distribution of the nerves in the juxtaglomerular region were unsettled. With the advent of electron microscopy, some of these questions were soon

answered. It was possible, for example, to rule out the presence
of myelinated nerves in the hilus of the glomerulus and the pene-
tration of nerves into the glomerular tufts, two points of considerable debate among histologists. An early electron microscopic
study of the innervation of the glomerular arterioles of monkey and
rat showed that they were extensively innervated by unmyelinated
nerves (Barajas, 1964). Nerves were seen in association with granular as well as agranular smooth muscle cells of the vascular component of the juxtaglomerular apparatus. Axons with the ultrastructural features characteristic of adrenergic nerves were described.

A. The Juxtaglomerular Nerves by Catecholamine Fluorescent
Histochemistry

When the histochemical fluorescence method for biogenic mono-
amines (Falck, Hillarp, Thieme, and Thorp, 1962) is applied to the
kidney, an adrenergic innervation of the glomerular arterioles can
be demonstrated in the monkey, rat (Figure 10), and other species
(Nilsson, 1965; McKenna and Angelakos, 1968b; Wagermark, Ungerstedt,
and Ljundqvist, 1968; Munkacsi, 1969). In the monkey, a distinct
tubular innervation also can be seen (Müller and Barajas, 1972),
which consists of nerve bundles arising from the perivascular nerves
and following the contour of proximal and distal tubules. In the
rat, tubular adrenergic innervation is confined to the juxtaglomerular region, except for occasional areas of catecholamine fluorescence attached to the wall of tubules located at some distance from
the glomerular arterioles (Barajas, 1978). The advantages provided
by the specificity of the fluorescent techniques are marred by problems of anatomic interpretation, stemming from the darkness of the
background structures when observed under the fluorescence microscope, the great thickness of the sections required for the visuali-
zation of the nerves, and the relatively low resolution of the light
microscope. It is, therefore, of great value to obtain electron
microscopic verification of the findings provided by fluorescence
histochemistry.

B. The Juxtaglomerular Nerves by Localization of
Acetylcholinesterase

Another light microscopic method useful in the study of the
juxtaglomerular nerves is that of Koelle and Friedenwald (1949) or
its modification by Karnovsky and Roots (1964), for the demonstration
of acetylcholinesterase (Ballantyne, 1959; McKenna and Angelakos,
1968b; Wagermark, Ungerstedt, and Ljundqvist, 1968; Munkacsi, 1969).
In the monkey, a distinct tubular innervation also can be seen
(Müller and Barajas, 1972). This method can be used at the ultrastructural level (Barajas, Silverman, and Müller, 1974; Barajas,
Wang, and De Santis, 1976). The distribution and extent of acetyl-

cholinesterase-positive innervation of the juxtaglomerular apparatus
parallel that observed with catecholamine fluorescence (Figure 11).
The histochemical demonstration of acetylcholinesterase in the renal
nerves has been considered to indicate the existence of a cholinergic
innervation. This possibility was investigated using 6-hydroxydopa-
mine, a drug that selectively destroys adrenergic nerves (Thoenen
and Tranzer, 1968; Barajas and Wang, 1975). We examined kidneys
from rats after administration of 6-hydroxydopamine, by combining
light microscopic histochemical techniques with electron microscopy.
Both the fluorescence and the acetylcholinesterase precipitate decreased concomitantly from the glomerular arterioles after one injection of the drug and disappeared almost totally after two injections
(Barajas and Wang, 1975). By electron microscopy, only degenerating
nerves were observed in association with the glomerular arterioles
in these animals. Since 6-hydroxydopamine destroys only adrenergic
nerve endings, it was concluded that the glomerular arterioles of
the rat are innervated by adrenergic nerves which display acetylcholinesterase activity.

            C.   The Juxtaglomerular Nerves by Electron Microscopy

       The higher resolution provided by the electron microscope allows
study of the fine structure of the nerve bundles, the axoplasm and
its contents, and the precise relationships between nerves and the
components of the juxtaglomerular apparatus (Barajas, 1964; Simpson
and Devine, 1966). Ultrastructurally, the nerve bundles are seen
to be composed of axons partially or totally surrounded by Schwann
cells. Along their course, the axons present dilated segments
(varicosities) containing vesicles. Microtubules are observed in
the axons, predominantly in the intervaricose regions.

       Four types of vesicles were encountered in the renal nerves:
small granular dense-cored vesicles that averaged about 500 Å,
small agranular (clear) vesicles, large (average 900 Å) granular
vesicles, and large agranular vesicles. The small dense-cored
vesicles are thought to be characteristic of adrenergic nerves and
might contain norepinephrine. They disappear from the renal nerves
after the administration of reserpine, coinciding with the depletion
of tissue catecholamines and the abolition of monoamine fluorescence
(Silverman and Barajas, 1974). Varicosities establish contact with
agranular (including smooth muscle) cells and with granular cells of
the vascular component (Figure 12) and less frequently with distal
and proximal tubular cells in the juxtaglomerular region (Barajas
and Müller, 1973; Gorgas, 1978). It must be mentioned that the
nerves do not penetrate the wall of the vascular component or the
area of tubulo-vascular contact, at least in the area of fixed contact. If we define the macula densa as the portion of the distal
tubule in contact with the vascular component, no nerves are seen
in contact with the macula densa. They are seen, however, touching

the free wall of the distal tubule (Figure 13) near the macula densa.
The varicosities in contact with effector cells are sometimes referred
to as "nerve endings" or "nerve terminals". It is assumed that at the
sites of contact, a neuroeffector junction is established and that
neural transmission occurs. The varicosities, containing combinations
of all of the types of vesicles mentioned above, are separated from
the cells of the vascular or tubular component of the juxtaglomerular
apparatus by a 1000-2000 Å space containing basement membrane material
(Figures 12 and 13).

D.   The Juxtaglomerular Nerves by Serial Section Electron
                         Microscopy

        To establish the relationships of the nerves with the different
components of the juxtaglomerular apparatus, the technique of serial
section electron microscopy was particularly useful (Barajas and
Müller, 1973). It was applied in conjunction with the three-
dimensional study mentioned above. The results showed that about
one-third of the cells of the vascular component of the juxtaglomerular apparatus were innervated and that the majority of the innervated
cells were in contact with varicosities belonging to more than one
axon. How the neural stimulus reaches the noninnervated cells is a
matter of speculation. Gap junctions, thought to be sites of low
resistance allowing electrical coupling, are frequent between cells
of the vascular component (Boll, Forssman, and Taugner, 1975).
Therefore, the noninnervated cells may be electrically coupled to
innervated cells. Another possibility is that a high enough concentration of the neurotransmitter released from the varicosities in the
interstitial space may reach the noninnervated cell to stimulate it.

        As individual axons were followed, a complex pattern of inner-
vation emerged (Figure 14). Individual axons were observed to establish contact along their path with granular and agranular cells of
the afferent and efferent arteriole and extraglomerular mesangium.
Of considerable interest was the observation of individual axons
establishing contact along their path with both vascular and tubular
cells. It appears that innervation by the same axon of granular and
smooth muscle cells of the afferent arteriole and of the distal tubule may take place. Therefore, activity of an individual axon could
affect renin secretion, vasoconstriction of the arterioles, and tubular resorption of sodium, thus providing functional integration of
the various components of the juxtaglomerular apparatus.

        All axons followed through the serial sections contained at one
point or another small dense-cored vesicles which are considered
characteristic of adrenergic nerves. This finding supports the view
that the innervation of the juxtaglomerular region is exclusively
adrenergic.

In addition to the well established physiological significance
of the renal vascular innervation, there is physiological evidence
in support of participation of the renal nerves in the control of
renin secretion (Davis and Freeman, 1976). Furthermore, recent
studies suggest that the tubular nerves exert an influence on the
proximal tubular resorption of sodium (Slick, Aguilera, Zambraski,
et al., 1975; Bello-Reuss, Trevino, and Gottschalk, 1976). The
renal nerves, therefore, appear to play a significant role in the
control of renal function.

E. Nerves in a Juxtaglomerular Cell Tumor

In a recent study, neural elements were observed in a juxtaglomerular cell tumor of a 15-year-old girl with hypertension
(Barajas, Bennett, Connor, and Lindstrom, 1977). The axons
observed in the tumor contained the small dense-cored vesicles
characteristic of adrenergic nerves. Nerve terminals contacted
juxtaglomerular tumor cells (Figure 15). A significant difference
between the contact of nerves with juxtaglomerular tumor cells and
the contact of nerves and the juxtaglomerular cells in the juxtaglomerular apparatus was observed. In the tumor, direct contact of
the nerve terminals with the juxtaglomerular cells took place,
without any intervening basement membrane and with a gap between
the two plasma membranes of only approximately 150 Å. In the
juxtaglomerular apparatus, on the other hand, basement membrane is
always present between the plasma membrane of the nerve terminal
and that of the juxtaglomerular cell, with a gap between the two
membranes many times greater than that seen in the tumor. The
presence of sympathetic fibers in the juxtaglomerular cell tumor
underscores the close biological relationship between the sympathetic and the renin-angiotensin systems.

VIII. SUMMARY

The juxtaglomerular apparatus consists of a tubular and a
vascular component. The vascular component includes portions of
the afferent and efferent arterioles proximal to the glomerulus
and the extraglomerular mesangium (also referred to as Polkissen,
lacis, or juxtaglomerular body). This region, situated between the
two arterioles at the hilus of the glomerulus, is continuous with
the intraglomerular mesangium. The tubular component includes the
macula densa and consists of a portion of the distal tubule, which
establishes contact with the vascular component. Two morphologically different types of contact have been described: one is
thought to be permanent and the other reversible. A model for the
control of renin secretion based on variation in contact between
the tubular and vascular component has been proposed.

Cells containing membrane-bound secretory granules (juxta-glomerular cells) are observed in all parts of the vascular compo-nent and are the source of renin. The juxtaglomerular cell has functional and anatomical features of endocrine cells while still retaining structures characteristic of smooth muscle cells, such as fibrillar bundles and attachment bodies. They can, therefore, be considered to be modified smooth muscle cells. It has been proposed that the mature amorphous juxtaglomerular granules develop from crystalline protogranules observed in the Golgi cisternae.

The cells of the macula densa are packed closer together than contiguous parts of the distal tubule. Other differences from the other cells of the distal tubule are the basal location of the Golgi system and lesser development of the infoldings of the plasma membrane.

Fluorescence histochemistry shows a rich adrenergic innervation of the juxtaglomerular region. With the electron microscope, unmyeli-nated nerves are seen in association with glomerular arterioles and renal tubules of the region. Axons contain small dense-cored vesicles, implying adrenergic function. Distinct neuro-vascular and neuro-tubular junctions, anatomically consistent with being the sites of synaptic transmission, are observed. They occur on juxta-glomerular cells, on smooth muscle cells, on the distal tubular cells at the level of the macula densa, and on the proximal tubules of the region. In a juxtaglomerular cell tumor, adrenergic nerve fibers with axons in direct contact with the juxtaglomerular tumor cells are found. These observations underscore the close biological relation-ship between the renin-angiotensin and the sympathetic systems.

REFERENCES

Ballantyne, B. (1959). The neurohistology of mammalian kidney.
    Univ. Leeds Med. J. 8: 50-59.
Barajas, L. (1964). The innervation of the juxtaglomerular
    apparatus. An electron microscopic study of the innervation
    of the glomerular arterioles. Lab. Invest. 13: 916-929.
Barajas, L. (1966). The development and ultrastructure of the juxta-
    glomerular cell granule. J. Ultrastruct. Res. 15: 400-413
Barajas, L. (1970). The ultrastructure of the juxtaglomerular
    apparatus as disclosed by three-dimensional reconstructions
    from serial sections: The anatomical relationship between the
    tubular and vascular components. J. Ultrastruct. Res. 33:
    116-147.
Barajas, L. (1971). Renin secretion: An anatomical basis for
    tubular control. Science 172: 485-487.
Barajas, L. (1972). Anatomical considerations in the control of
    renin secretion. In: *Control of Renin Secretion*. (Assaykeen,
    T. A., ed.), pp. 1-16, Plenum Publishing Corp., New York.

Barajas, L. (1978). Innervation of the renal cortex. Fed. Proc.
    37: 1192-1201.

Barajas, L., Bennett, C., Connor, G., and Lindstrom, R. (1977).
    Structure of a juxtaglomerular cell tumor: The presence of a
    neural component. A light and electron microscopic study.
    Lab. Invest. 37: 357-368.

Barajas, L. and Latta, H. (1963a). A three-dimensional study of
    the juxtaglomerular apparatus in the rat. Light and electron
    microscopic observations. Lab. Invest. 12: 257-269.

Barajas, L. and Latta, H. (1963b). The juxtaglomerular apparatus
    in adrenalectomized rats. Light and electron microscopic
    observations. Lab. Invest. 12: 1046-1059.

Barajas, L. and Latta, H. (1965). The development of the juxta-
    glomerular cell granule. Anat. Rec. 151: 321.

Barajas, L. and Latta, H. (1967). Structure of the juxtaglomerular
    apparatus. Circ. Res. 21 (Suppl. 2): 15-28.

Barajas, L. and Müller, J. (1973). The innervation of the juxta-
    glomerular apparatus and surrounding tubules: A quantitative
    analysis by serial section electron microscopy. J. Ultrastruct.
    Res. 43: 107-132.

Barajas, L., Sampson, R. J., and Latta, H. (1965). The juxta-
    glomerular apparatus of patients with renovascular hypertension,
    a light and electron microscopic study. Fed. Proc. 24: 435.

Barajas, L., Silverman, A. J., and Müller, J. (1974). Ultrastruc-
    tural localization of acetylcholinesterase in the renal nerves.
    J. Ultrastruct. Res. 49: 297-311.

Barajas, L. and Wang, P. (1975). Demonstration of acetylcholin-
    esterase in the adrenergic nerves of the renal glomerular
    arterioles. J. Ultrastruct. Res. 53: 244-253.

Barajas, L., Wang, P., and De Santis, S. (1976). Light and electron
    microscopic localization of acetylcholinesterase activity in
    the rat renal nerves. Am. J. Anat. 147: 219-233.

Bello-Reuss, E., Trevino, D. L., and Gottschalk, C. W. (1976).
    Effect of renal sympathetic nerve stimulation on proximal water
    and sodium reabsorption. J. Clin. Invest. 57: 1104-1107.

Biava, C. G. and West, M. (1965). Lipofuscin-like granules in
    vascular smooth muscle and juxtaglomerular cells of human
    kidneys. Am. J. Pathol. 47: 287-313.

Biava, C. G. and West, M. (1966). Fine morphology of human JG cells
    in patients with benign essential hypertension. Lab. Invest.
    15: 1902-1920.

Bohle, H. A. (1959). Elektronenmikroskopische Untersuchungen uber
    die Struktur des Gefabpois der Niere. Verh. Dtsch. Ges. Path.
    43: 219-225.

Boll, H. U., Forssmann, W., and Taugner, R. (1975). Studies on the
    juxtaglomerular apparatus. IV. Freeze-fracturing of membrane
    surfaces. Cell Tissue Res. 161: 459-469.

Chandra, S., Hubbard, J. C., Skelton, F. R., Bernadis, L. I., and
Kamura, S. (1965). Genesis of juxtaglomerular cell granules.
A physiologic light and electron microscopic study concerning
experimental renal hypertension. Lab. Invest. 14: 1835-1842.

Christensen, J., Meyer, D., and Bohle, A. (1975). The structure of
the human juxtaglomerular apparatus. A morphometric light
microscopic study on serial sections. Virchows Arch. [Pathol.
Anat.] 367: 83-92.

Cook, W. F. (1971). Cellular localization of renin. In: *Hormones
and the Kidney*. (Fisher, J. W., ed.), pp. 117-128, Academic
Press, New York.

Cook, W. F. and Pickering, G. W. (1959). The location of renin
within the kidney. J. Physiol. (Lond.) 149: 526-536.

Davis, J. O. and Freeman, R. H. (1976). Mechanisms regulating
renin release. Physiol. Rev. 56: 1-56.

DeMuylder, C. G. (1952). *The "Neurility" of the Kidney. A Mono-
graph on Nerve Supply to the Kidney*. Charles C. Thomas,
Springfield, IL

Edelman, R. and Hartroft, P. M. (1961). Localization of renin in
juxtaglomerular cells of rabbit and dog through use of fluorescent antibody technique. Circ. Res. 9: 1069-1077.

Faarup, P. (1964). Morphology of the juxtaglomerular apparatus.
In: *Proceedings of the Second International Congress of
Nephrology*. (Vortil, Y. and Richet, G., eds.), p. 427,
Excerpta Medica Foundation, New York.

Faarup, P. (1967). Renin location in the different parts of the
juxtaglomerular apparatus in the cat kidney. I. The afferent
arteriole and the macula densa. Acta Pathol. Microbiol. Scand.
71: 509-521.

Faarup, P. (1968). Renin location in the different parts of the
juxtaglomerular apparatus in the cat kidney. II. Fractions
of the afferent arteriole, the cell group of Goormaghtigh, the
efferent arteriole, and the glomerulus. Acta Pathol. Microbiol.
Scand. 72: 109-117.

Falck, B., Hillarp, A., Thieme, G., and Thorp, A. (1962). Fluorescence of catecholamines and related compounds condensed with
formaldehyde. J. Histochem. Cytochem. 10: 348-354.

Gorgas, K. (1978). Innervation of the juxtaglomerular apparatus.
In: *Peripheral Neuroendocrine Interaction*. (Coupland, R. E.
and Forssmann, W. G., eds.), pp. 144-152, Springer-Verlag,
New York.

Goormaghtigh, N. (1939). Existence of an endocrine gland in the
media of the renal arterioles. Proc. Soc. Exp. Biol. Med.
42: 688-689.

Goormaghtigh, N. (1945). La fonction endocrine des arterioles
renales: Son role dans la pathogenie de l'hypertension
arterielle. Rev. Belge Sci. Med. 16: 65-155.

Guyton, A. C., Langston, J. B., and Navar, G. (1964). Theory for
renal autoregulation by feedback at the juxtaglomerular
apparatus. Circ. Res. 15 (Suppl. 1): 187-197.

Hartroft, P. M. (1968). The juxtaglomerular complex as an endocrine gland. In: *Endocrine Pathology*. (Bloodworth, J. M. B., ed.), pp. 641-677, Williams and Wilkins, Baltimore.

Hartroft, P. and Newmark, L. N. (1961). Electron microscopy of renal juxtaglomerular cells. Anat. Rec. 139: 185-199.

Karnovsky, M. J. and Roots, L. (1964). A direct-coloring thiocholine method for cholinesterases. J. Histochem. Cytochem. 12: 219-221.

Koelle, G. B. and Friedenwald, J. S. (1949). A histochemical method localizing cholinesterase activity. Proc. Soc. Exp. Biol. Med. 70: 617-622.

Lacy, P. E. (1975). Endocrine secretory mechanisms. Am. J. Pathol. 79: 170-188.

Latta, H. and Johnston, W. H. (1978). Granular and agranular cell counts in the juxtaglomerular apparatuses of rats with unilateral renovascular hypertension. Lab. Invest. 39: 219-224.

Latta, H. and Maunsbach, A. B. (1962). The juxtaglomerular apparatus as studied electron microscopically. J. Ultrastruct. Res. 6: 547-561.

Lee, J. C., Hurley, S., and Hopper, J., Jr. (1966). Secretory activity of the juxtaglomerular granular cells of the mouse: Morphologic and enzyme histochemical observations. Lab. Invest. 15: 1459-1476.

MacCallum, D. K., Conn, J. W., and Baker, B. L. (1973). Ultrastructure of a renin-secreting juxtaglomerular cell tumor of the kidney. Invest. Urol. 11: 65-74.

McKenna, O. C. and Angelakos, E. T. (1968a). Acetylcholinesterase-containing nerve fibers in the canine kidney. Circ. Res. 23: 645-651.

McKenna, O. C. and Angelakos, E. T. (1968b). Adrenergic innervation of the canine kidney. Circ. Res. 22: 345-354.

McManus, J. F. A. (1943). Apparent reversal of position of the Golgi element in the renal tubule. Nature 152: 417.

Müller, J. and Barajas, L. (1972). Electron microscopic and histochemical evidence for a tubular innervation in the renal cortex of the monkey. J. Ultrastruct. Res. 41: 533-549.

Munkacsi, I. (1969). Distribution of the intrarenal monoaminergic nerves in the kidneys of the desert rat (*Dipodomys merriami*) and the white rat (*Rattus norvegicus*). Acta Anat. 73: 56-68.

Nilsson, O. (1965). The adrenergic innervation of the kidney. Lab. Invest. 14: 1392-1395.

Oberling, C. and Hatt, P. Y. (1960). Etude de l'appareil juxtaglomerulaire du rat au microscope electronique. Ann. Anat. Pathol. (Paris) 5: 411-474.

Peter, S. (1976). Ultrastructural studies on the secretory process in the epitheloid cells of the juxtaglomerular apparatus. Cell Tissue Res. 168: 45-53.

Silverman, A. J. and Barajas, L. (1974). Effect of reserpine on the juxtaglomerular granular cells and renal nerves. Lab. Invest. 30: 723-731.

Simpson, F. O. and Devine, C. E. (1966). The fine structure of autonomic neuromuscular contacts in arterioles of sheep renal cortex. J. Anat. 100: 127-137.

Slick, G. L., Aguilera, A. J., Zambraski, E. J., Dibona, G. F., and Kaloyanides, G. J. (1975). Renal neuroadrenergic transmission. Am. J. Physiol. 229: 60-65.

Sokabe, H. (1974). Phylogeny of the renal effects of angiotensin. Kidney Int. 6: 263-271.

Sokabe, H. and Ogawa, M. (1974). Comparative studies of the juxta-glomerular apparatus. Int. Rev. Cytol. 37: 271-327.

Taugner, R., Forssmann, W. G., Billich, H., Boll, U., Ganten, D., and Seller, H. (1978). Innervation of the juxtaglomerular apparatus and the effects of renal nerve stimulation. In: *Peripheral Neuroendocrine Interaction.* (Coupland, R. E. and Forssmann, W. G., eds.), pp. 153-163, Springer-Verlag, New York.

Thoenen, H. and Tranzer, J. P. (1968). Chemical sympathectomy by selective destruction of adrenergic nerve endings with 6-hydroxydopamine. Naunyn Schmiedebergs Arch. Pharmacol. 261: 271-288.

Thurau, K. (1964). Renal hemodynamics. Am. J. Med. 36: 698-719.

Vander, A. J. and Miller, R. (1964). Control of renin secretion in the anesthetized dog. Am. J. Physiol. 207: 537-545.

Wägermark, J., Ungerstedt, U., and Ljundqvist, A. (1968). Sympa-thetic innervation of the juxtaglomerular cells of the kidney. Circ. Res. 22: 149-153.

Wolfe, D. E., Potter, L. T., Richardson, K. C., and Axelrod, J. (1962). Localizing tritiated norepinephrine in sympathetic axons by electron microscopic autoradiography. Science 138: 440-442.

Wright, F. S. and Briggs, J. P. (1979). Feedback control of glomerular blood flow, pressure, and filtration rate. Physiol. Rev. 59: 958-1006.

Zimmermann, K. W. (1933). Über den Bau des Glomerulus der Saugerniere. Z. Mikrosk. Anat. Forsch. 32: 176-278.

ACKNOWLEDGMENTS

The authors thank Dennis Gross for his contribution in the preparation of the solid model, and Dr. Michael Lubran for his suggestions regarding the manuscript. We thank Ms. Astara Mayeda for her skilled typing of the manuscript.

Figure 1.   *Photomicrograph of hypergranulated juxtaglomerular apparatus from ischemic kidney of a rat with reno-vascular hypertension. Paraffin embedded tissue stained with the Bowie method. A, afferent arteriole; E, efferent arteriole; MD, macula densa. x 750.*

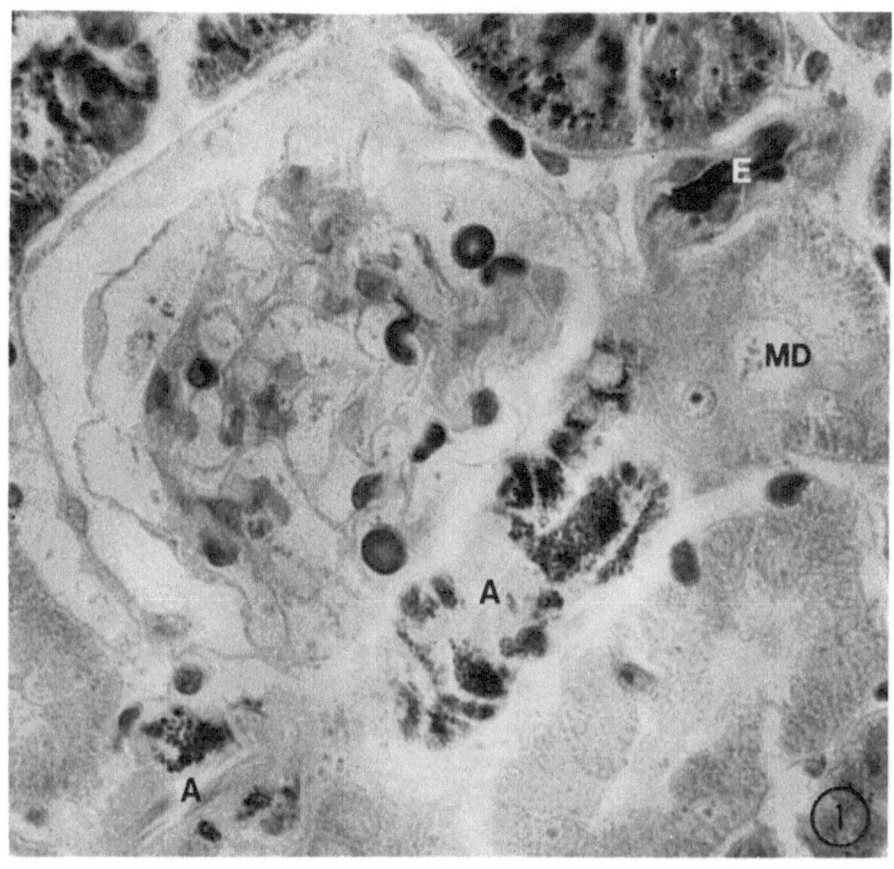

Figure 2.   *Portion of cytoplasm of a rat juxtaglomerular cell.*
The characteristic large, irregular, amorphous granules
occupy much of the cytoplasmic space.   A sac containing
a small protogranule (P) is observed near the nucleus
(N).   x 55,000.

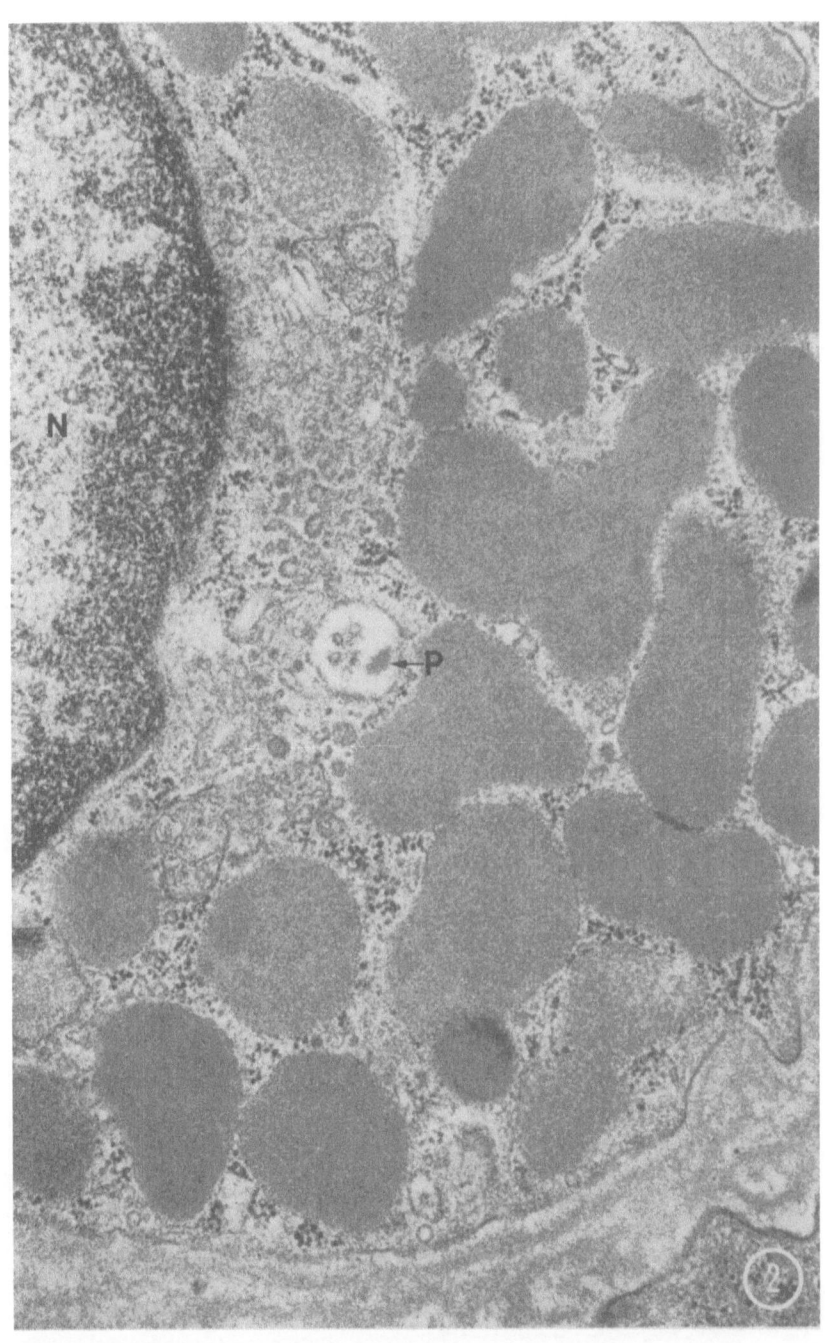

Figure 3. *Two crystalline protogranules (arrows) are noted within distended cisternae of the Golgi apparatus (GA) of a juxtaglomerular granular cell. At the upper right corner a smooth membranous sac (S) containing several protogranules and vesicles is shown. Mature granules (G) are also seen. From a juxtaglomerular apparatus of the rat kidney with constricted renal artery, x 50,000. Figs. a and b. Enlargements of Fig. 3. The periodicity of the crystalline layers is observed in all protogranules. Fig. 3b also shows protogranules and vesicles in a smooth membranous sac. Periodicities in two directions are visible in one of the protogranules in the sac. Fig. 3a x 130,000. Fig. 3b x 110,000. From Barajas, L. (1966). J. Ultrastruct. Res. 15: 400-413.*

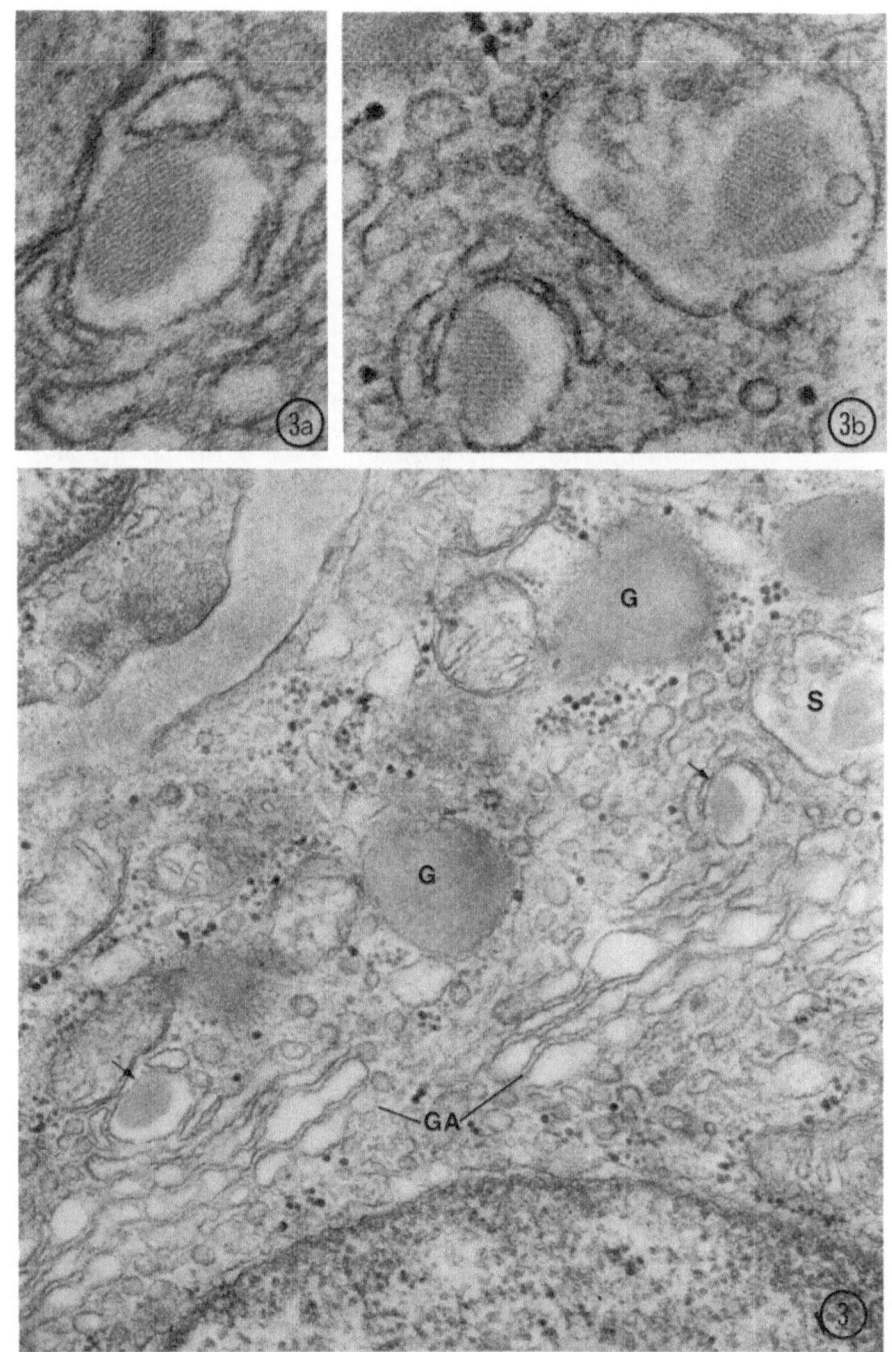

Figure 4. *A conglomerate of protogranules showing independent crystalline patterns. Vesicles are in the left mid portion of the conglomerate. From a rat with constricted renal artery, x 110,000. From Barajas, L. (1966). J. Ultrastruct. Res. 15: 400-413.*

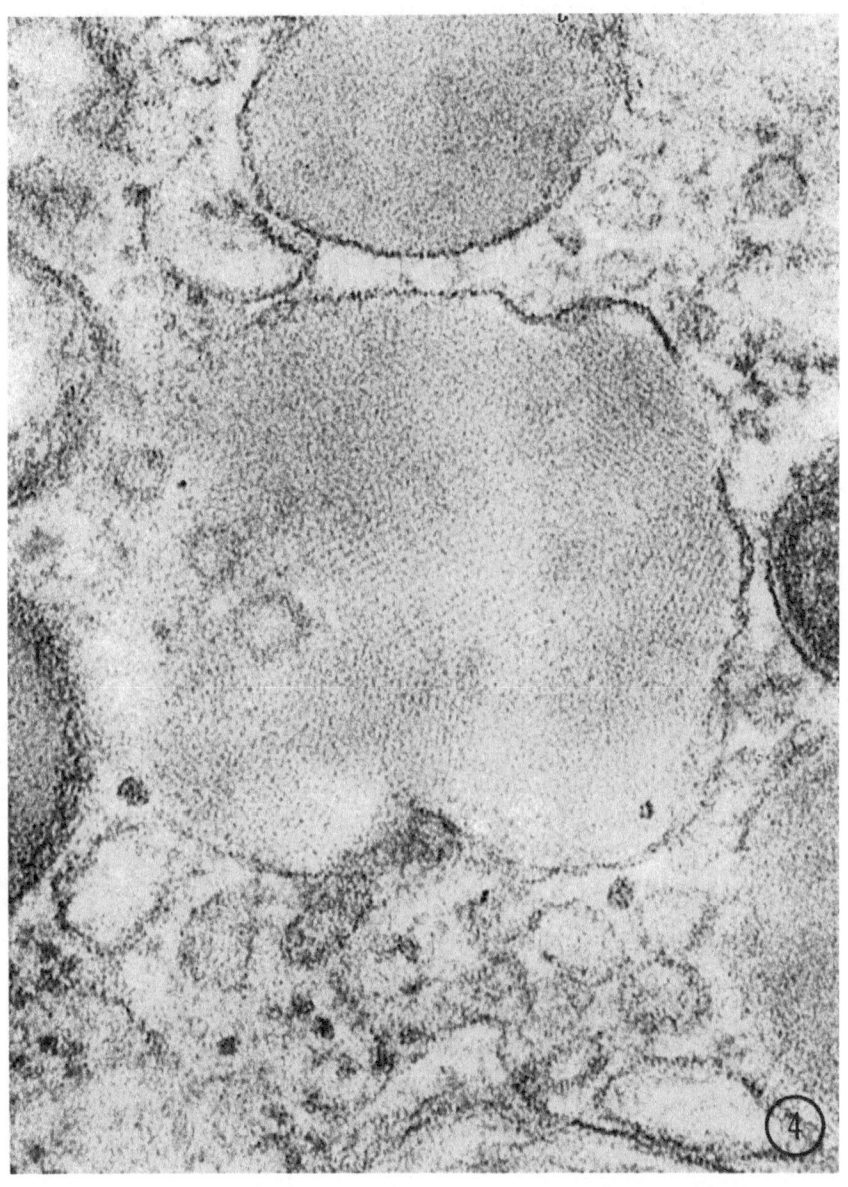

Figure 5.   *Drawing representing the proposed sequence of formation*
             of juxtaglomerular cell granule in the rat. From rat
             with constricted renal artery. From Barajas, L. (1966).
             J. Ultrastruct. Res. 15: 400-413.

Figure 6.   *Macula densa (MD), extraglomerular mesangium (EM), and*
             efferent arteriole (E). The Golgi apparatus (GA) lies
             at the base of the cells, and appears abundant. Extra-
             cellular compartments (EC) are frequently found near
             the base of cells of the macula densa. Lateral processes
             (LP) also are found near the base of the cells. Projec-
             tions (P) of the macula densa cells extend down toward
             the extraglomerular mesangium and efferent arteriole.
             Microvilli are more prominent in the angles between
             cells. Several junctional complexes (JC) are noted.
             Agranular cell processes lie in a moderately dense
             matrix. x 9,000. From Barajas, L. and Latta, H.
             (1963a). Lab. Invest. 12: 257-269.

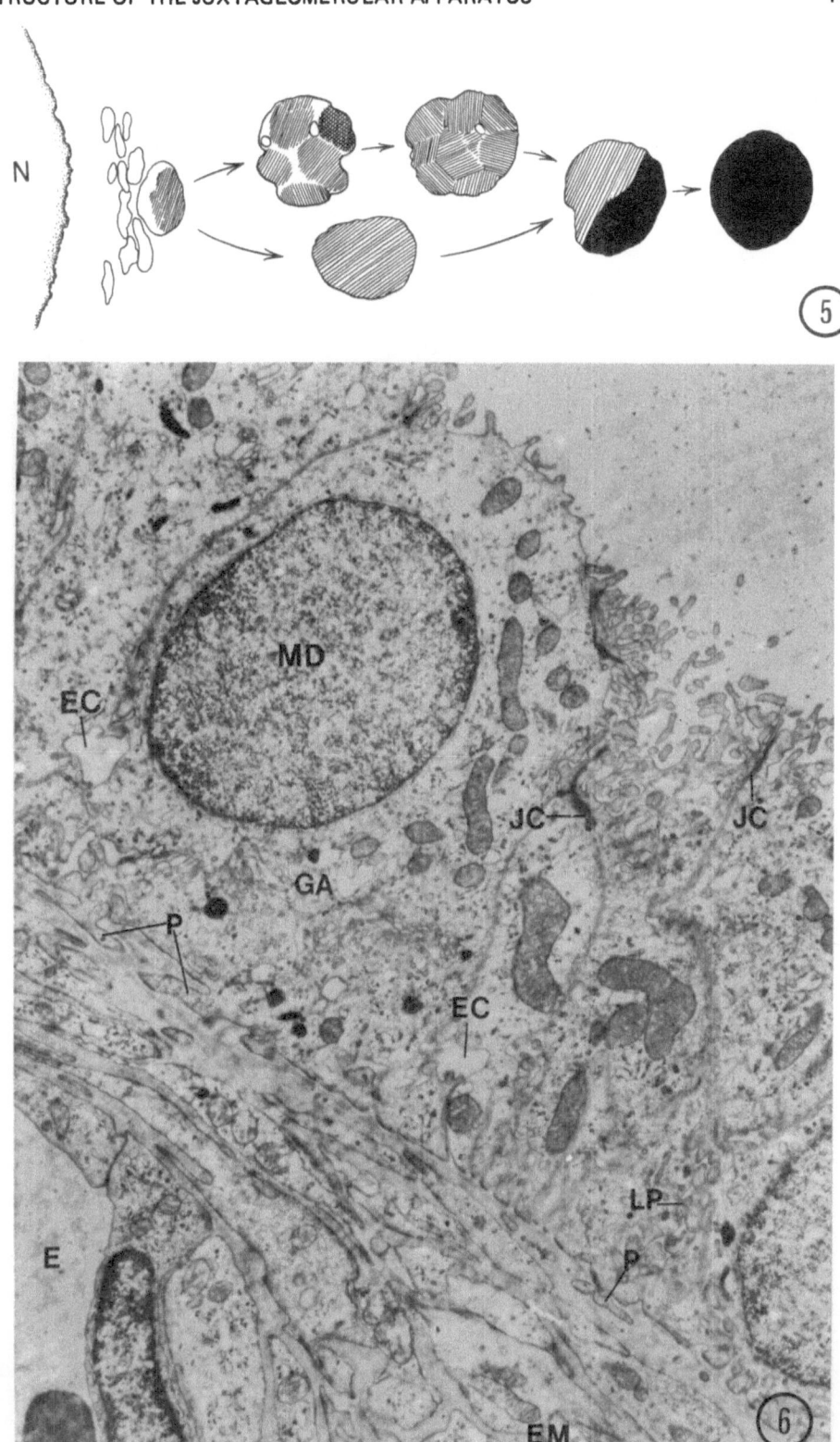

Figure 7.   *Clay model reconstructed from light micrography of*
            serial sections two microns in thickness. The distal
            tubule (D) is associated over a long distance with the
            efferent arterioles (E). It runs between this and the
            afferent arteriole (A) at the hilus of the glomerulus.
            The extent of the contact with the afferent arteriole
            appears very small. The glomerulus is represented by
            a large round mass and the origin of the proximal
            convoluted tubule by the projection at the lower right.
            From Barajas, L. and Latta, H. (1963a). Lab. Invest.
            12: 257-269.

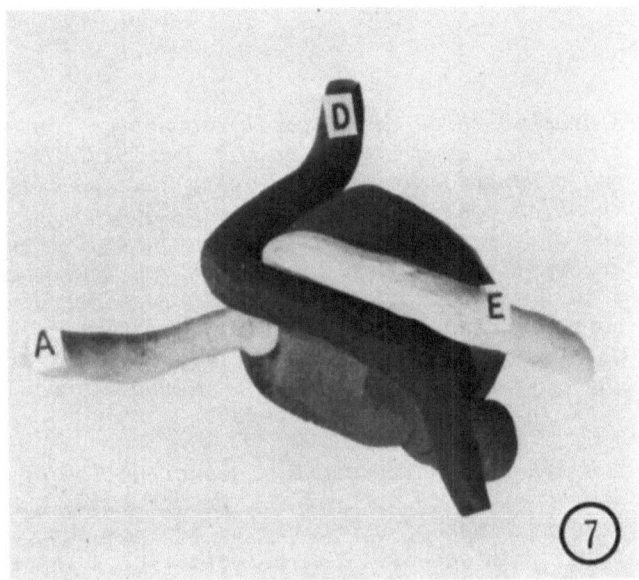

Figure 8a.   *A graphic three-dimensional reconstruction of a juxta-*
             glomerular apparatus. It was constructed by superimpos-
             ing schematic drawings of every 18th section. The areas
             in which contact occurs are represented by thick lines;
             the different components of the juxtaglomerular apparatus
             are outlined in thin lines. In the lower portion of the
             illustration the lines are numbered according to their
             corresponding sections. Distal tubule (dt), extra-
             glomerular mesangial region (m), afferent arteriole (aa),
             and efferent arteriole (ea). x 900.   From Barajas, L.
             (1971). Science 172: 485-487.

Figure 8b.   *A solid three-dimensional reconstruction of the same*
             juxtaglomerular apparatus. It was built up from out-
             line tracings of every eighth section cut out of ure-
             thane foam sheets. The orientation of the solid model
             is the same as that of the graphic model shown in Fig.
             8a. Afferent arteriole (aa), efferent arteriole (ea),
             distal tubule (dt), and extraglomerular mesangial
             region (m).

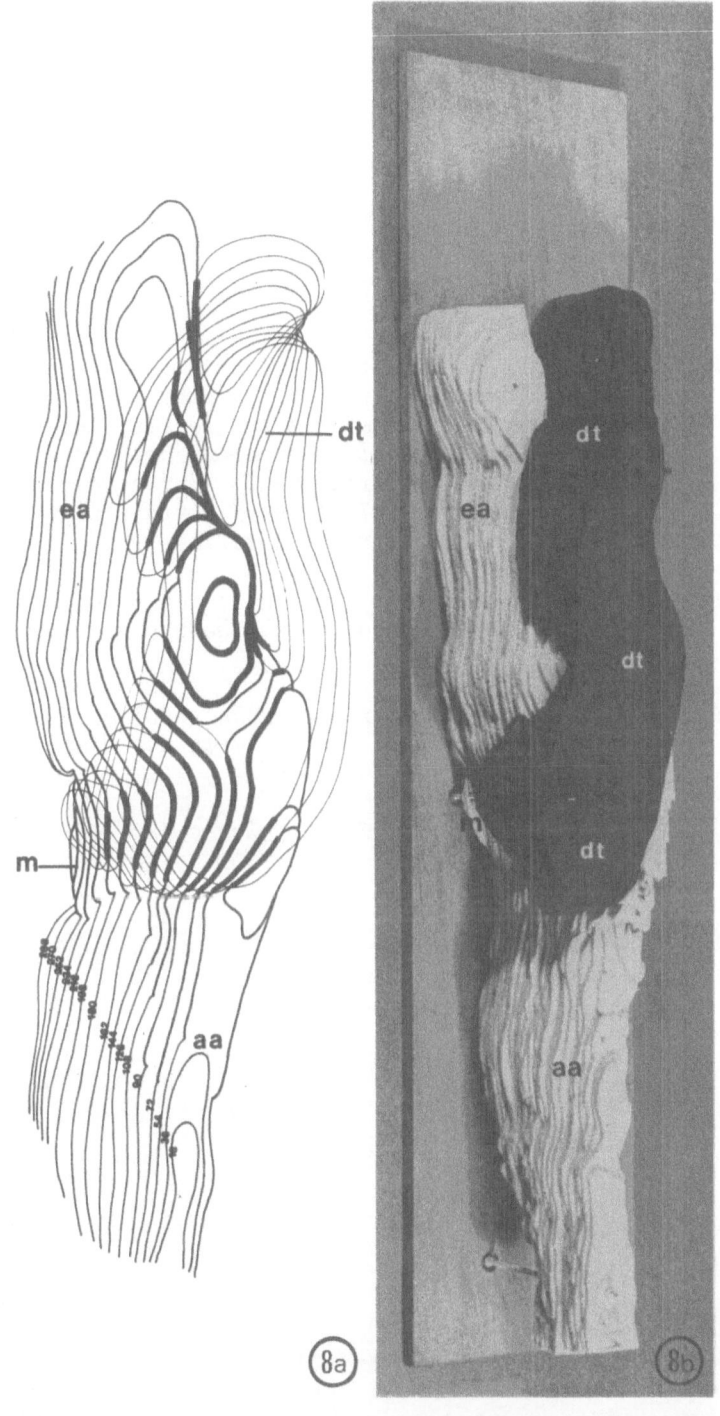

Figure 9.   A simplified schematic representation of the proposed
             functional model of the juxtaglomerular apparatus. The
             contact between the distal tubule (dt) and the mesangial
             region (m) and the hilar efferent arteriole (ea) which
             is interpreted as permanent is represented by wavy lines,
             whereas the reversible type of contact is represented
             by heavy lines. Afferent arteriole (aa).

Figure 9a.   As the distal tubule expands (lines B and C) the area
             of "reversible" contact with the vascular components
             increases.

Figure 9b.   As the afferent arteriole expands (lines B and C) the
             area of "reversible" contact with the distal tubule
             increases.

             From Barajas, L. (1971). Science 172: 485-487.

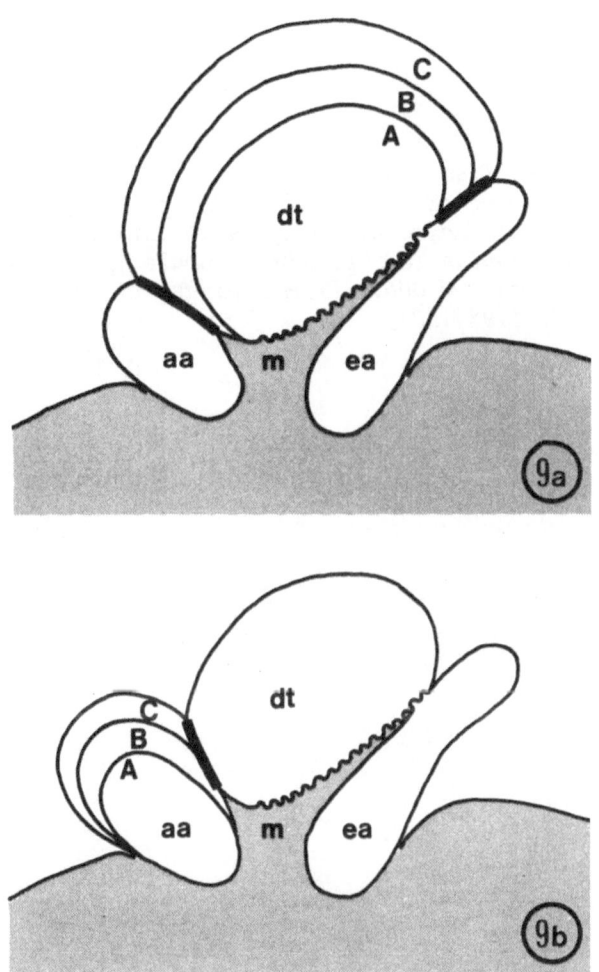

Figure 10. *Nerve fibers are seen along the afferent (A) and*
            efferent (E) arterioles. A spot of fluorescence
            appears adjacent to a distal (dt) tubule (arrows).
            Glomerulus (G), proximal tubule (pt). From rat
            kidney. x 400. From Barajas, L. (1978). Fed. Proc.
            37: 1192-1201.

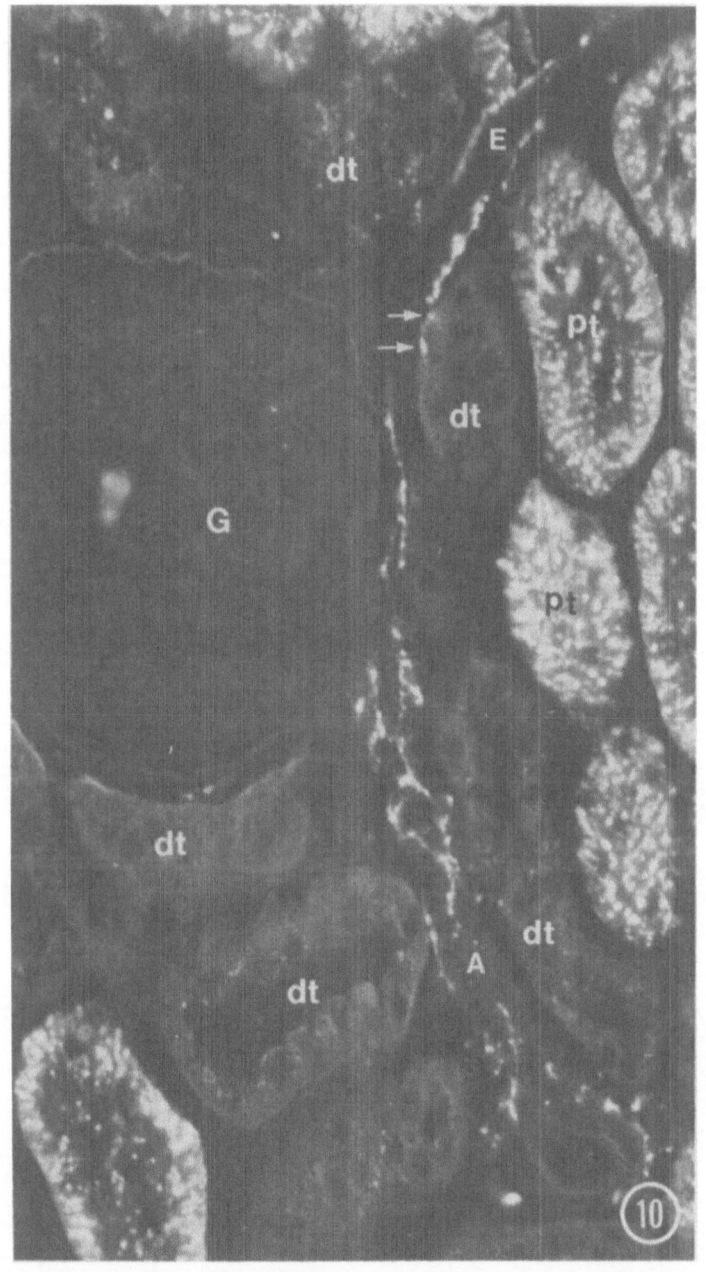

Figure 11. *Acetylcholinesterase-positive nerves along an afferent arteriole (A) departing from a larger interlobular artery (I) and extending to the efferent arteriole (E). Some nerve bundles are present between the arteriolar wall and the proximal (pt) and distal (dt) tubules. Glomerulus (G). From monkey. x 350. From Barajas, L. (1978). Fed. Proc. 37: 1192-1201.*

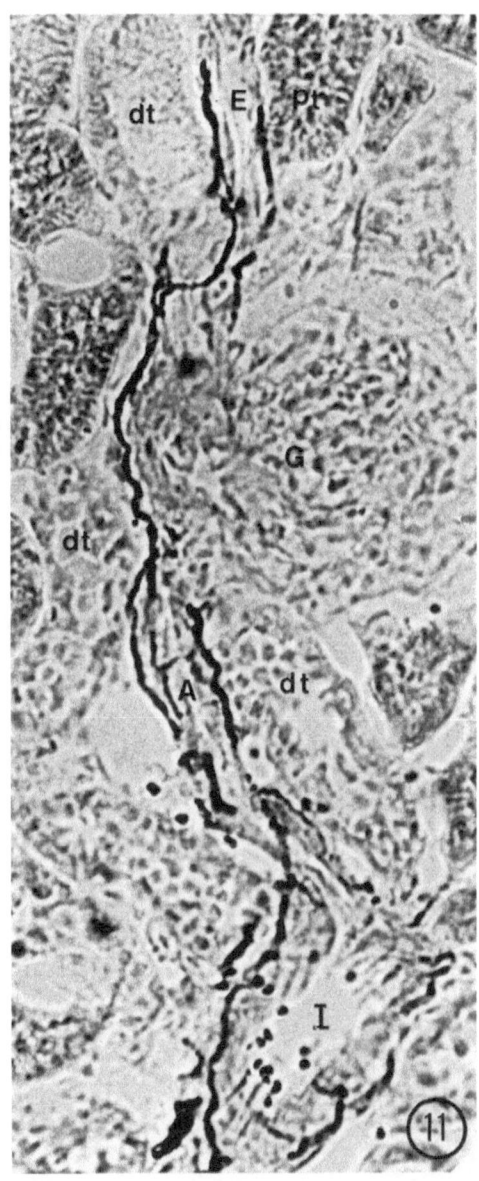

Figure 12.   *A nerve ending (NE) associated with a juxtaglomerular*
granular cell (GC) of an afferent arteriole.   The
axoplasm contains several mitochondria and small
densely cored vesicles.   A space 1,000-1,800 Å wide
separates the plasma membrane of the nerve from that
of the granular cell.   From monkey.   x 63,000.   From
Barajas, L. (1964).   Lab. Invest. 13: 916-929.

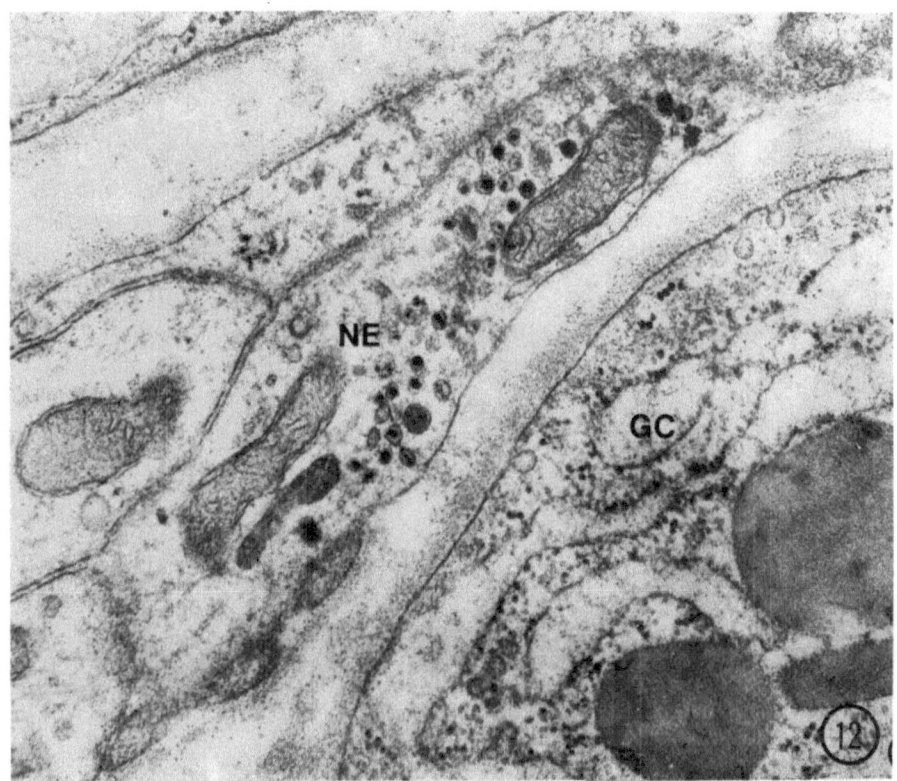

Figure 13.　*Two nerve endings (NE) contacting the distal tubule*
(DT) at the hilus of the glomerulus. The dense-
cored vesicles are of the type associated with
adrenergic nerves. From rat kidney. x 36,000.
From Barajas, L. (1972). In: Control of Renin
Secretion. Assaykeen, T. A. (ed.), pp. 1-16.
Plenum Publishing Corp., New York.

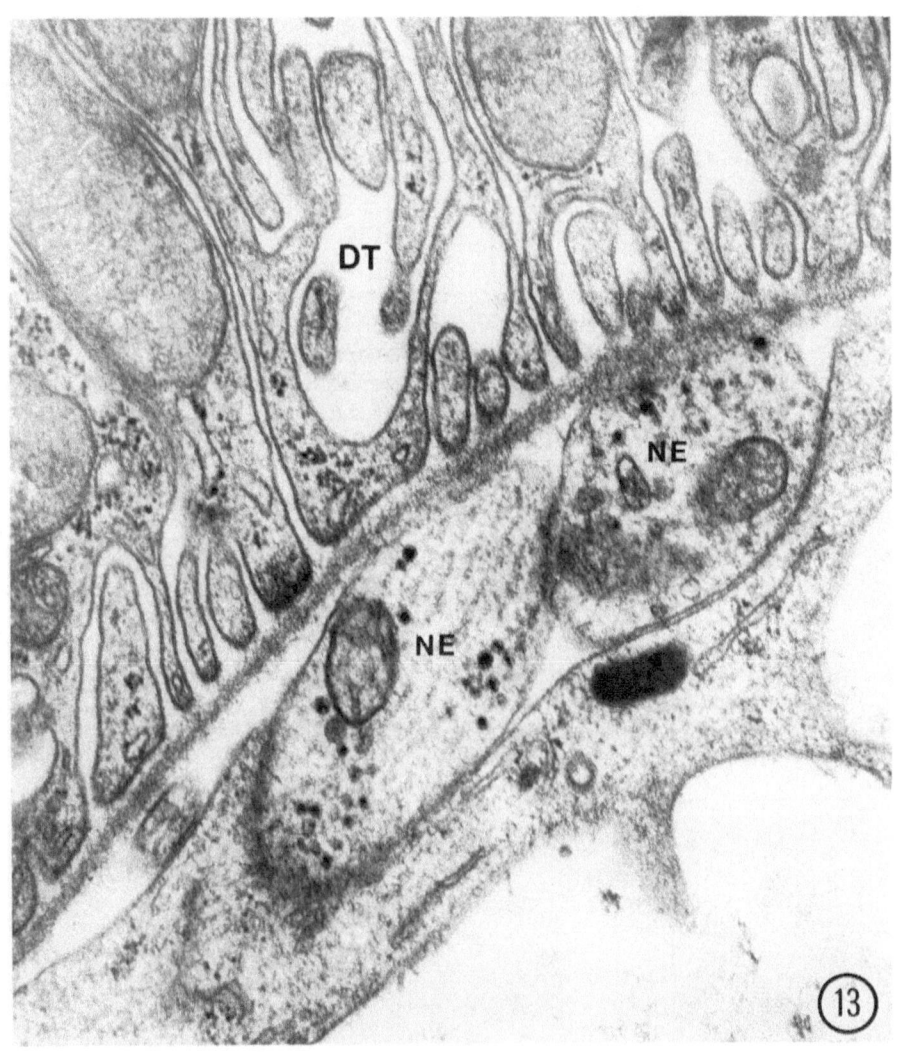

Figure 14.   *Schematic representation of the different patterns of*
innervation of a juxtaglomerular apparatus. Axon
segments were traced which: (A) span from afferent
arteriole (AA) to extraglomerular mesangium (M) and
efferent arteriole (EA), establishing contact with
cells in the three parts of the vascular component;
(B) contact cells of the efferent arteriole;
(C) contact cells of the afferent arteriole;
(D) contact cells of the afferent arteriole and
distal tubule (DT); (E) contact cells of the efferent
arteriole and proximal tubule (PT); (F) contact only
the proximal tubule. The granular cells in the vascu-
lar component are filled with small circles. Filled
circles in the axon segments represent varicosities;
clear triangles are nerve endings in contact with the
indicated structures. From Barajas, L. and Müller, J.
(1973). J. Ultrastruct. Res. 43: 107-132.

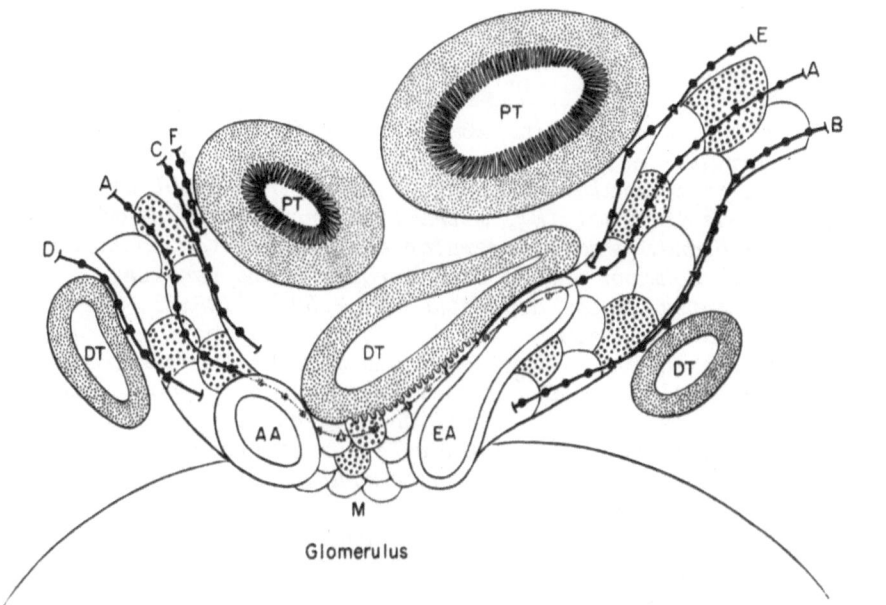

Figure 15. *Close relationship between tumor juxtaglomerular*
granular cell and nerve bundle is seen. A tongue of
juxtaglomerular cell cytoplasm is in contact with the
nerve terminal (N), without intervening basement
membrane. Juxtaglomerular cell (JGC), Varicosities
(v), Schwann cell (SC). Arrows, protogranules;
asterisk, Golgi apparatus. x 7,500. INSERT: Area
of contact between the juxtaglomerular cell and the
nerve ending. The two plasma membranes are separated
by less than 200 Å and no intervening basement mem-
brane is present. Small densely cored vesicles
characteristic of adrenergic nerves are seen in the
nerve ending. The juxtaglomerular cell cytoplasm in
the region adjacent to the area of contact with the
nerve has a sac containing crystalline protogranule
(P). Nerve ending (N). Asterisk, Golgi apparatus.
x 26,000. From Barajas, L., Bennett, C., Connor, G.,
and Lindstrom, R. (1977). Lab. Invest. 37: 357-368.

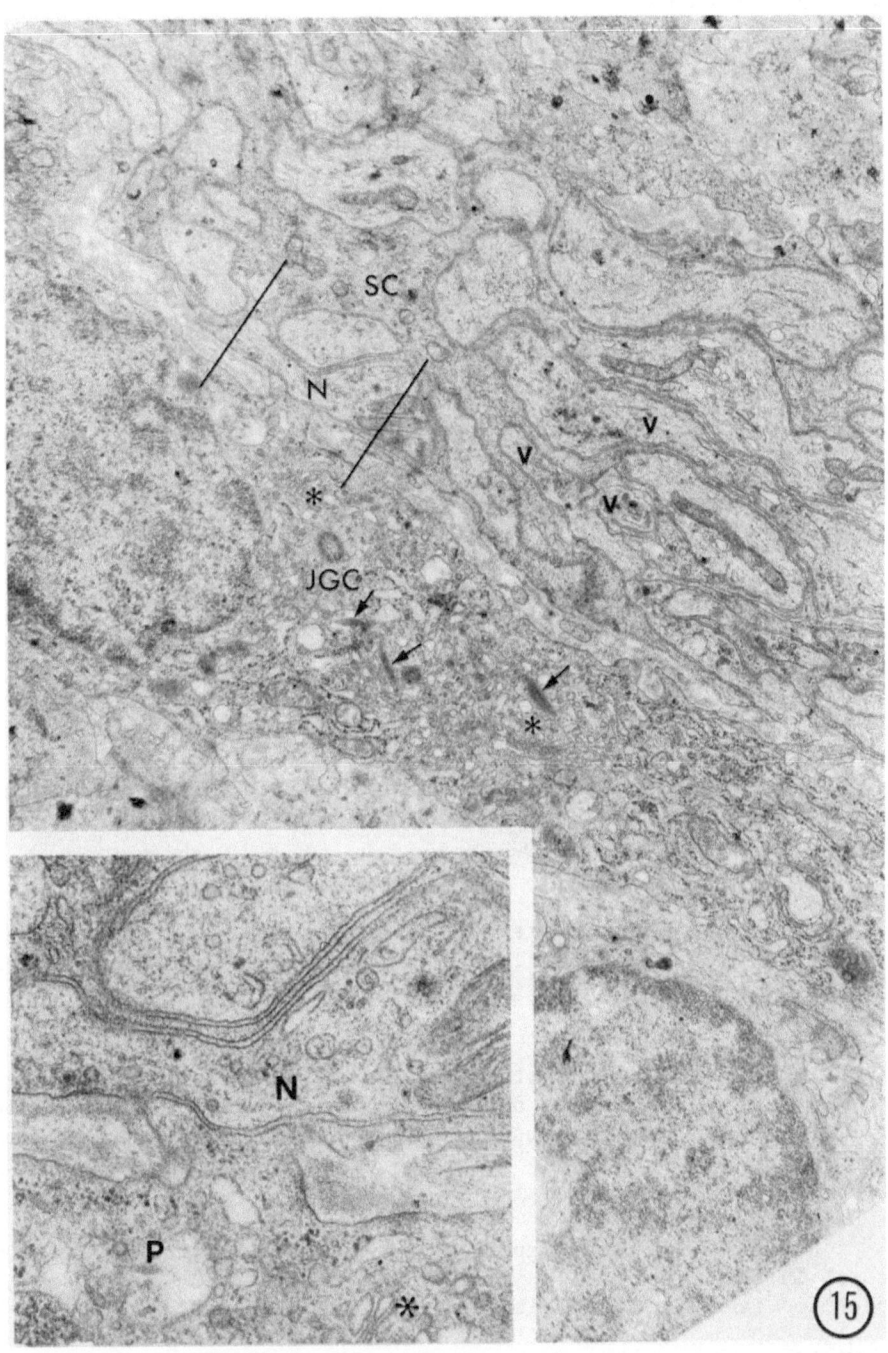

DISCUSSION AFTER DR. BARAJAS' PAPER

Dr. Davis

I thought that was a very interesting case, the last one you showed. Is there any evidence from the clinical history that the sympathetic nerves were controlling the release of renin from that tumor?

Dr. Barajas

To my knowledge, they didn't study the tumor from that standpoint. However, the patient did respond to propranolol, which is a beta-adrenergic blocking drug. Now that we have shown that this type of tumor exists, whenever the diagnosis of a renin-secreting tumor is made maybe further tests should be integrated into the workup of the patient to study the role of the renal nerves in the excess renin secretion.

Dr. Davis

I was thinking more about the episodic secretion of renin such as is seen in a patient with a pheochromocytoma. This was not noted, I gather, in the clinical history.

Dr. Barajas

No, it was not, to my knowledge.

Dr. Nishimura

Regarding the juxtaglomerular granules, did I understand you correctly in saying that you can recognize both the mature and the smaller crystalline granules?

Dr. Barajas

Yes, they are very different. The protogranules, which have a crystalline shape, are small, and they usually are seen in the Golgi region or near the Golgi region.

Dr. Nishimura

Do you have any observations, such as, if you give a stimulation to cause renin release do the mature granules disappear first, and if the stimulation is sustained then are the protogranules also gone?

Dr. Barajas

I haven't done those experiments. However, protogranules are present in larger amounts in kidneys of rats with increased renin production, such as those with constriction of the renal artery.

Dr. Nishimura

I am asking this because in one of my studies in fishes, I observed that when I repeatedly gave a strong stimulation to cause

renin release, it appeared that a biochemically different form of
renin was released.

Dr. Barajas
   That is very interesting. People have speculated that the
small granules may be a different form of renin. It would be
interesting to investigate those kidneys with the electron microscope. These particular granules are too small to be visible otherwise; they can be seen only with the electron microscope.

Dr. Klachko
   Dr. Barajas, I believe you said that these are modified smooth
muscle cells, and you showed some elongated structures. Do they
have remnants of smooth muscle characteristics in them?

Dr. Barajas
   Yes, they do. These elongated structures were myofibrils and
attachment bodies which can be seen inside the cytoplasm often
attached to the plasma membrane.

Dr. Klachko
   What I'm leading up to is, do you think that these cells may
have built-in stretch receptors of their own and that these fibrils
could be a part of the signal mechanism? Is there any relationship
between the length of stretch of these fibrils and the number of
granules?

Dr. Barajas
   I think you can say that the more the granules, the less the
fibrils. This is my impression. You can perhaps measure their
cross-section, but measuring their length would be very difficult
because they are so thin and are not oriented with any apparent
order.

Dr. Klachko
   Perhaps the longer they are, the narrower they are, if they
are from that same fiber that is stretched out. It might be of
interest to see if there is any correlation between numbers of
granules and the length or cross-section of these fibers.

Dr. Davis
   I would like to ask you about the incidence of granules in the
efferent arterioles in other species. Are these studies you reported all in the rat?

Dr. Barajas
   Yes.

Dr. Davis

Have you studied other species? Are there as many granules in the efferent arteriole in other species as there are in the efferent arteriole of the rat?

Dr. Barajas

I have not studied any other species to the extent that I have studied the rat, but I have seen granular cells in the efferent arterioles in the mouse, monkey, and in man. My impression is that they are easier to find in hypergranulated juxtaglomerular apparatuses.

Dr. Goetz

Getting back to your case of the renin-secreting tumor, I think Conn has shown that patients who have this tumor do respond with an increase in renin secretion to the upright posture, but they do not respond to things like sodium deprivation. I think his explanation has been that the circulating levels of catecholamines might be responsible for the response to the upright posture. But in light of your evidence, perhaps it might be a direct sympathetic stimulation of the tumor.

Dr. Barajas

That is very interesting. Possibly it is both. The tumor is very vascularized, and circulating catecholamines might reach it as well.

DISCUSSION REFERENCES

Conn, J. W., Cohen, E. L., Lucas, C. P., McDonald, W. J., Mayor, G. H., Blough, Jr., W. M., Eveland, W. C., Bookstein, J. J. and Lapides, J. (1972). Primary reninism. Hypertension, hyper-reninemia, and secondary aldosteronism due to renin-producing juxtaglomerular cell tumors. Arch. Int. Med. 130: 682-696.

MECHANISMS CONTROLLING RENIN RELEASE

J. E. Zehr, K. D. Kurz, A. A. Seymour and H. D. Schultz[1]

Department of Physiology and Biophysics
University of Illinois
Urbana, IL   61801

OUTLINE

I.   INTRODUCTION

Despite the fact that the renin-angiotensin system has been extensively studied for many years, it still remains the center of

[1]Research originating from the authors' laboratory was supported by NIH Grants HL 15307 and 5TI-GM 07143 and a Grant from the Illinois Heart Association.

much experimental and clinical investigation. A central focus of
this work has been directed toward underlying mechanisms controlling
renin release, and although many fundamental factors have been
defined, considerable gaps in our understanding still remain.

Space limitations do not permit a compregensive review of all
of the work reported concerning renin release. For this the
interested reader is referred to recent reviews (Davis and Freeman,
1976; Reid, Morris, and Ganong, 1978). The present discussion will
be limited to a brief overview of basic concepts with emphasis on
experimental data to support more recent advances in the field.

Mechanisms controlling renin release can be broadly classified
into two major groups: (1) Intrarenal factors, whose primary
signals arise from within and are inherent to the renal mass itself,
and (2) Extrarenal factors, arising from without the renal mass but
whose signals are imposed directly or indirectly on renal secretory
processes. It is doubtful whether under normal physiological conditions these factors ever act completely independent from each
other in their control of renin secretion. This interdependence has
been a major complication in achieving a full understanding of renin
secretory mechanisms. However, it has been possible, at least in
part, to isolate individual factors for experimental study and
analysis.

II.   INTRARENAL MECHANISMS CONTROLLING RENIN RELEASE

A substantial body of evidence has been accumulated indicating
that intrarenal-dependent renin release is modified by an afferent
arteriolar baroreceptor and by a tubular, probably macula densa,
component. In addition, recent evidence has been developed indicating that components of the renal medullary lipids modify renin
release by complex and as yet undefined mechanisms.

A.   Intrarenal Baroreceptor Control of Renin

It is generally accepted that reduced renal perfusion pressure
triggers an independent afferent arteriolar receptor to stimulate
prompt increases in renin release. The large body of evidence to
support this fundamental concept has been reviewed comprehensively
by Davis and Freeman (1976) and will not be reported here. The
prevailing data suggest that the receptor is activated by changes
in the tensile status of the afferent arteriolar vascular tree.
Definitive data for this concept were obtained in the nonfiltering
kidney model (Blaine, Davis, and Witty, 1970). Reduction in renal
perfusion pressure resulted in increased renin output despite the
absence of sympathetic or tubular influences (Blaine, Davis, and
Prewitt, 1971). Since this increased renin output was blocked by

renal vascular paralysis with papaverine (Witty, Davis, Johnson, and Prewitt, 1971) the conclusion that the renal baroreceptor responds to changes in arteriolar wall tension seems justified. However, precise cellular events linking altered arteriolar wall tension with release of renin are undefined.

B. Macula Densa Control of Renin

It has been recognized for many years that alterations in tubular ionic events are associated with modifications in juxtaglomerular granularity and renin output. The early suggestion of Goormaghtigh (1939, 1945) that the highly differentiated macula densa cells of the renal tubules may interact with specialized juxtaglomerular cells of the renal afferent arterioles has enjoyed wide acceptance. A discussion of supporting evidence for a macula densa component in the control of renin release is a topic of the recent review by Davis and Freeman (1976).

Despite intense investigation into the precise signal perceived by the macula densa, fundamental mechanisms remain to be defined. The most widely accepted view has been that renin release is centered around some function of tubular sodium. However, in the recent past the role of sodium has been challanged. Kotchen, Galla, and Luke (1976) concluded that because plasma renin activity and renal renin content are suppressed in rats by both sodium and potassium chloride, but not by sodium and potassium bicarbonate, the determining factor modifying renin must have been chloride. This idea was strengthened further by additional studies in which salt depleted rats were repleted either with sodium chloride or with sodium salts other than chloride (Kotchen, Galla, and Luke, 1978). In these experiments, renin activity was not suppressed in animals loaded with sodium acetate, sodium nitrate, or sodium thiocyanate when compared to those loaded with sodium chloride. In addition, rats loaded with choline chloride exhibited markedly suppressed renins, while rats loaded with choline bicarbonate did not. Taken together, these data were interpreted to indicate that chloride rather than sodium was the crucial factor in the modification of renin release. On the other hand, Stephens, Davis, Freeman, and Watkins (1978) recently demonstrated that the rate of renin release in dogs with thoracic caval constriction is suppressed by intra-renal infusion of sodium and potassium lactate to a degree similar to that seen during sodium chloride infusion. Since sodium lactate infusion was accompanied by decreased chloride excretion, it was concluded that the renin response was not primarily chloride mediated. Additional work is needed to clarify the precise role that both cations and anions play in renin secretory processes.

III. INFLUENCE OF CALCIUM ON RENIN RELEASE

Since ionized calcium has been implicated in several secretory processes, it has come under increasing scrutiny with respect to renin secretory processes as well. Kotchen, Maull, Luke, *et al.* (1974) demonstrated that infusion of calcium into the renal artery of anesthetized dogs suppressed renin release. Kisch, Dluhy, and Williams (1976) reported that $CaCl_2$ infusion suppressed renin in normal man. However, in view of the uncertainties surrounding Cl^-, it was not clear whether this reduction was due to Cl^- or possibly secondary to altered renal handling of Na^+. This was clarified further by the experiments of Watkins, Davis, Lohmeier, and Freeman (1976) who demonstrated that intrarenal infusion of Ca^{++} suppresses renin both in filtering and in nonfiltering kidneys in dogs. Since this response was present even in the absence of Cl^- as the accompanying anion, the conclusion was drawn that Ca^{++} exerts a direct action on juxtaglomerular cells to modify renin release.

There have been several recent reports concerning the influence of Ca^{++} on renin release in isolated perfused kidneys (Fray, 1977; Lester and Rubin, 1977) and in isolated superfused glomeruli (Baumbach and Leyssac, 1977). Most reports are consistent with the idea that renin release is inversely related to perfusate Ca^{++} concentrations. The very recent report of Harada and Rubin (1978) supports a concept that mobilization of Ca^{++} from intracellular sites may be involved in the renin secretory process. This is based on their observation that either infusion of norepinephrine into the renal artery or renal nerve stimulation in isolated perfused cat kidneys resulted in parallel increases in renin release and the release of preloaded $^{45}Ca^{++}$ from the kidney. In addition, intrarenal propranolol administration prevented both the increased renin release and the increased renal $^{45}Ca^{++}$ efflux during norepinephrine treatment. Although this appears to imply that renin secretory processes are associated with movement of Ca^{++} from intracellular stores, the question remains open since there is no assurance that the Ca^{++} efflux measured from the whole kidney is a valid index of its efflux from the juxtaglomerular cells.

Several laboratories have reported recently that alterations in the cellular compartmentalization of calcium by the use of Ca^{++} specific ionophores modify renin release (Baumbach and Leyssac, 1977; Fynn, Onamakpome, and Peart, 1977). In the perfused cat kidney, addition of the Ca^{++} ionophore A-23187 to a Ca^{++} free perfusate resulted in an actual increase in renin output. Again, this appears to be consistent with the idea that renin release is influenced by some function of membrane Ca^{++} flux or possibly by intracellular Ca^{++} concentration or binding.

Additional support for this idea comes from studies by Baumbach and Leyssac (1977) who reported that renin release from a superfused, isolated rat glomeruli preparation was increased by graded reductions in Ca^{++} in the perfusate. This preparation, of course, limits the Ca^{++} effects to a direct action on the renin secretory cells. Reports concerning the effects of Ca^{++} on *in vitro* renal cortical slices have been contradictory and are inconclusive (Aoi, Wade, Rosner, and Weinberger, 1974; Corsini, Crosslan, and Bailie, 1974; Michelakis, 1971; Saruta and Matsuki, 1975; Yamamoto, Iwao, Abe, and Morimoto, 1974). Precisely how Ca^{++} influences renin secretion is open for considerable further clarification and should provide a fertile field for future study.

IV. INTRARENAL PROSTAGLANDINS AND RENIN RELEASE

Over the past few years considerable interest has arisen concerning the influence of intrarenal medullary lipids on renin secretion, with the prostaglandins and their synthetic intermediates receiving particular attention. This renewed interest has been a result of the observation that inhibitors of the renal cyclooxygenase-dependent conversion of arachidonic acid to prostaglandins also suppress renin release in a variety of species, including man (Larsson, Weber, and Anggård, 1974; Romero and Strong, 1977; Yun, Kelly, Bartter, and Smith, 1977; Frolich, Hollifield, Dormois, *et al.*, 1976; Romero, Dunlap, and Strong, 1976). In addition, the rate at which renin is released from *in vitro* renal cortical slices has been shown to be enhanced by arachidonic acid and by both natural and synthetic prostaglandin endoperoxides (Weber, Larsson, Anggård, *et al.*, 1976). While studies such as these imply that prostaglandin synthetic events may modify renin secretory mechanisms, it is not known how this may be accomplished *in vivo*. Conceivably the renal prostaglandins or their synthetic intermediates could modify renin secretion by altering renal hemodynamics or renal blood flow distribution, or they could alter renal electrolyte handling; also, they could modify renal sympathetic pathways or they might influence renin by acting directly on the juxtaglomerular cells. Of special interest is the possibility that Ca^{++} linked events may be involved, because of the influence of prostaglandins on membrane Ca^{++} flux and intracellular binding.

To investigate these several possibilities, a series of studies were undertaken in our laboratory in both filtering and nonfiltering kidneys of anesthetized dogs (Seymour and Zehr, 1977; Seymour and Zehr, 1978). To avoid neural influences, renal denervation of the experimental kidney was carried out several days prior to all procedures. The contralateral kidney was removed to restrict the response to only the experimental kidney. In this preparation a twenty minute infusion (0.1 mg/kg/min) of indomethasin, a non-steroidal cyclooxygenase inhibitor, directly into the renal artery resulted in a 50% reduction in both plasma renin activity and in the rate of prostaglandin efflux from the renal vein (Table 1).

This route of indomethacin administration was chosen to minimize
systemic effects. It was assumed throughout that renal prostaglandin efflux (ng/min) was a valid index for qualitative monitoring
of the intrarenal prostaglandin synthetic events during activation
of known renin control mechanisms. To test whether prostaglandin
synthesis was capable of modifying the usual increase in renin
release during activation of the intrarenal baroreceptor, a series
of dogs was studied for their response to a 50% reduction in renal
perfusion pressure by suprarenal aortic constriction both with and
without intrarenal indomethacin infusion. Renin output was similar
in both groups despite the fact that during reduced renal perfusion
pressure the prostaglandin efflux was suppressed to levels less
than 10% of those of the untreated group (Table 2). From this we
infer that prostaglandin synthetic events do not act primarily via
intrarenal baroreceptor mechanisms, although altered tubular mechanisms secondary to decreased glomerular filtration rate could not be
ruled out. To test whether prostaglandin synthetic processes are
acting on renin release through macula densa or tubular pathways,
furosemide was administered intravenously to control dogs and to
dogs receiving indomethacin directly into the renal artery. The
indomethacin-treated group exhibited a statistically significant
reduction in their response to furosemide (Table 3). These data
are consistent with others (Romero, Dunlap, and Strong, 1976;

*Table 1.   ARTERIAL PRESSURE AND RENAL RESPONSES TO 60 MINUTES OF
            INDOMETHACIN DIRECTLY INTO THE SOLE REMAINING DENERVATED
            KIDNEY OF ANESTHETIZED DOGS (n = 6).   VALUES ARE MEANS
            ± SEM.*

	Control	Indomethacin (0.1 mg/kg/min)
Arterial Pressure mm Hg	135.3 ±5.3	127.1 ±6.0
Renal Blood Flow ml/min	132.4 ±13.8	101.8 ±14.4*
Plasma Renin Activity ng/ml/hr	10.7 ±2.7	3.0 ±1.1*
Prostaglandin Efflux ng/min	235.7 ±71.0	60.7 ±53.6*

*P<0.01

Table 2. RESPONSES TO SUPRARENAL AORTIC CONSTRICTION IN CONTROL DOGS AND IN DOGS RECEIVING INDOMETHACIN (0.1 mg/Kg/min) DIRECTLY INTO A SOLE, REMAINING DENERVATED KIDNEY. VALUES ARE MEANS ± SEM

	Untreated (n = 6)		Indomethacin (n = 6)	
	Control	Experimental	Control	Experimental
Arterial Pressure mmHg	118.0 ± 7.5	135.3 ± 12.0	126.3 ± 12.0	144.4 ± 9.0†
Renal Perfusion Pressure mmHg	115.8 ± 7.5	58.6 ± 2.3*	124.8 ± 12.8	57.1 ± 3.0*
Renal Blood Flow ml/min	178.4 ± 33.9	88.3 ± 16.0*	218.9 ± 27.3	79.6 ± 10.8*
Plasma Renin Activity ng/ml/hr	3.7 ± 2.0	15.8 ± 4.5†	4.8 ± 1.0	13.8 ± 4.4†
Prostaglandin Efflux ng/min	434.0 ± 139.0	507.0 ± 192.0	169.0 ± 87.0	34.0 ± 13.0*

*P < 0.01--Compares experimental vs respective control

†P < 0.05--Compares experimental vs respective control

Table 3. RESPONSES TO FUROSEMIDE ADMINISTRATION IN CONTROL DOGS AND IN DOGS RECEIVING INDOMETHACIN (0.1 mg/Kg/min) DIRECTLY INTO A SOLE, REMAINING DENERVATED KIDNEY. VALUES ARE MEANS ± SEM.

	Untreated (n = 6)		Indomethacin (n = 6)	
	Control	Furosemide	Control	Furosemide
Arterial Pressure mmHg	121.8 ± 6.0	118.8 ± 9.0	130.8 ± 12.0	129.3 ± 11.3
Renal Blood Flow ml/min	193.8 ± 10.5	198.2 ± 26.2	171.4 ± 35.4	166.0 ± 43.4
Plasma Renin Activity ng/ml/hr	3.2 ± 0.9	18.3 ± 5.8*	1.0 ± 0.2	6.1 ± 1.7*†
Prostaglandin Efflux ng/min	537.0 ± 279.0	457.0 ± 311.0	182.0 ± 123.0	254.0 ± 215.0

*$P < 0.05$--Compares experimental values with the respective control.

†$P < 0.02$--Compares response between the two groups.

Frolich, Hollifield, Dormois, *et al.*, 1976) and initially suggested that prostaglandins modify tubular electrolyte handling which in turn alter renin via macula densa mechanisms, although a cause and effect relationship could not be established. Alternative explanations must be considered since furosemide has been shown to stimulate renin secretion in the nonfiltering kidney through renal baroreceptor mechanisms, independent of tubular events (Corsini, Hook and Bailie, 1975). In addition, furosemide elicits parallel increases in renin and free arachidonic acid, the fatty acid precursor for prostaglandin synthesis (Weber, Scherer, and Larsson, 1977) and it was proposed that an accompanying increase in prostaglandin synthesis is a primary mechanism underlying the renin response to the diuretic. To test whether *in vivo* enhancement or depression of prostaglandin synthesis may affect renin secretion by direct action on the juxtaglomerular cells, we undertook a series of studies in dogs with nonfiltering, denervated kidneys. Indomethacin (0.1 mg/kg/min) infusion into the renal artery of these nonfiltering kidneys again resulted in a 50% reduction in the rate of renin secretion after twenty minutes (Table 4). Thus, it appeared that direct, but undefined prostaglandin action on the juxtaglomerular cells *in vivo* was a valid hypothesis. To test this idea further, arachidonic acid, which is the primary precursor for prostaglandin synthesis, was infused directly into the renal artery of nonfiltering kidneys. After twenty minutes, control samples were drawn after which indomethacin was infused into the renal artery in addition to the continued infusion of arachidonic acid. This procedure resulted in large increases in renin and prostaglandin secretion during arachidonic acid alone and depressions of both prostaglandin cyclooxygenase inhibition, despite continued excess prostaglandin substrate

Table 4. RESPONSE TO 60 MINUTES INTRARENAL INDOMETHACIN INFUSION (0.1 mg/Kg/min) DIRECTLY INTO SINGLE DENERVATED NONFILTERING KIDNEYS (n = 5). VALUES ARE MEANS ± SEM

	Control	Indomethacin
Arterial Pressure mm Hg	95.0 ±5.8	82.2 ±7.7
Renal Blood Flow ml/min	54.6 ±7.2	25.4 ±7.6*
Renin Secretion ng/min	83.7 ±38.2	23.9 ±16.2*

*$P < 0.025$

Table 5. *RESPONSES TO INTRARENAL ARACHIDONIC ACID (AA) INFUSION*
(15 µg/Kg/min) ALONE AND IN COMBINATION WITH INDOMETHACIN
(0.1 mg/Kg/min). VALUES ARE MEANS ±SEM.

	Control	AA	AA + Indomethacin
Arterial Pressure mm Hg	103.6 ±12.8	96.0 ±14.9	97.6 ±16.1
Renal Blood Flow ml/min	68.5 ±12.7	91.7 ±23.7	73.3 ±21.3
Renin Secretion ng/min	16.2 ±4.4	78.9 ±24.3*	31.2 ±10.4
Prostaglandin Efflux ng/min	952 ±357	2074 ±1415	621 ±188

*$P < 0.05$

(Table 5). This again suggested that prostaglandin synthetic events
have direct actions on juxtaglcmerular cells to affect renin release,
although in this instance modification of renal vascular events could
not be ruled out completely. In order to eliminate possible hemodynamic changes, a similar study was conducted in nonfiltering kidneys but with concomitant renal vascular paralysis with papaverine
(4 mg/ min). Under these conditions both renin and prostaglandin
secretion rates again were increased by arachidonic acid (Table 6);
however, indomethacin failed to suppress renin secretion even though
prostaglandin secretion was reduced. Although it is unclear as to
precisely why indomethacin failed to suppress renin secretion during
papaverine infusion, it was clear that increased renin secretion was
associated with enhanced prostaglandin synthesis even in the absence
of functional renal tubules and renal baroreceptors, in kidneys
devoid of sympathetic nerves.

By exclusion, these data imply that prostaglandin synthetic
events affect renin secretion by a direct action on juxtaglomerular
cells. In a recent paper, Data, Gerber, Crump, *et al.* (1978) reported that in nonfiltering kidneys indomethacin was effective in blocking the renin response to aortic constriction and concluded that the
prostaglandins modify renin release through renal baroreceptor mechanisms. This was not tested directly, however, by prior paralysis
of the renal baroreceptor.

There appear to be several synthetic products of the arachidonic acid-cyclooxygenase system involved in renin release. In
general, the endoperoxides (Weber, Larsson, Änggård, *et al.*, 1976),

Table 6. *RESPONSES TO INTRARENAL ARACHIDONIC ACID (AA) INFUSION
(15 µg/Kg/min) ALONE AND IN COMBINATION WITH INDOMETHACIN
(0.1 mg/Kg/min) IN PAPAVERINIZED, NONFILTERING KIDNEYS.
VALUES ARE MEANS ±SEM.*

	Control	AA	AA + Indomethacin
Arterial Pressure mm Hg	115.8 ±6.2	102.0 ±6.4	95.2 ±9.6*
Renal Blood Flow ml/min	143.4 ±21.8	141.7 ±20.4	115.8 ±19.8
Renin Secretion ng/min	87.6 ±32.8	348.0 ±162.7*	312.9 ±176.7**
Prostaglandin Efflux ng/min	252 ±101	1716 ±1082*	62 ±31

*$P < 0.05$ **$P < 0.025$

prostacyclin (PGI_2) (Gerber, Branch, Nies, *et al.*, 1978) and PGE_2
(Gerber, Branch, Nies, *et al.*, 1978; Yun, Kelly, Bartter, and Smith,
1977) have been reported to enhance renin release in animals and
from cortical slices. On the other hand, PGD_2 has been reported to
be ineffective (Gerber, Branch, Nies, *et al.*, 1978) and $PGF_2\alpha$ to
be suppressive to renin release (Weber, Larsson, Änggård, *et al.*,
1976). Additional work will be required to verify these observations.
Precise cellular influence and the physiological control of renal
prostaglandin-renin interactions remain as important and fertile
areas for further research.

V. CONTROL OF RENIN BY THE NERVOUS SYSTEM

It is now widely accepted that the sympathetic nervous system
is capable of modulating renin release both by a direction action
through innervation of the juxtaglomerular cells and by indirect
actions imposed on other intrarenal and hormonal factors known to
control renin. The evidence to support these conclusions has been
comprehensively reviewed by Davis and Freeman (1976). A number of
studies have demonstrated that renal sympathetic nerves terminate
directly on juxtaglomerular cells (Barajas, 1964; Wagermark, Ungerstedt, and Ljungqvist, 1968; Hartroft, 1966). Under controlled experimental conditions these can be shown to stimulate renin release
independent of vascular or tubular actions (Johnson, Davis, and
Witty, 1971).

Considerable effort has been expended in an effort to characterize the JG membrane receptors involved in renin release. A pre-
ponderance of experimental evidence supports the concept of an
intrarenal beta-adrenergic receptor (Vandongen, Peart, and Boyd,
1973; Johnson, Davis, Gotshall, *et al.*, 1976), although an extrarenal site of action also has been hypothesized (Reid, Schrier,
ane Earley, 1972). An intrarenal alpha-adrenergic receptor has
also been proposed but despite intensive investigation a clear
physiological role has yet to be established (Pettinger, Keeton,
Campbell, *et al.*, 1976; Vandongen and Peart, 1974; Winer, Chokshi,
and Walkenhorst, 1971).

Since propranolol, a widely used beta-adrenergic blocker, is
lipid soluble and is concentrated in brain tissue, it was proposed
that a central site of action may, in part, be responsible for the
ability of this compound to reduce renin activity. A recent preliminary report (Schultz and Zehr, 1977) tested this idea directly
by administering propranolol intravenously or through the III and
IV cerebroventricles during reflex activation of renin by mild
hemorrhage. In a group of control dogs, the III and IV cerebroventricles were perfused with artificial cerebrospinal fluid during
imposition of a mild nonhypotensive hemorrhage. Careful monitoring
of arterial pressure assured that reductions of renal perfusion
were not present. The renin response in this group was then compared with the response in dogs receiving propranolol either intravenously or directly into the III and IV cerebroventricles. To
verify the partition of the drug between the serum and cerebrospinal fluid, propranolol concentrations were monitored in these
compartments through all experimental procedures. The results of
these studies (Table 7) indicate that propranolol is rapidly concentrated in cerebrospinal fluid but that, despite this, the usual
pattern of renin release is unaffected so long as serum propranolol
concentrations are minimal; the implication is that central beta
adrenergic receptors bathed by cerebrospinal fluid are not responsible for the action of this drug.

Even though it has been shown experimentally that direct electrical stimulation of the central nervous system (Passo, Assaykeen,
Otsuka, *et al.*, 1971; Ueda, Yasudo, Takabatake, *et al.*, 1967;
Richardson, Stella, Leonetti, *et al.*, 1974; Zehr and Feigl, 1973)
or the renal sympathetic nerves (Johnson, Davis, and Witty, 1971;
Coote, Johns, Macleod, and Singer, 1972) modifies renin secretion,
the more crucial questions are whether neural mechanisms are involved
in moment control of renin secretion, particularly in pathophysio-
logic states. It would be of great interest if it could be shown
experimentally that the central nervous system *selectively* modulates
renin release through direct sympathetic pathways under normal,
unanesthetized conditions. However, changes in renin release
resulting from electrical stimulation of central structures invariably are accompanied by vascular responses, and no reports have been

Table 7. THE RENIN RESPONSE TO NONHYPOTENSIVE HEMORRHAGE DURING EITHER INTRAVENOUS (IV) OR INTRACEREBROVENTRICULAR (ICV) ADMINISTRATION OF PROPRANOLOL. VALUES ARE MEANS ± SEM

	No Propranolol administration n = 8		Propranolol 1 mg/Kg i.v. n = 6		Propranolol 20 µg/Kg i.c.v. n = 6	
	Control	Hemmorhage	Control	Hemmorhage	Control	Hemmorhage
Mean Arterial Pressure (mmHg)	105.0 ± 7.0	105.0 ± 7.2	122.0 ± 5.0	120.6 ± 6.5	112.0 ± 5.6	115.0 ± 5.3
Plasma Renin Activity (% of Control)	100.0 ± 5.0	256.0 ± 44.3	100.0 ± 7.0	110.0 ± 11.9	100.0 ± 25.8	229.0 ± 60.1
Propranolol Concentration Serum (ng/ml)	---	---	424.0 ± 57.0	301.0 ± 47.0	20.0 ± 6.0	30.0 ± 7.1
Propranolol Concentration CSF (ng/ml)	---	---	231.0 ± 56.1	475.0 ± 26.1	23,000.0 ± 3,000.0	26,000.0 ± 5,600.0

published which show conclusively that renin release is directly
under independent neural control. However, indirect evidence has
accumulated which, when taken as a whole, strongly suggests that
some fraction of the basal renin level is under tonic sympathetic
influences. This concept stems from several facts: (1) Experimental animals exhibit suppressed renins for extended periods following renal denervation (Mogil, Itskovitz, Ressell, and Murphy,
1969; Reid, MacDonald, Pachnis, and Ganong, 1975; Zehr and Feigl,
1973) although they will still respond to other stimuli; (2) Propranolol and other beta adrenergic blocking drugs reduce renin
levels in experimental animals (Johnson, Davis, Gotshall, *et al.*,
1976; Assaykeen, Clayton, Goldfien, and Ganong, 1970; Weber, Stokes,
and Gain, 1974) and man (Michelakis and McAllister, 1972); (3) Stimulation of suprabulbar inhibitory structures in the central nervous
system results in reduced renin release, a response shown to be
mediated by the renal sympathetic nerves (Zehr and Feigl, 1973);
(4) Centrally acting drugs, such as clonidine, which suppress peripheral sympathetic outflow, reduce renin release despite a paradox-
ical decrease in arterial pressure (Reid, MacDonald, Pachnis, and
Ganong, 1975; Onesti, Schwartz, Kim, *et al.*, 1971). Therefore, it
seems reasonable to hypothesize that some fraction of basal renin
output is a result of a balance between central nervous excitatory
and inhibitory drives, and that peripheral reflex mechanisms may
act through these drives to adjust the rate of renin secretion.

A. Evidence for Cardiopulmonary Reflex Control of Renin Release

     Evidence from a number of sources has led to speculation that
low pressure cardiopulmonary receptors may reflexively modify renin
release as a part of volume homeostatic mechanisms. Fundamental to
the development of this idea was the recognition that tonic drive
to renal sympathetic nerves is under the restraining influence of
these vagally mediated cardiopulmonary receptors (Mancia, Shepherd,
and Donald, 1975; Karim, Kidd, and Malpus, 1972; Kahl, Fling, and
Szidon, 1974; Clement, Pelletier, and Shepherd, 1972) and that
tonic sympathetic outflow to the renal vasculature and juxtaglomerular cells is one component of renin control mechanisms. A number of
studies have shown that a very modest nonhypotensive hemorrhage
results in increased renin release (Claybaugh and Share, 1973; Weber,
Thornell, and Stokes, 1974). This suggested that low pressure receptors might very early detect small blood volume changes to which
arterial receptors are insensitive and thus increase renin release
as a compensatory response to volume reduction. The fact that renal
denervation and ganglionic or beta adrenergic blockade prevents the
nonhypotensive hemorrhage response (Weber, Thornell, and Stokes,
1974; Zehr and Feigl, 1972) lent additional credence to the basic
hypothesis that neural reflex pathways were involved. Figure 1
illustrates the renin response to nonhypotensive hemorrhage both

with and without beta receptor blockade in the same unanesthetized
dogs. Recent evidence in unanesthetized dogs (Grandjean, Annat,
Vincent, and Sassard, 1978) and anesthetized cats (Stella and Zanchetti, 1977) undergoing passive head-up tilting reconfirms that
neural pathways are involved in the renin response to this maneuver
as well. More direct evidence that cardiopulmonary receptors are
involved was provided recently (Mancia, Romero, and Shepherd, 1975;
Zehr, Hasbargen, and Kurz, 1966). Mancia, Romero, and Shepherd
(1975) reported that bilateral cervical vagal cooling resulted in
prompt elevations in renin secretion, a response dependent upon
intact renal nerves. The conclusion was drawn that blockage of
vagal restraint placed upon centrally mediated sympathetic drive
resulted in an increase in renin secretion. Zehr, Hasbargen, and
Kurz (1976) confirmed this basic concept by converse experiments
during which small elevations of left atrial-pulmonary vein pressure
were imposed in salt-restricted, chloralose-anesthetized dogs. Renin
secretion was suppressed so long as both renal sympathetic and cervical vagi were intact (Table 8); thus, it was concluded that cardiopulmonary receptors reflexively modulate renin output via vagal afferent and renal sympathetic efferent pathways. Further support for
this basic concept was provided by a recent report (Brosnihan and
Bravo, 1978) showing that graded decreases in right atrial pressure
were accompanied by graded increases in renin secretion despite no
changes in renal perfusion pressure or flow. In addition to atrial-
pulmonary sites, receptors residing in the coronary arterial tree
also have been implicated. Bolus injections of cryptenamine into the
coronary artery of anesthetized dogs resulted in dramatic reductions
in the rate of renin secretion within four minutes, despite a para-
doxical reduction in arterial pressure (Thames, 1977). Since this
response was abolished by vagotomy, the conclusion was drawn that
vagally mediated chemo-sensitive cardiac receptors were responsible.
The bradycardiac and hypotensive response (Bezold-Jarisch reflex)
to intracoronaly veratrum alkaloid injection is generally accepted
to be the result of reduced peripheral sympathetic drive which led
the author to conclude that a reduction of renal sympathetic activity
was the mechanism responsible for the suppression of renin release;
however, this conclusion was not tested directly in denervated
kidneys.

More recent evidence suggests that cardiopulmonary receptors
express their maximal influence on renin secretion in both experimental animals (Thames, Jarecki, and Donald, 1978) and man (Mark,
Abboud, and Fitz, 1978) only if concomitant modulation by arterial
baroreceptors is held constant or is absent.

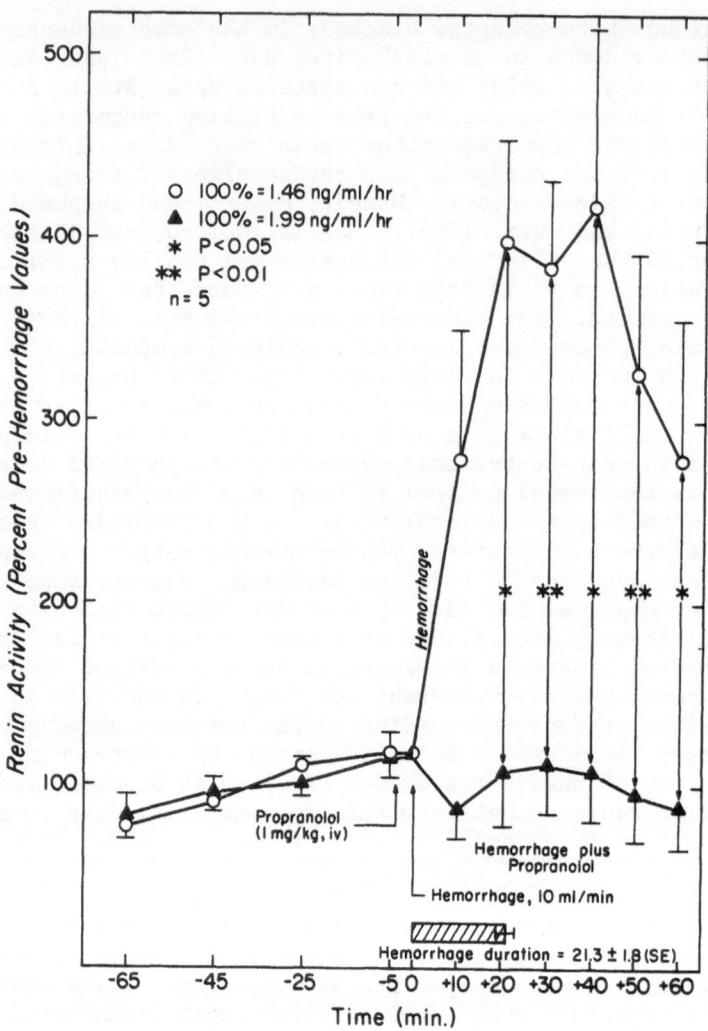

Figure 1.   *The effect of propranolol on the renin response following*
            nonhypotensive hemorrhage is shown.   Data for both
            experimental conditions were obtained in the same five
            unanesthetized, trained dogs.   Each data point is
            expressed as a percentage of the average of the four pre-
            hemorrhage control samples.   Under both conditions a
            controlled hemorrhage of 10.4 ml/min was begun at time 0
            and continued until 16 ml blood/Kg had been removed.
            Propranolol (1 mg/Kg, iv) effectively prevented the
            acute rise in plasma renin activity brought on by
            hemorrhage.   Control renin level was 1.46 ng/ml/hr for
            the hemorrhage alone and 1.99 ng/ml/hr for the hemorrhage
            plus propranolol.   One standard error of the mean is
            indicated.

Table 8. CARDIOVASCULAR AND RENIN SECRETION RESPONSES TO LEFT ATRIAL DISTENTION IN CHLORALOSE ANESTHETIZED DOGS. VALUES ARE MEANS.

Response to Atrial Distention	Intact Vagi Intact Renal Nerves n = 7	Intact Vagi Unilateral Renal Denervation n = 10	Vagotomized Intact Renal Nerves n = 6
ΔHeart Rate (bpm)	+ 15.7	+ 22.2	+ 3.7
ΔAortic Pressure (mmHg)	− 3.4	− 1.6	− 1.2
ΔCentral Venous Pressure (cm H_2O)	− 0.2	− 0.1	+ 0.2
ΔLAP−ITP (cm H_2O)	+ 5.4	+ 5.9	+ 5.4
ΔRenal Blood Flow (ml/min)	− 3.7 (Intact) (Denervated)	− 2.4 (Intact) − 3.1 (Denervated)	− 4.0
ΔRenin Secretion (ng AI/min)	−116.0 (Intact) (Denervated)	−183.0* (Intact) + 80.0 (Denervated)	+56.0

LAP = Left atrial pressure

ITP = Intrathoracic pressure

*$P < 0.001$--Compares intact vs denervated response

B. Evidence for Arterial Baroreceptor Control of Renin Release

Since renin control is intimately tied to vascular volume and
pressure regulation, and since renin has been dempnstrated to be
modified by sympathetic influences, it is not surprising that evidence for arterial baroreceptor control of renin has been sought.
Data to support this idea have been controversial with some studies
indicating that carotid sinus baroreceptors affect changes in renin
(Hodge, Lowe, and Vane, 1966; McPhee and Lakey, 1971; Reid and
Jones, 1976) while others (Brosnihan and Travis, 1976; Brennan,
Henninger, Jochim, and Malvin, 1974; Skinner, McCubbin, and Page,
1964) have reported negative results in this regard. A part of
this inconsistency may stem from a lack of attention to the impact
on renin secretion of renal vascular and cardiopulmonary responses
to manipulation of arterial pressoreceptors. The most recent
studies (Reid and Jones, 1976; Cunningham, Feigl, and Scher, 1978;
Thames, Jarecki, and Donald, 1978; Jarecki, Thoren, and Donald,
1978) have suggested that if cardiopulmonary neural input and renal
perfusion pressure are controlled, carotid sinus hypotension results
in reproducible elevations in renin secretion.

To test this idea more fully, a series of studies was undertaken in our laboratory, during which an isolated carotid sinus
preparation was combined with an arterial pressure clamp to dis-
sociate carotid sinus pressures from arterial pressure responses.
With this preparation, pressure in the carotid sinus baroreceptors
could be manipulated abruptly during constant sinus flow, while
systemic arterial pressure could either be allowed to express its
usual response or be held constant. Under these carefully controlled conditions, carotid sinus hypotension resulted in increased
renin release when systemic arterial pressure was held constant;
however, when arterial pressure was allowed to rise, the renin
response was absent. All experiments were conducted in anesthetized
dogs which had been maintained on 45 meq/day of dietary sodium
intake and whose cervical vagi were transected to avoid aortic arch
and cardiopulmonary influences. A partial summary of these data is
shown in Tables 9 and 10. Since this response was abolished by
renal denervation (Table 10), it seems apparent that arterial
baroreceptors must now also be considered a part of the integrated
reflex control system for renin release.

Although the data cited above show that under limited experimental conditions cardiopulmonary and arterial receptors can be
shown to modify renin release acutely, it is not clear precisely
what homeostatic role they might play, particularly as related
to disturbances which compromise the overall control system.

Table 9. RENIN AND CARDIOVASCULAR RESPONSES TO ISOLATED CAROTID SINUS HYPOTENSION DURING BOTH CONTROLLED AND UNCONTROLLED SYSTEMIC ARTERIAL PRESSURE. VALUES ARE MEANS $\pm$ SEM

	Arterial Pressure Clamped		Arterial Pressure Uncontrolled	
	Control	Carotid Sinus Hypotension	Control	Carotid Sinus Hypotension
Carotid Sinus Pressure (mmHg)	187 ± 1.9	29 ± 1.1	185 ± 2.0	30 ± 1.0
Mean Arterial Pressure (mmHg)	102 ± 1.9	106 ± 5.3	101 ± 4.0	160 ± 9.5
Heart Rate (bpm)	137 ± 6.4	170 ± 3.7	141 ± 6.2	160 ± 4.6
Plasma Renin Activity % of Control	100 ± 3.9	162 ± 31.5	100 ± 2.7	101 ± 6.8

$n = 8$

Table 10. RENIN AND CARDIOVASCULAR RESPONSE TO ISOLATED CAROTID SINUS HYPOTENSION DURING BOTH CONTROLLED AND UNCONTROLLED SYSTEMIC ARTERIAL PRESSURE IN DOGS WITH DENERVATED KIDNEYS. VALUES ARE MEANS ± SEM.

	Arterial Pressure Clamped		Arterial Pressure Uncontrolled	
	Control	Carotid Sinus Hypotension	Control	Carotid Sinus Hypotension
Carotid Sinus Pressure mmHg	182 ± 3.1	27 ± 2.5	181 ± 2.0	24 ± 1.7
Mean Arterial Pressure mmHg	115 ± 10.5	116 ± 10.4	94 ± 10.8	167 ± 20.4
Heart Rate bpm	163 ± 4.3	179 ± 8.4	140 ± 2.4	170 ± 6.3
Plasma Renin Activity % of Control	100 ± 4.1	105 ± 6.3	100 ± 4.9	91 ± 7.8

$n = 6$

C. Physiological Activation of Neural Pathways Controlling Renin
Release

Even though experimental data indicate that renin release can
be modified by reflex pathways, our understanding of the significance of this in the day-to-day control of renin release is still
primitive. The more important aspectes of this area involve questions related to mechanisms by which renin release is activated
during pathophysiological conditions or periods of psychologically
induced stress, and particularly what role these may play as a
precipitating factor in renin-related disease states.

To study questions such as these, we recently examined mechanisms surrounding the release of renin during acute respiratory
acidosis (Kurz and Zehr, 1978). The impetus for this study was a
report (Anderson, Datta, and Samols, 1976) that patients suffering
acute bouts of respiratory insufficiency also exhibit elevated
plasma renin activity. To test the mechanisms underlying this
observation, acute dogs undergoing controlled CO_2 inhalation were
studied. Figure 2 shows that a dose-dependent and reversible
increase in plasma renin activity is present during graded increases
of inspired CO_2. Further studies in denervated and in adrenalectomized dogs indicated that while adrenal activation was a major
factor, renal sympathetic influences also contributed to the renin
response. In addition, it was shown (Kurz and Zehr, 1978) that the
renin response was dependent on the arterial CO_2 pressure ($PaCO_2$)
rather than secondary to the accompanying fall in arterial pH. This
conclusion was drawn from the observation that the renin response
was present during elevated $PaCO_2$ even though arterial pH was held
constant by concomitant THAM infusion (Figure 3). On the other hand,
depressed arterial pH during constant $PaCO_2$ failed to elicit the
renin response (Figure 4). From this it was hypothesized that
elevated $PaCO_2$ during constant pH results in a relative intracellular
acidosis which may act either on neural sensory sites, directly on
juxtaglomerular cells, or on renal electrolyte handling which in turn
might modify macula densa mechanisms. The possible role of altered
tubular mechanisms was tested in dogs with nonfiltering kidneys.
A preliminary report (Kurz, Heath, and Zehr, 1977) indicates that
a slowly acting renin response to respiratory acidosis was blunted
in adrenalectomized dogs with denervated nonfiltering kidneys, and
a tentative proposal was advanced that one component of the long-
term renin response is mediated via macula densa mechanisms, possibly
secondary to altered renal bicarbonate or chloride handling. Thus,
it appears that several components of the redundant renin control
system are recruited and probably act in concert to combat the hypotension often observed during acute respiratory acidosis.

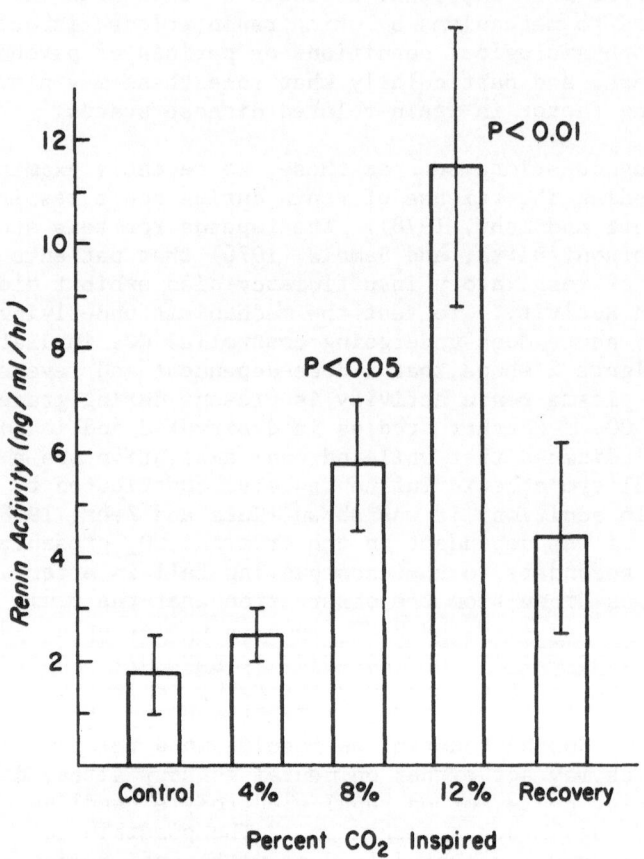

Figure 2.   *The renin response to graded CO_2 inhalation in chloralose-anesthetized dogs is shown. A dose-dependent and reversible increase in renin is present during controlled hypercapnia (n = 8). (Kurz and Zehr, Am. J. Physiol. 234:H575-581, 1978-by permission).*

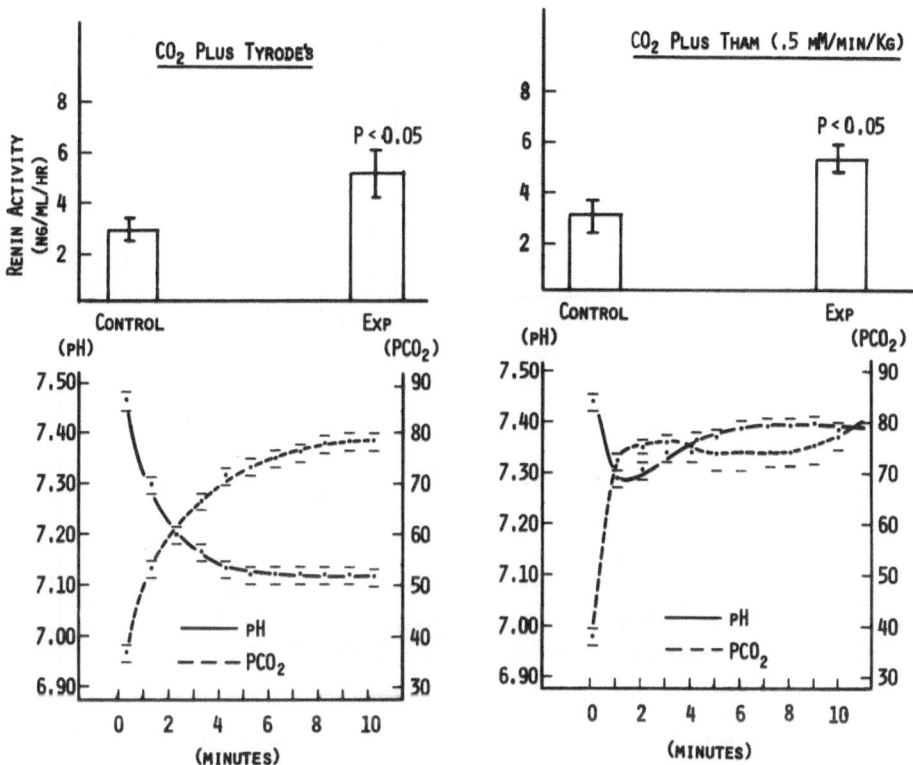

Figure 3. A comparison of the renin response to 10 min CO_2 inhalation prior to and during blood buffering with iv THAM infusion. A similar renin response was present during elevated $PaCO_2$ despite a relatively constant arterial pH (n = 6). (Kurz and Zehr, Am. J. Physiol. 234:H573-581, 1978-by permission).

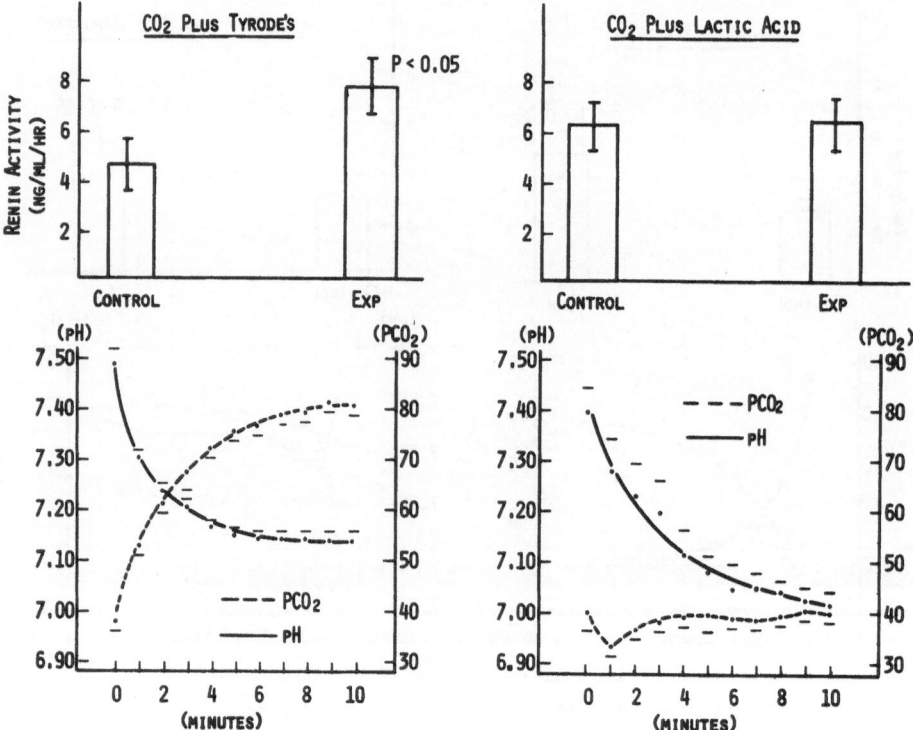

*Figure 4.   Comparison of the renin response during acidosis
              produced by CO$_2$ inhalation with that produced by
              lactic acid infusion.   When PaCO$_2$ was held constant
              during lactic acid infusion, the renin response was
              lost despite reduction in arterial pH (n = 6).
              (Kurz and Zehr, Am. J. Physiol.   234:H573-581, 1978
              by permission).*

Several interesting reports recently have appeared to the effect that psychologically stressful stimuli are associated with increased plasma renin. Clamage, Sanford, Vander, and Mouw (1976) reported that plasma renin activity is elevated in caged rats after exposure to a hungry cat or during exposure to a novel environment. Vander, Kay, Dugan, and Mouw (1977) reported that broadband noise of 100-115 dB intensity also produced significant increases of plasma renin in rats. The same laboratory (Vander, Henry, Stephens, *et al.*, 1978) recently reported that mice reared under conditions of a high level of social interaction and competition had elevated plasma renins when compared to siblings reared in isolation. Interestingly, the stressed group exhibited concomitantly elevated systolic pressures. In another report Blair, Feigl, and Smith (1976) demonstrated that three hours of Sidman avoidance conditioning would elicit a rise in peripheral renin in chaired baboons. Apparently under these conditions, the psychological stresses associated with work performance and avoidance of electrical shock were sufficient to trigger renin release.

While there is a lack of definitive proof in any of these studies that activation of the central nervous system was the precipitating factor, it seems reasonable at least to hypothesize that it was involved in some major way. Central neuronal pools and neural transmitters involved in the translation of information stemming from peripheral receptors or psychological stresses is a challenging area for future research. The long-term implications of psychological stresses are uncertain, particularly as they may relate to renin-dependent hypertensive disease.

VI. SUMMARY

Mechanisms controlling renin are redundant and interactive and may be broadly classified into intra- and extrarenal groups. Classic intrarenal factors have involved the renal baroreceptor and the macula densa, while extrarenal factors are considered to be the sympathetic nervous system and circulating blood-borne constituents.

The precise signal perceived by the macula densa remains unclear; however, chloride has received increasing attention as a possible regulator of renin via this pathway. Although calcium has also been shown to influence renin secretion, probably by directly affecting juxtaglomerular cells, considerable work remains before a cellular basis for calcium effects can be established.

Recent evidence suggests that intrarenal products of arachidonic acid and cyclooxygenase interaction may also be involved. Although the precise manner by which prostaglandins and their synthetic intermediates influence renin is unclear, evidence is accumulating to suggest their direct effect on juxtaglomerular cells.

A substantial body of experimental evidence indicates that the sympathetic nervous system is a contributor to renin control, either directly or through other of the redundant mechanisms influencing renin release. Recent data suggest that release of renin may be reflexively influenced both by carotid sinus arterial baroreceptors and by vagally mediated cardiopulmonary receptors. In addition, psychological stresses result in enhanced renin output in experimental animals. The long-term implications of these observations are unclear. Thus, despite the fact that fundamental mechanisms underlying renin release have been the object of intensive investigation for many years, it can be expected that new insights will continue to evolve. Particular attention undoubtedly will be focused on a hypothesized, but elusive, "final common signal" responsible for renin release.

REFERENCES

Anderson, W. H., Datta, J., and Samols, E. (1976). The renin angio-
    tensin system in patients with acute respiratory insufficiency.
    Chest 69 (Suppl.): 309-310.
Aoi, W., Wade, M. B., Rosner, D. R., and Weinberger, M. H. (1974).
    Renin release by rat kidney slices *in vitro*: Effects of
    cations and catecholamines. Am. J. Physiol. 227: 630-634.
Assaykeen, T. A., Clayton, P. L., Goldfien, A., and Ganong, W. F.
    (1970). Effect of alpha- and beta-adrenergic blocking agents
    on the renin response to hypoglycemia and epinephrine in dogs.
    Endocrinology 87: 1318-1322.
Barajas, L. (1964). The innervation of the juxtaglomerular appara-
    tus. An electron microscopic study of the innervation of the
    glomerular arterioles. Lab. Invest. 13: 916-929.
Baumbach, L. and Leyssac, P. P. (1977). Studies on the mechanism
    of renin release from isolated superfused rat glomeruli:
    Effects of calcium, calcium ionophore, and lanthanum. J.
    Physiol. (Lond.) 273: 745-764.
Blaine, E. H., Davis, J. O., and Prewitt, R. L. (1971). Evidence
    for a renal vascular receptor in control of renin secretion.
    Am. J. Physiol. 220: 1593-1597.
Blaine, E. H., Davis, J. O., and Witty, R. T. (1970). Renin release
    after hemorrhage and after suprarenal aortic constriction in
    dogs without sodium delivery to the macula densa. Circ. Res.
    27: 1081-1089.
Blair, M. L., Feigl, E. O., and Smith, O. A. (1976). Elevation of
    plasma renin activity during avoidance performance in baboons.
    Am. J. Physiol. 231: 772-776.
Brennan, L. A., Henninger, A. L., Jochim, K. E., and Malvin, R. L.
    (1974). Relationship between carotid sinus pressure and plasma
    renin level. Am. J. Physiol. 227: 295-299.

Brosnihan, K. B. and Bravo, E. L. (1978). Graded reductions of
    atrial pressure and renin release. Am. J. Physiol. 235: H175-
    H181.
Brosnihan, K. B. and Travis, R. H. (1976). Influence of the vagus
    and carotid sinus nerves on plasma renin in the cat. J. Endo-
    crinol. 71: 59-65.
Clamage, D. M., Sanford, C. S., Vander, A. J., and Mouw, D. (1976).
    Effects of psycosocial stimuli on plasma renin activity in rats.
    Am. J. Physiol. 231: 1290-1294.
Claybaugh, J. R. and Share, L. (1973). Vasopressin, renin, and
    cardiovascular responses to continuous slow hemorrhage. Am. J.
    Physiol. 222: 519-523.
Clement, D. L., Pelletier, C. L., and Shepherd, J. T. (1972). Role
    of vagal afferents in the control of renal sympathetic nerve
    activity in the rabbit. Circ. Res. 31: 824-830.
Coote, J. H., Johns, E. J., Macleod, V. H., and Singer, B. (1972).
    Effect of renal nerve stimulation, renal blood flow, and
    adrenergic blockage on plasma renin activity in the cat.
    J. Physiol. (Lond.) 226: 15-36.
Corsini, W. A., Crosslan, K. L., and Bailie, M. D. (1974). Renin
    secretion by rat kidney slices in $vitro$. Proc. Soc. Exp.
    Biol. Med. 145: 403-406.
Corsini, W. A., Hook, J. B., and Bailie, M. D. (1975). Control of
    renin secretion in the dog: Effects of furosemide on the
    vascular and macula densa receptors. Circ. Res. 37: 464-470.
Cunningham, S. G., Feigl, E. O., and Scher, A. M. (1978). Carotid
    sinus reflex influence on plasma renin activity. Am. J.
    Physiol. 234: H670-H678.
Data, J. L., Gerber, J. G., Crump, W. J., Frolich, J. C., Hollifield,
    J. W., and Nies, A. S. (1978). The prostaglandin system.
    A role in canine baroreceptor control of renin release.
    Circ. Res. 42: 454-458.
Davis, J. O. and Freeman, R. H. (1976). Mechanisms controlling
    renin release. Physiol. Rev. 56: 1-56.
Fray, J. C. S. (1977). Stimulation of renin release in perfused
    kidney by low calcium and high magnesium. Am. J. Physiol.
    232: F377-F382.
Frolich, J. C., Hollifield, J. W., Dormois, J. C., Frolich, B. L.,
    Seyberth, H., Michelakis, A. M., and Oates, J. A. (1976).
    Suppression of plasma renin activity by indomethacin in man.
    Circ. Res. 39: 447-452.
Fynn, M., Onamakpome, N., and Peart, W. S. (1977). The effects of
    ionophores (A-23187 and RO2-2985) on renin secretion and renal
    vasoconstriction. Proc. R. Soc. London (Biol.) 199: 199-212.
Gerber, J. G., Branch, R. A., Nies, A. S., Gerkens, J. F., Shand,
    D. G., Hollifield, J. and Oates, J. A. (1978). Prostaglandins
    and renin release: II. Assessment of renin secretion following
    infusion of PGI_2, E_2, and D_2 into the renal artery of anesthe-
    tized dogs. Prostaglandins 15: 81-88.

Goormaghtigh, N. (1939). Existence of an endocrine gland in the
    media of the renal arterioles. Proc. Soc. Exp. Biol. Med. 42:
    688–689.
Goormaghtigh, N. (1945). Facts in favor of an endocrine function
    of the renal arterioles. J. Pathol. Microbiol. 57: 392–393.
Grandjean, B., Annat, G., Vincent, M., and Sassard, J. (1978).
    Influence of renal nerves on renin secretion in the conscious
    dog. Pflugers Arch. 373: 161–165.
Harada, E. and Rubin, R. P. (1978). Stimulation of renin secretion
    and calcium efflux from the isolated perfused cat kidney by
    noradrenaline after prolonged calcium deprivation. J. Physiol.
    (Lond.) 274: 367–379.
Hartroft, P. M. (1966). Electron microscopy nerve endings associated
    with juxtaglomerular (JG) cells and macula densa. Lab. Invest.
    15: 1127–1128.
Hodge, R. L., Lowe, R. D., and Vane, J. R. (1966). Increased angio-
    tensin formation in response to carotid occlusion in the dog.
    Nature 211: 491–493.
Jarecki, M., Thoren, P. N., and Donald, D. E. (1978). Release of
    renin by the carotid sinus baroreflex in anesthetized dogs.
    Circ. Res. 42: 614–619.
Johnson, J. A., Davis, J. O., Gotshall, R. W., Lohmeier, T. E.,
    Davis, J. L., Braverman, B., and Tempel, G. E. (1976).
    Evidence for an intrarenal beta receptor in control of renin
    release. Am. J. Physiol. 230: 410–418.
Johnson, J. A., Davis, J. O., and Witty, R. T. (1971). Effects of
    catecholamine and renal nerve stimulation on renin release in
    the nonfiltering kidney. Circ. Res. 29: 646–653.
Kahl, F. R., Flint, J. F., and Szidon, J. P. (1974). Influence of
    left atrial distention on renal vasomotor tone. Am. J. Physiol.
    226: 240–246.
Karim, F., Kidd, C., Malpus, C. M., and Penna, P. E. (1972). The
    effects of stimulation of the left atrial receptors on sympa-
    thetic efferent nerve activity. J. Physiol. (Lond.) 227: 243–
    260.
Kisch, E. S., Dluhy, R. G., and Williams, G. H. (1976). Regulation
    of renin release by calcium and ammonium ions in normal man.
    J. Clin. Endocrinol. Metab. 43: 1343–1350.
Kotchen, T. A., Galla, J. H., and Luke, R. G. (1976). Failure of
    $NaHCO_3$ and $KHCO_3$ to inhibit renin in the rat. Am. J. Physiol.
    231: 1050–1056.
Kotchen, T. A., Galla, J. H., and Luke, R. G. (1978). Contribution
    of chloride to the inhibition of plasma renin by sodium
    chloride in the rat. Kidney Int. 13: 201–207.
Kotchen, T. A., Maull, K. I., Luke, R., Rees, D., and Flamenbaum, W.
    (1974). Effect of acute and chronic calcium administration on
    plasma renin. J. Clin. Invest. 54: 1279–1286.
Kurz, K. D., Heath, J. E., and Zehr, J. E. (1977). Effects of res-
    piratory acidosis on circulating renin in dogs with filtering
    and nonfiltering kidneys. Fed. Proc. 36: 482 (Abstract).

Kurz, K. D. and Zehr, J. E. (1978). Mechanisms of enhanced renin secretion during CO_2 retention in dogs. Am. J. Physiol. 234: H537-H581.

Larsson, C., Weber, P., and Änggård, E. (1974). Arachidonic acid increases and indomethacin decreases plasma renin activity in the rabbit. Eur. J. Pharmacol. 28: 391-394.

Lester, G. E. and Rubin, R. P. (1977). The role of calcium in renin secretion from the isolated perfused cat kidney. J. Physiol. (Lond.) 269: 93-108.

Mancia, G., Romero, J. C., and Shepherd, J. T. (1975). Continuous inhibition of renin release in dogs by vagally innervated receptors in the cardiopulmonary region. Circ. Res. 36: 529-535.

Mancia, G., Shepherd, J. T., and Donald, D. E. (1975). Role of cardiac, pulmonary, and carotid mechanoreceptors in the control of hind-limb and renal circulation in dogs. Circ. Res. 37: 200-208.

Mark, A. L., Abboud, F. M., and Fitz, A. E. (1978). Influence of low- and high-pressure baroreceptors on plasma renin activity in humans. Am. J. Physiol. 235: H29-H33.

McPhee, M. S. and Lakey, W. H. (1971). Neurologic release of renin in mongrel dogs. Can. J. Surg. 14: 142-147.

Michelakis, A. M. (1971). The effect of sodium and calcium on renin release *in vitro*. Proc. Soc. Exp. Biol. Med. 137: 833-836.

Michelakis, A. M. and McAllister, R. G. (1972). The effect of chronic adrenergic receptor blockade on plasma renin activity in man. J. Clin. Endocrinol. Metab. 34: 386-394.

Mogil, R. A., Itskovitz, H. D., Russell, J. H., and Murphy, J. J. (1969). Renal innervation and renin activity in salt metabolism and hypertension. Am. J. Physiol. 216: 693-697.

Onesti, G., Schwartz, A. B., Kim, K. E., Paz-Martinez, V., and Schwartz, C. (1971). Antihypertensive effect of clonidine. Circ. Res. 28-29 (Suppl.): 53-69.

Passo, S. S., Assaykeen, T. A., Otsuka, K., Wise, B. L., Goldfien, A., and Ganong, W. F. (1971). Effect of stimulation of the medulla oblongata on renin secretion in dogs. Neuroendocrinology 7: 1-10.

Pettinger, W. A., Keeton, T. K., Campbell, W. B., and Harper, D. C. (1976). Evidence for a renal alpha-adrenergic receptor inhibiting renin release. Circ. Res. 38: 338-346.

Reid, I. A. and Jones, A. (1976). Effects of carotid occlusion and clonidine on renin secretion in anesthetized dogs. Clin. Sci. Mol. Med. 51: 109s-111s.

Reid, I. A., MacDonald, D. M., Pachnis, B., and Ganong, W. F. (1975). Studies concerning the mechanisms of suppression of renin secretion by clonidine. J. Pharmacol. Exp. Ther. 192: 713-721.

Reid, I. A., Morris, B. J., and Ganong, W. F. (1978). The renin-angiotensin system. Ann. Rev. Physiol. 40: 370-410.

Reid, I. A., Schrier, R. W., and Earley, L. E. (1972). Effect of
    extrarenal beta-adrenergic stimulation on the release of renin.
    J. Clin. Invest. 51: 1861-1869.
Richardson, D., Stella, A., Leonetti, G., Bartonelli, A., and
    Zanchetti, A. (1974). Mechanisms of renal release of renin by
    electrical stimulation of the brainstem in the cat. Circ. Res.
    34: 425-434.
Romero, J. C., Dunlap, C. L., and Strong, C. G. (1976). The effect
    of indomethacin and other anti-inflamatory drugs on the renin-
    angiotensin system. J. Clin. Invest. 58: 282-288.
Romero, J. C. and Strong, C. G. (1977). The effect of indomethacin
    blockade of prostaglandin synthesis on blood pressure of normal
    rabbits and rabbits with renovascular hypertension. Circ. Res.
    40: 35-41.
Saruta, T. and Matuki, S. (1975). The effects of cyclic AMP,
    theophylline, angiotensin II, and electrolytes upon renin
    release from rat kidney slices. Endocrinol. Jpn. 22: 137-140.
Schultz, H. D. and Zehr, J. E. (1977). Effect of central and
    peripheral beta adrenergic blockage on renin release during
    hemorrhage. Physiologist 20: 84 (Abstract).
Seymour, A. A. and Zehr, J. E. (1977). Renin response to suprarenal
    aortic clamp and to furosemide in indomethacin-treated dogs.
    Fed. Proc. 36: 458 (Abstract).
Seymour, A. A. and Zehr, J. E. (1978). Renin response to intrarenal
    indomethacin and arachidonic acid infusions into denervated
    non-filtering kidneys. Fed. Proc. 37: 306 (Abstract).
Skinner, S. L., McCubbin, J. W., and Page, I. H. (1964). Control
    of renin secretion. Circ. Res. 15: 64-76.
Stella, A. and Zanchetti, A. (1977). Effects of renal denervation
    on renin release in response to tilting and furosemide. Am. J.
    Physiol. 232: H500-H507.
Stephens, G. A., Davis, J. O., Freeman, R. H., and Watkins, B. E.
    (1978). Effects of sodium and potassium salts with anions
    other than chloride on renin secretion in the dog. Am. J.
    Physiol. 234: F10-F15.
Thames, M. D. (1977). Reflex suppression of renin release by
    ventricular receptors with vagal afferents. Am. J. Physiol.
    233: H181-H184.
Thames, M. D., Jarecki, M., and Donald, D. E. (1978). Neural
    control of renin secretion in anesthetized dogs. Circ. Res.
    42: 237-245.
Ueda, H., Yasuda, H., Takabatake, Y., Iizuka, M., Iizuka, T.,
    Ihori, M., Yamamoto, M., and Sakamoto, Y. (1967). Increased
    renin release evoked by mesencephalic stimulation in the dog.
    Jpn. Heart J. 8: 498-506.
Vander, A. J., Henry, J. P., Stephens, P. M., Kay, L. L., and
    Mouw, D. R. (1978). Plasma renin activity in psycosocial
    hypertension of DBA mice. Circ. Res. 42: 496-502.

Vander, A. J., Kay, L. L., Dugan, M. E., and Mouw, D. R. (1977).
    Effects of noise on plasma renin activity in rats. Proc. Soc.
    Exp. Biol. Med. 156: 24-26.
Vandongen, R. and Peart, W. S. (1974). The inhibition of renin
    secretion by alpha-adrenergic stimulation in the isolated
    rat kidney. Clin. Sci. Mol. Med. 47: 471-479.
Vandongen, R., Peart, W. S., and Boyd, G. W. (1973). Adrenergic
    stimulation of renin secretion in the isolated perfused rat
    kidney. Circ. Res. 32: 290-296.
Wagermark, J., Ungerstedt, W., and Ljungqvist, A. (1968). Sympa-
    thetic innervation of the juxtaglomerular cells of the kidney.
    Circ. Res. 22: 149-153.
Watkins, B. E., Davis, J. O., Lohmeier, T. E., and Freeman, R. H.
    (1976). Intrarenal site of action of calcium on renin secre-
    tion in dogs. Circ. Res. 39: 847-853.
Weber, M. A., Stokes, G. S., and Gain, M. J. (1974). Comparison of
    the effects on renin release of beta adrenergic antagonists
    with differing properties. J. Clin. Invest. 54: 1413-1419.
Weber, M. A., Thornell, I. R., and Stokes, G. S. (1974). Effects
    of beta adrenergic blocking agents on plasma renin activity
    in the conscious rabbit. J. Pharmacol. Exp. Ther. 188: 234-
    240.
Weber, P. C., Larsson, C., Änggård, E., Hamberg, M., Corey, E. J.,
    Nicolaou, K. C., and Samuelsson, B. (1976). Stimulation of
    renin release from rabbit renal cortex by arachidonic acid
    and prostaglandin endoperoxides. Circ. Res. 39: 868-873.
Weber, P. C., Scherer, B., and Larsson, C. (1977). Increase of
    free arachidonic acid by furosemide in man as the cause of
    prostaglandin and renin release. Eur. J. Pharmacol. 41: 329-
    332.
Winer, N., Chokshi, D. S., and Walkenhorst, W. G. (1971). Effects
    of cyclic AMP, sympathomimetic amines, and adrenergic receptor
    antagonists on renin secretion. Circ. Res. 29: 239-248.
Witty, R. T., Davis, J. O., Johnson, J. A., and Prewitt, R. L.
    (1971). Effects of papaverine and hemorrhage on renin
    secretion in the nonfiltering kidney. Am. J. Physiol. 221:
    1666-1671.
Yamamoto, K., Iwao, H., Abe, Y., and Morimoto, S. (1974). Effect
    of Ca^{++} on renin release *in vitro* and *in vivo*. Jpn. Circ. J.
    38: 1127-1131.
Yun, J. C. H., Kelly, G., Bartter, F. C., and Smith, H. C. (1977).
    Role of prostaglandins in the control of renin secretion in
    the dog. Circ. Res. 40: 459-464.
Zehr, J. E. and Feigl, E. O. (1972). Attenuation of renin activity
    by beta receptor blockade. Fed. Proc. 31: 825 (Abstract).
Zehr, J. E. and Feigl, E. O. (1973). Suppression of renin activity
    by hypothalamic stimulation. Circ. Res. 32-33 (Suppl. 1):
    17-27.

Zehr, J. E., Hasbargen, J. A. and Kurz, K. D.   (1976).   Reflex
    suppression of renin secretion during the distention of
    cardiopulmonary receptors in dogs.   Circ. Res.   38:232-239.

DISCUSSION AFTER DR. ZEHR'S PAPER

Mr. Ray
    I have two unrelated questions.   First, a few years ago
Zanchetti and Stella (1975) reported a study in cats with unilateral
renal denervation, and they found that low doses of furosemide
produced increases in renin release only from innervated kidneys--
not from the denervated kidneys.   With larger doses of furosemide
they saw increased renin release also from the denervated kidneys,
which possibly could have been through macula densa mechanisms.
What is your opinion of these findings?

Dr. Zehr
    I am familiar with that paper.   I think it is unclear exactly
why the low doses of furosemide failed to increase renin release
in the denervated kidneys.   A study from Mike Bailie's laboratory
at Michigan State (Corsini, Hook, and Bailie, 1975) would suggest
that furosemide triggers intrarenal baroreceptor mechanisms as
well.   I think that when large doses of furosemide are administered,
probably both the renal baroreceptor and tubular mechanisms are
affected.   How denervation of the kidney acts to blunt the response
to furosemide is not clear, at least to me.   Possibly over longer
periods of time there may be the cumulative effects of volume
depletion, but it seems very unlikely that this would have been a
factor in the studies to which you referred.

Mr. Ray
    Secondly, I would like to ask one thing regarding Dr. Mancia's
work (Mancia, Shepherd, and Donald, 1976) which I read recently in
the American Journal of Physiology, concerning the idea of cross-
talk between the barostatic reflex and the cardiopulmonary reflex.
I was wondering, in your work with this, what pressures did you
start out with?   Apparently when high pressures are seen by the
barostatic reflex, it acts more or less like a parameter.

Dr. Zehr
    I also am familiar with that work.   By the way, their con-
clusions are in agreement with the study to which I referred from
the University of Iowa (Mark, Abboud, and Fitz, 1978).   The basic
conclusion from that study in man was that in order to observe the
maximum response to lower body negative pressure, both reflexes

must work together. I can't give you the precise arterial pressure
in our studies, but it was in no way changed or altered during our
maneuvers. I think it is of significance that prior sodium deprivation was required to elicit the response reproducibly. I would
presume that under these conditions the system had a somewhat
different sensitivity. I think this is consistent with virtually
every other study in this area. It takes prior sodium deprivation
to see the response consistently. This raises a question as to the
functional role of this reflex in normal homeostasis. At least,
the reflex is there under specialized conditions.

Dr. Poisner
     I would like to point out another aspect of the role of calcium
in the control of renin release. Several years ago Dr. Chen and I
(Chen and Poisner, 1976) reported that renin release was evoked from
kidney slices by reintroducing calcium after a period of calcium
deprivation, and this was subsequently confirmed by Lester and Rubin
(1977) using the isolated cat kidney. We interpreted this to mean
that the reintroduction of calcium into the inside of the cell was
sufficient to cause renin secretion. I think some of the conflicting results in the literature are attributable not only to the
different types of preparations that have been used, but also to
lumping the types of stimuli which have been used for evoking renin
release. It is not known whether spontaneous renin release occurs
by the same mechanism as that evoked by isoproterenol or by some
other mechanism. There is a precedent for that. I could cite the
fact that in muscle contraction, where we all know that calcium is
required, there are vast differences in the sensitivities of various
types of muscle, depending on the type of muscle and the type of
stimulation, insofar as their sensitivity to calcium is involved.

Dr. Zehr
     I think that is absolutely correct. At the present time the
relationship between isoproterenol and calcium is very unclear.

Dr. Goetz
     John, I might just summarize some work which I think agrees
with what you are saying, except that one may even see a mild renin
response without sodium depletion. We have recently completed a
study in conscious dogs in which we prehydrated them with 200-300 ml.
of saline to insure that they were not sodium depleted while in the
kennels; one day later they were brought to the laboratory and were
hydrated slightly. We then anesthetized the surface of either the
right or left atrial epicardium in the conscious dog with lidocaine.
When we added lidocaine to either the right or left side, thereby
wiping out the afferent impulses from the heart, we observed an
increase in plasma renin activity of about 50 to 100 percent. It
should be emphasized that this procedure produced a very marked
decrease in atrial receptor discharge; it was almost totally
abolished in the studies in which we recorded afferent nerve

activity. For this reason we don't know whether the response is
really of physiological significance. In any case, the response was
observed in a conscious animal that probably was not sodium depleted.

Dr. Zehr

How long did you see the renin elevation when compared to the
relief from local anesthetic? Is there any correlation? Was renin
maintained during the entire period of time when the lidocaine was
effective?

Dr. Goetz

We haven't looked at that closely. In our experiments we have
a 30-minute control period in which the surface of the epicardium
is perfused with saline. Then we switch to a 30 minute perfusion
with lidocaine, and finally, back to saline for 30 minutes. Our
neural recordings indicate that it takes anywhere from 3 to 7
minutes to cause a marked reduction in atrial receptor activity.
When we switch back to saline sometimes it takes even longer than
that before receptor activity returns. We find that after 25 minutes
of lidocaine the plasma renin is up, and after 25 minutes in the
recovery period the renin is still up. We're not sure exactly why
this is, but it probably is because some of the receptors are
quieter after the lidocaine than they were before.

Just one other quick comment. As far as whether this means
anything physiologically, I have the same answer as you--I don't
know. We have a very preliminary series of experiments in which
we've taken two groups of dogs and denervated the hearts in one
group by the Geis-Randall-Kaye method. We have performed either
volume expansion or hemorrhage in these animals and compared the
results with those from a group of sham operated, control dogs.
On the basis of very preliminary evidence, they both responded in
precisely the same way; that is, plasma renin activity was reduced
by volume expansion and was increased by hemorrhaging. So animals
certainly can respond very well after cardiac denervation.

Dr. Peach

Maybe this is my ignorance about prostaglandins. I feel
there's prost-another-one coming next week. I really don't know
what people are hypothesizing who are throwing indomethacin into
the kidney. I don't find it unusual that the kidney might make
prostaglandins when obviously cell walls must change to move renin
from an intracellular compartment to an extracellular compartment.
I'm not exactly sure how this occurs. Maybe Dr. Poisner could help
us to understand how renin blasts through the cell wall. Certainly,
in changing the constituents of a cell wall one of the easiest things
to do is play around with phospholipids, and if you could prevent
that from occurring, then perhaps you could play havoc with the
ability of renin to leave the cell. Since you work in this area,
what is your bias as to the role of prostaglandins in renin release?

Dr. Zehr

I can only give you my bias. I like the fundamental hypothesis that prostaglandins probably act through some function of calcium, but of course I really don't know if this will prove to be true. With regard to indomethacin, it is virtually impossible to conduct an indomethacin study and show that indomethacin itself is not having an independent and direct effect. Also, we can't give indomethacin without changing the prostaglandins, so it is quite difficult to do these experiments and draw final conclusions. The use of other cyclooxygenase inhibitors tends to produce the same general reduction in renin release, so we suspect that the effect is prostaglandin mediated. I don't know what the final cellular mechanism is, but there must be one somewhere down the line. I suspect that some day we may discover that it is calcium--calcium flux, intracellular calcium concentration or binding, or something such as this.

Dr. Nishimura

Regarding the prostaglandins, if I remember correctly, prosta-cyclin has also been shown to be present in the vascular wall of the blood vessels of the kidney. Do you think they may possibly interact at the juxtaglomerular cell site and may be an intra-cellular mediator for a renin release mechanism?

Dr. Zehr

I think that is very possible. It could act through cyclic-AMP mechanisms or related events.

Dr. Freeman

John, you didn't say anything about the short-loop feedback mechanism, which I think is very important physiologically. We know that angiotensin releases prostaglandins and that calcium is involved in this. How do you think the calcium and the prosta-glandins fit into the physiological short-loop feedback?

Dr. Zehr

I don't know. Does anyone? A lot of work needs to be done at this level as well.

DISCUSSION REFERENCES

Chen, D. S. and Poisner, A. M. (1976). Direct stimulation of renin release by calcium. Proc. Soc. Exp. Biol. Med. 152: 565-567.
Corsini, W. A., Hook, J. B., and Bailie, M. D. (1975). Control of renin secretion in the dog. Effects of furosemide on the vascular and macula densa receptors. Circ. Res. 37: 464-470.

Lester, G. E. and Rubin, R. P. (1977). The role of calcium in
    renin secretion from the isolated perfused cat kidney. J.
    Physiol. (Lond.) 269: 93-108.
Mancia, G., Shepherd, J. T., and Donald, D. E. (1976). Interplay
    among carotid sinus, cardiopulmonary, and carotid body
    reflexes in dogs. Am. J. Physiol. 230: 19-24.
Mark, A. L., Abboud, F. M., and Fitz, A. E. (1978). Influence of
    low- and high-pressure baroreceptors on plasma renin activity
    in humans. Am. J. Physiol. 235: H29-H33.
Zanchetti, A. and Stella, A. (1975). Neural control of renin
    release. Clin. Sci. Mol. Med. 48 (Suppl. 2): 215s-223s.

MOLECULAR APPROACHES TO THE STUDY OF ANGIOTENSIN RECEPTORS

Michael J. Peach and Nigel R. Levens

Department of Pharmacology and the Hypertension Unit
University of Virginia School of Medicine
Charlottesville, VA 22908

OUTLINE

I. Introduction

II. Methods used to study angiotensin receptors

A. Structure-activity relationships

B. Radioligand studies of angiotensin receptors

C. Cellular location of angiotensin receptors

I. INTRODUCTION

An understanding of the mode of action of any hormone requires an approach at the molecular level (see Table 1). Hormones such as angiotensin can induce a response only by interacting their molecular structure with specific receptor molecules in sensitive tissues. The molecular properties of the hormone, therefore, determine its action and activity, and hence a relationship exists between structure and activity. Considerable effort has been directed toward determining the molecular interaction of angiotensin with its receptors, in order to obtain a better understanding of its mode of action. From these investigations the molecular composition of receptor sites can be determined, leading ultimately to their solubilization. Once purified, an antibody to the receptor could be generated which would have great potential for studying the location of angiotensin receptor sites. This approach to studying receptors, linked to radioreceptor binding studies, generates the potential for deriving and utilizing models to design drugs. Indeed,

Table 1.   WHY STUDY ANGIOTENSIN RECEPTORS ?

Studying angiotensin receptors:

a)   Promotes a better understanding of the mode of action of
     the hormone.

b)   Leads to a determination of the molecular composition of
     the receptor site and its solubilization, subsequently
     allowing antibodies to be developed for mapping angioten-
     sin receptors in sensitive tissues.

c)   Has utility in designing drugs, leading to a determination
     of the mechanism of angiotensin action in disease states.

---

these methods could be used to derive low molecular weight compounds
which could have considerable utility in modulating the activity of
the renin-angiotensin system. Recently it has been suggested that
changes in receptors or receptor coupling to second messengers may
play an important role in disease states. Therefore, a thorough
understanding of the interaction between the angiotensin molecule
and its receptor, and the induced intracellular process could have
great utility in understanding and controlling angiotensin-induced
pathological changes. These reasons for investigating receptors
have resulted in the development of specific methodologies for
their study.

II.   METHODS USED TO STUDY ANGIOTENSIN RECEPTORS

Historically, knowledge of receptors has been derived from
structure-activity studies, using agonists and antagonists of a
particular response in a particular effector organ. From the first
synthesis of angiotensin by Bumpus, Schwartz, and Page (1957)
numerous structural-activity studies have been performed with analogues of angiotensin that have either full agonistic activity, or
analogues which are antagonistic to the response of the parent peptide (see Table 2). Another method of investigating receptors is
by radioligand studies. This technique, which examines the interaction of radiolabelled compounds with sensitive tissues, has been
used widely to determine the kinetics of binding, association-
dissociation constants, the number of receptor sites per cell, and
the concentration of receptors in a given tissue. Radioligand
studies with angiotensin have been confined mainly to intact tissues
removed from animals following the administration of labelled peptides. However, cell suspensions of tissues, such as the adrenal
zona glomerulosa, and membranes isolated by differential centrifugation also have been investigated. Ultimately it is possible
that comparable studies can be performed with a receptor macro-
molecule that has been solubilized from cell membrane components.

Table 2.   HOW HAVE ANGIOTENSIN RECEPTORS BEEN STUDIED ?

Angiotensin receptors have been studied by:

1)   Structure-activity relationships

   using a)   agonists

          b)   antagonists

2)   Radioligand studies

   in   a)   tissues

         b)   cells

         c)   membranes (ultimately after receptor
              solubilization)

3)   Receptor distribution and cellular location

   by   a)   autoradiography

         b)   macromolecular analogues

         c)   immunofluorescence

In many cases these radioligand studies cannot be correlated with a
response; for example, it is very difficult to monitor a response to
angiotensin in membranes obtained by differential centrifugation.
Therefore, the bulk of the receptor studies are based on the use of
analogues of angiotensin which are known to mimic or to compete with
the parent peptide in intact tissues where a response can be measured.
Hence, the positioning of competitive curves between an analogue and
radioactive angiotensin has become the basis for these studies, and
it is assumed that the receptors are not altered by disrupting the
integrity of the tissue. Finally, the distribution and cellular
location of specific receptor sites can be investigated by autoradiography, immunofluorescence techniques, product precipitation,
and by the use of macromolecular analogues of angiotensin which
should be confined to the extracellular compartment.

Just as alpha and beta receptors for catecholamines, and H_1 and
H_2 receptors for histamine have been characterized, many investigators have considered the possibility that in the same species there
may be different receptors for endogenous angiotensin. One of the
simplist conditions would be represented by one peptide, for example
angiotensin II, interacting with one receptor type, regardless of
the effector organ or the response being monitored. Alternatively,
it is possible to have angiotensins I, II, and III all interacting
with a single type of receptor in all tissues and organs. Thirdly,
one peptide, such as angiotensin II, could interact with multiple

Table 3. *ARE THERE DIFFERENT ANGIOTENSIN RECEPTORS IN THE SAME*
SPECIES ?

If there are, then the following possibilities exist:

1) One peptide interacting with one receptor type.

2) Multiple peptides interacting with one receptor type.

3) One peptide interacting with multiple receptor types.

4) Multiple peptides interacting with multiple receptor types.

---

receptor types, which could vary depending upon the tissue studied.
Lastly, all of the angiotensin peptides could couple with multiple
receptor types (see Table 3). In reviewing the literature it is
immediately obvious that every investigator and laboratory has a
bias towards one of these possibilities. On the available evidence,
we favor the possibility of multiple peptides interacting with multiple receptor types.

Having discussed the general methodology used for studying
receptors, this review next will assess the literature to indicate
how each of these techniques has been used to characterize the
interaction of angiotensin with its receptors.

A. Structure-activity Relationships

Numerous structure-activity studies have been performed in a
variety of sensitive tissues by the use of differing structural
analogues of angiotensin. The majority of these investigations
have used contractile responses in vascular and nonvascular contractile systems or have used blood pressure responses in intact
animals. A good example of the differences in structure-activity
relationships among sensitive tissues is illustrated by a comparison of the structural requirements for the action of angiotensin
on an end organ which contracts in response to the hormone, with
the structural requirements for a neurogenic response or for the
stimulation of salt and water transfer across epithelial tissues.
Clearly the pressor and myotropic systems have an absolute requirement for phenylalanine as the 8th amino acid of the octapeptide
chain; however, aliphatic substitutions can be made for phenylalanine without greatly affecting the activity of the molecule on
the sympathetic nervous system or the ability to stimulate salt and
water transfer. These observations lead to the conclusion that
there are at least two different types of angiotensin receptors,
differing mainly in their requirements for phenylalanine in position
8 of the molecule. Representative tissues and the properties of
each of these receptors are described in Table 4.

Table 4. MOLECULAR PROPERTIES OF THE TWO TYPES OF ANGIOTENSIN RECEPTORS

Locations of each receptor type:

Receptor Type 1

Pressor systems	(Khosla et al., 1974)
Myotropic systems	(Khosla et al., 1974)
Vasopressin release	(Gagnon et al., 1973)
Thirst	(Fitzsimons, 1975)

Receptor Type 2

Adrenal medulla	(Peach & Ober, 1974)
Sympathetic nerve endings	(Peach et al., 1972)
Frog skin	(Wideman et al., 1972)
Intestinal salt & water transfer	(Bumpus et al., 1976)
Renal tubules	(Freedlender, 1977)

Angiotensin properties for each receptor type:

Receptor Type 1

Positions 4 and 6 necessary for binding.
Phenylalanine at position 8.
Free $-COOH^-$ necessary at position 3.
Angiotensin I acts via angiotensin II.

Receptor Type 2

Positions 4 and 6 necessary for binding.
Aliphatic possible at position 8.
Free $-COOH^-$ unnecessary at position 8.
Angiotensin I directly active.

Although the structural requirements for the action of angiotensin have been characterized extensively for the majority of sensitive tissues, too little consideration has been directed at either
the purity or the stability of the peptides used in these investigations. Conversely, radioligand and radioreceptor binding studies
generally have been performed under conditions where much attention
has been directed to the stability of the radiolabelled peptide in
the tissue or subcellular fraction used as the source of binding
sites. The assumption, therefore, can be made that the radiolabelled angiotensin II and the various analogues used to compete
with the parent peptide are stable under the conditions of these
studies. However, as with the majority of structure-activity studies, little attention has been directed at determining the purity
of the peptides used in any of the radioligand studies.

B. Radioligand Studies of Angiotensin Receptors

An example of the dangers of applying structure-activity relationship studies to radioreceptor ligand studies can be illustrated
by investigations performed in our laboratory with [Ala7]-substituted
analogues of angiotensin. Due to its biochemical structure, it is
generally assumed that proline in position 7 of the octapeptide
chain imparts a rigidifying effect on the peptide backbone, undergoing trans isomerization to produce a preferred conformation of the
peptide in solution. Substitution of aliphatic residues for proline
leads to analogues of angiotensin which are poor agonists, with
little or no intrinsic activity. It is well documented that angiotensin converting enzyme is unable to hydrolyze any peptide containing a penultimate proline residue. Thus, converting enzyme is devoid
of hydrolytic activity against angiotensin II, as proline is the
penultimate residue in this peptide. Replacement of proline by
alanine as the 7th amino acid in the octapeptide chain results in a
compound that is a superb substrate for converting enzyme. We have
performed a series of investigations in rabbit atria, a tissue which
is rich in converting enzyme, and in rabbit aorta, which is usually
accepted to be a tissue with low converting enzyme activity. In
tissues pretreated with teprotide (SQ 20,881), an inhibitor of converting enzyme activity, we found that the activities of the [Ala7]
angiotensins were potentiated dramatically. Interestingly, the
[Ala7] analogues also had activity in rabbit aorta, which was
observed primarily after converting enzyme inhibition (Figure 1).

Based on the available knowledge of angiotensin structure-
activity relationships reported in the literature, [Ala7] angiotensin II would be a compound that could be used in radioligand studies
as an example of an angiotensin analogue devoid of activity and
unable to compete for binding. As our findings presented above indicate, if [Ala7] angiotensin II were studied under the classical

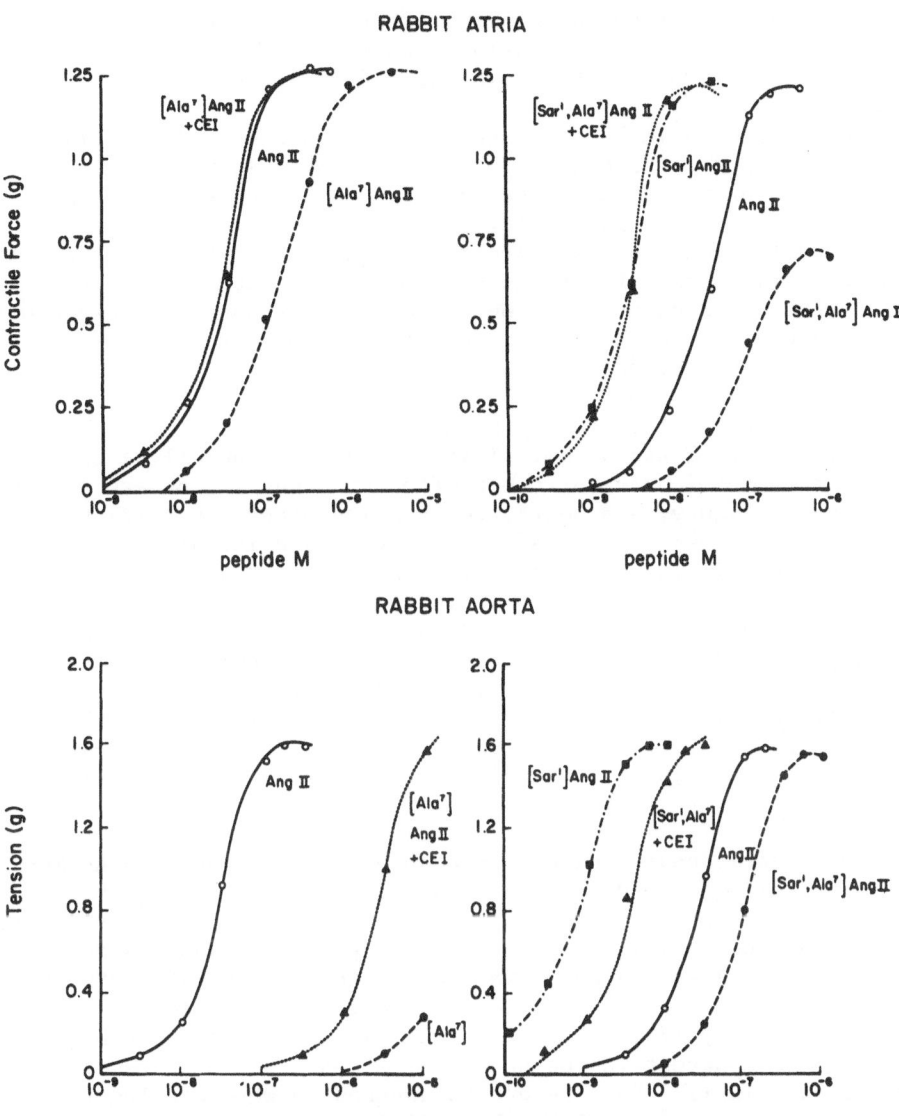

Figure 1. Effect of converting enzyme inhibitor (CEI) 10 μg/ml.
on the response of rabbit atria to [Ala⁷]-Ang. II and
[Sar¹, Ala⁷]-Ang. II. Each point represents the mean of
8-12 experimental observations. Isometric contractions
were recorded from a base of 1 gm. resting tension.
Doses of each peptide are shown as molar concentrations
for ease of comparison. Pretreatment with CEI had no
effect on responses induced by [Sar¹]-Ang. II or Ang. II
(curves omitted).

conditions of radioreceptor binding, where most proteolytic enzyme activity is inhibited, this analogue would have considerable activity and would compete with radiolabelled angiotensin II for binding.

Summarized in Table 5 are the many tissues used in binding studies with radioactive angiotensin II. Investigations have been performed in preparations of vascular and nonvascular smooth muscle, adrenal cortex, renal glomeruli, various regions of the central nervous system, and in dispersed fetal chick ventricle. Intact tissues or microsomal fractions of homogenized tissues have been used as the basis of many of these studies, although investigations of the adrenal cortex have used cell suspensions or primary isolates of the zona glomerulosa.

In smooth muscle, binding sites can be demonstrated having an affinity between 5 and 50 nM. This is a value generally comparable to that reported in several other effector organs. Conversely, in the adrenal, kidney, and heart, two binding sites are evident from Scatchard analyses: a high affinity site and a low affinity site, which possess binding constants of less than 1 nM and between 8 and 100 nM, respectively. The low affinity site in these tissues appears generally comparable to the arbitrarily defined "high affinity" site perviously described in smooth muscle. Interestingly, the adrenal, in addition to the brain, kidney, and heart possesses a high affinity site exhibiting a much greater affinity than the single binding site identified in smooth muscle. This suggests a rather arbitrary definition of the angiotensin II binding site in smooth muscle.

We recently have studied the binding of radiolabelled angiotensin to collagenase-dispersed cardiac ventricular cells obtained from fertilized chick eggs 13-18 days of age. In these experiments, an apparent low affinity angiotensin receptor site was characterized in 13-15 day chicks and which was unable to discriminate between angiotensin I and II, as both peptides demonstrated similar binding kinetics. By day 17-18 of development, a second site with higher affinity was apparent in the heart cells, and this site was specific for angiotensin II. Both receptors apparently were coupled for contractile responses. Although Goodfriend, Fyhrquist, Gutmann, *et al*. (1972) also have reported the binding of radiolabelled angiotensin to subcellular fractions of fetal bovine kidneys and adrenals, very few investigators have tackled the problems of angiotensin binding in fetal tissues. Our data in chick heart suggest that the properties of angiotensin and peptide binding in development and maturation studies may be a potentially exciting area of investigation.

Although the existence of specific angiotensin II receptor sites generally is accepted, of considerable debate over the last

Table 5. PROPERTIES OF ANGIOTENSIN BINDING SITES IN SENSITIVE TISSUES

Tissue	Radioactive Label	High Affinity Site (K_1)	Low Affinity Site (K_2)	Reference
Aortic plasma membrane				
rabbit	^3H	6 nM	----	Devynck & Meyer (1976)
guinea pig	^{14}C	20-50 nM	----	LeMorvan & Palaic (1975)
Uterine plasma membrane				
rat	^3H	8-20 nM	----	Devynck et al. (1976)
	^{125}I	----	----	Aguilera et al.
Adrenal cortex				
bovine particulate fraction	^3H	2 nM	83 nM	Glossman et al. (1974)
rat particulate fraction	^{125}I	0.2-0.5 nM	8 nM	Glossman et al.
rat zona glomerulosa cells	^{125}I	1.5-2 nM	80 nM	Douglas & Catt (1976)
	^3H	3-5 nM	25 nM	Pernollet et al. (1977)
rabbit zona glomerulosa cells	^3H	29 nM	----	Gurchinkoff et al. (1976)
canine glomerul. cells	^{125}I	0.5 nM	25 nM	Bravo et al. (1976)
Kidney				
rat glomerular membranes	^{125}I	0.05-0.07 nM	2 nM	Beaufils et al. (1976)
	^3H	----	----	Srauer et al. (1977)
rat dispersed tubules	^{125}I	6 nM	60 nM	Freedlender & Goodfriend (1977)
Brain				
calf cerebral cortex	^{125}I	0.2 nM	----	Bennett & Snyder (1976)
rat hypothalamus medulla	^{125}I	0.9 nM	----	Sirett et al. (1977)
Heart				
dispersed fetal chick ventricle	^3H	0.5 nM	100 nM	Peach (unpublished)

few years has been the suggestion that there also might be specific
receptors for angiotensin III. Some recent studies suggest that
there is selectivity of the heptapeptide for receptor sites in some
tissues. In this respect Dr. Meyer's laboratory in Paris (Devynck
and Meyer, 1978) has investigated the binding of ^{3}H-angiotensin II
and III to homogenates of the adrenal zona glomerulosa. These
investigators found that although angiotensin III bound to this
tissue, angiotensin II was unable to compete for the binding of the
heptapeptide, suggesting a specific receptor site for angiotensin III
in the adrenal. A second angiotensin binding site also was characterized in these studies which alternatively exhibited selectivity for
angiotensin II, as unlabeled angiotensin II was a better competitor
for the binding of labelled octapeptide than was angiotensin III.
On the other hand, Aguilera, Hauer, and Catt (1978) could find no
evidence in the rat adrenal of a selective or specific site for
the binding of ^{125}I-angiotensin III. They suggested that the difference between these studies could be due to the much higher specific
activity of their ^{125}I-angiotensin III compared with the ^{3}H-peptide
used in the studies of Devynck and Meyer (1978).

Although there is confusion over the existence of specific
binding sites for radiolabeled angiotensin III in the adrenal cortex,
structural-activity studies suggest that this tissue may contain
different receptors for the heptapeptide than those found in other
tissues. In vascular smooth muscle, substituted analogues of the
heptapeptide, such as [Ile[7]] angiotensin III, have very poor antagonistic action and weak, if any, agonistic activity. This is in
direct contrast to the adrenal cortex where these analogues possess
very high affinity and 10% of the potency of angiotensin II to stimulate steroidogenesis. These data suggest a preferential binding and
a high intrinsic activity for angiotensin III analogues in the
adrenal cortex. It will be imperative to wait for the involvement
of other laboratories before the existence of a specific angiotensin III receptor site can be accepted in this or any other tissue.

C. Cellular Location of Angiotensin Receptors

Having presented some of the binding properties and structural
requirements for angiotensin receptors, this review next will describe studies that have attempted to characterize the cellular
distribution and location of these receptors.

In 1971, Robertson and Khairallah administered ^{3}H-angiotensin II
into the left ventricle of anesthetized rats and then immediately
fixed the myocardium with glutaraldehyde. Subsequent electron microscopy of the heart showed a considerable increase in the number of
pinocytotic vesicles in endothelial cells of both the aorta and
coronary artery. Furthermore, autoradiography consistently demonstrated the presence of radioactivity in the nuclear zone of endo-

thelial cells as well as in the nuclei of smooth muscle cells of the
aorta and mitochondria of cardiac muscle. These data suggested to
these investigators that intact angiotensin II may have an action
on nuclear function. This hypothesis is consistent with the previous
work of Khairallah, Robertson, and Davila (1972) demonstrating that
angiotensin can stimulate nucleic acid synthesis in the myocardium
and the subsequent synthesis of protein by the ventricle. These
studies, therefore, are suggestive of a nuclear action of angiotensin, but cannot be considered as proof, for the identification
of tritium in the nuclear region by autoradiography does not show
that the radioactive material is intact angiotensin II.

    In addition to electron microscopy and autoradiography, the
location and distribution of angiotensin receptors also has been
studied by coupling the octapeptide to high molecular weight compounds. One of the first studies using this method was performed
in 1962 by Arakawa, Smeby, and Bumpus, at the Cleveland Clinic.
These investigators synthesized angiotensin II and coupled it to a
polymer of serine (MW 27,000) in which the hydroxyl groups were
o-acetylated. They found that this molecule of angiotensin II
still retained considerable activity in its ability to contract
smooth muscle, which suggested that in this tissue the angiotensin II
interacted with a receptor on the surface of the cell. Alternatively,
Goodfriend, Fyhrquist, Gutmann, *et al.* (1972) have suggested that
angiotensin II may have an intracellular site of action in the
heart. They demonstrated that the octapeptide tightened P/O ratios
in mitochondria isolated from the myocardium and postulated that the
positive inotropic action of angiotensin II in the heart may therefore be mediated through increased energy utilization and hence
increased efficiency of contraction of the heart. This is an interesting hypothesis when coupled to the previous work of Robertson and
Khairallah (1971), demonstrating binding of tritiated angiotensin II
to heart mitochondria.

    On the assumption that a high molecular weight angiotensin would
be unlikely to cross the cardiac cell membrane rapidly and thus would
not interact with myocardial mitochondria, we exposed cat papillary
muscles to the [poly-o-acetyl serine] angiotensin II previously
synthesized by Arakawa (Figure 2). This compound retained considerable activity in stimulating the heart (Peach, 1972). To determine
that this was not due to contamination of the preparation with free
angiotensin II, separate papillary muscles were exposed to either the
polymer or to the free octapeptide. At the peak of a sustained
contraction the bathing fluid was drained from the muscles and passed
through an Amicon UM2 membrane which allowed the passage of molecules
of less than 2,000 molecular weight. The collected filtrate from the
angiotensin II-treated preparation produced a dramatic positive inotropic response when administered to a naive (not previously treated)
papillary muscle. In contrast, the filtrate from the muscle treated
with [poly-o-acetyl-Seryl] angiotensin II failed to produce a

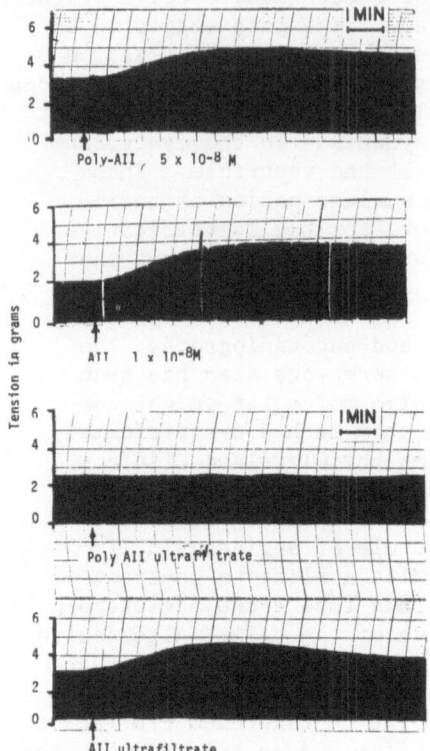

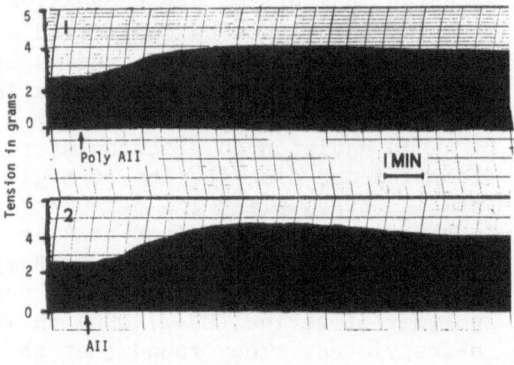

Figure 2.   Effect of an ED_{100} concentration of angiotensin II
            $(1 \times 10^{-8}$ Molar) and [poly-o-acetyl serine]-angiotensin II
            on myocardial contractility. Isometric contractions were
            recorded from maximum length-tension in isolated cat
            papillary muscles maintained at 35° C and paced by field
            stimulation at 60 beats/min. with twice threshold voltage.

            Upper left: Response of single papillary muscles to
            [poly-o-acetyl serine]-angiotensin II (Poly AII) and to
            angiotensin II (AII).

            Lower left: Response of naive papillary muscles to an
            ultrafiltrate of the bathing solution from muscles con-
            tracted with [poly-o-acetyl serine]-angiotensin II
            (Poly AII ultrafiltrate) and from muscles contracted
            with angiotensin II (AII ultrafiltrate).

            Right: Response of naive papillary muscles to unfiltered
            bathing fluid from muscles contracted with [poly-o-acetyl
            serine]-angiotensin II (Poly-AII) and from muscles con-
            tracted with angiotensin II (AII).

response, suggesting that the high molecular weight compound was not contaminated with the free octapeptide. Furthermore, the polymer had not been degraded or bound during exposure to the initial papillary muscle, as transferring the bathing fluid directly to another muscle produced an increase in contraction. In 1976, Bravo, Khosla, and Bumpus also showed that [poly-o-acetyl-Seryl] angiotensin II retained considerable activity as a steroidogenic agent in dog adrenal zona glomerulosa. It is interesting to speculate on the basis of our studies in the myocardium and the studies of Bravo *et al.* in the adrenal cortex, that in these two tissues the angiotensin receptor sites are located on the cell membrane. Such studies, however, do not rule out the possibility of intracellular receptors for angiotensins, but it seems unlikely that any intracellular receptor mediates the acute responses.

In 1971, Richardson and Beaulnes coupled ^{14}C-labeled angiotensin II to the enzymes horseradish peroxidase (MW 40,000) and cytochrome A (MW 12,000) by the use of 1% glutaraldehyde. In these studies a degree of coupling of 1:1 between angiotensin II and cytochrome A, and 1:1 or 2:1 between angiotensin II and horseradish peroxidase was determined by calculating the protein to ^{14}C-ratio. The activity of these two polymers was determined by the rat blood pressure assay and by the contractile responses produced by rat ascending colon and rabbit aortic strips. To determine the degree of contamination of the high molecular weight material with free angiotensin II, strips of rat colon were placed inside dialysis bags and were suspended in organ baths of 40 ml. volume. In this situation, angiotensin II or the polymer could be administered either inside or outside of the dialysis bag. Therefore, material administered outside the bag had to be dialyzable to come into contact with the tissue and thus to produce contraction. The colon strips contracted dramatically when either angiotensin II or the protein-coupled peptide was placed inside the dialysis bags. However, although angiotensin II, which is freely dialyzable, also produced contractions when added outside the dialysis membrane, the two high molecular weight compounds did not produce contractions when placed outside the dialysis bags, which suggested that they were not contaminated with the free octapeptide. These investigators also sought to determine the potency and duration of the contractile response of the rabbit aorta to angiotensin II and to the high molecular weight analogues by the oil immersion technique of Kalsner and Nickerson (1968). This method was used to determine the rate of relaxation of the aortic strips in oil and in Krebs' solution after first contracting the tissue with either angiotensin II or the polymers. In contrast to Krebs' solution, the rate of relaxation in oil is dependent on the rate of inactivation of angiotensin or the analogues by tissue enzymes, as these polypeptides are insoluble in oil and therefore are unable to diffuse from the microenvironment of the receptor. Using this technique, it was found that aortic strips which had been contracted with angiotensin II relaxed rapidly when

the bathing solution was replaced with either Krebs' solution or
oil, suggesting that angiotensin II is broken down rapidly in the
vicinity of the receptor. However, when these preparations were
contracted with angiotensin coupled to cytochrome A or horseradish
peroxidase and the bathing solutions were replaced by oil, the contractions were maintained for as long as 60 minutes, with no evidence
of relaxation. It is of interest that although the muscle treated
with horseradish peroxidase-angiotensin relaxed slowly when the oil
was replaced by Krebs' solution, the cytochrome A-angiotensin-
treated preparations failed to relax when returned to this buffer.
These data suggested that, in contrast to the free octapeptide, the
angiotensin II polymers were very slowly degraded, if at all, by the
tissue enzymes and that the high molecular weight angiotensins remained at the receptor sites, continually stimulating the tissue to
contract.

To test this hypothesis, Richardson and Beaulnes (1971) sought
to determine the intracellular and extracellular location of these
two polymers. In these experiments, mice were injected intravenously
with angiotensin II coupled to either cytochrome A or to horseradish
peroxidase. The animals then were decapitated at various times and
samples of tissues were removed and fixed in glutaraldehyde. Sections of tissues, plus aortic strips previously exposed to these
polymers, were prepared for light and electron microscopy and were
reacted with 3,3'-diaminobenzidine, which forms a dark complex with
both enzymes. Light microscopy of the aortic strips revealed the
reaction products of both enzyme-coupled angiotensins were located
in the endothelial region at the margins of the preparation and in
a few of the macrophages in the adventitia. The greater resolution
of electron microscopy showed that the enzymes were in fact located
primarily in small vesicles in the endothelial cells, with some
adherance to the cell surface. A loose collection of the enzyme
complex also was found in the subendothelial region of the aortic
strips that had been left in oil for longer than one hour. In those
strips where the integrity of the endothelial layer had been dis-
rupted following dissection or tissue preparation, a collection of
reaction products were found within the ground substance or adhering
to the internal elastic lamina. However, in no case could the enzyme
complex be seen in any of the aortic smooth muscle cells. In the
tissues removed from mice at various times after the intravenous
injection of the enzymes, reaction products were found in kidney,
liver, adrenal, and the choroid plexus. Interestingly, 30 seconds
after injection the enzyme complex was found in the lumen and endothelial vesicles of diaphragm capillaries. By $4\frac{1}{2}$ minutes later the
reaction products had entered the extracellular space close to the
smooth muscle cells. A similar distribution of high molecular weight
material also was found in arteries and arterioles obtained from the
choroid plexus and the lung. Location of these enzymes in the endothelium with no evidence of the appearance of this material on the
smooth muscle cells, even at the time of maximal response, suggested

that the contraction of smooth muscle initiated by angiotensin is mediated by the endothelium. Unfortunately, in these studies the authors were unable to show that dissociation of the angiotensin-enzyme complex was not occurring. Therefore, these studies could have been improved greatly if the enzyme-coupled angiotensin II had been radiolabeled with tritium of high specific activity. Localization of the enzyme by microscopy and of tritium by autoradiography would have greatly enhanced the postulated hypotheses of these authors.

In 1976 Fuxe, Ganten, Hokfelt, and Bolme labelled angiotensin II antibodies with a fluorescent probe, and by immuno-histochemical techniques they demonstrated angiotensin II-like immunoreactive material in the central nervous system. In these studies a high density of angiotensin-containing nerve terminals were located in the substantia gelatinosa and sympathetic lateral columns of the spinal cord, in the medulla oblongata of the brain stem, and in the locus coeruleus of the midbrain. Interestingly, these areas are known to be responsible for the changes in systemic blood pressure which occur when these peptides are introduced into the brain. These data are therefore consistent with the view that angiotensin of neural origin could play a major role in the control of blood pressure independent of changes in plasma angiotensin of renal origin. However, the occurrence of material within the central nervous system which is immunoreactive to angiotensin antibodies is suggestive but is not proof of the existence of the octapeptide. Although these areas of the brain which were shown by Fuxe *et al.* to contain angiotensin II correlate well with the distribution of binding sites for angiotensin II in subcellular particles obtained from different regions of the rat brain, clearly further investigations will have to be performed using more specific angiotensin II antibodies before these interesting observations can be fully appreciated.

This review next will consider some potential mechanisms for the action of angiotensin in a variety of end organs. These responses will be classified as being either biosynthetic or involving stimulus-contraction (or secretion) coupling (see Table 6).

In vascular and nonvascular smooth muscle the contractile response to angiotensin is dependent upon the generation of a calcium current across the plasma membrane, by the passage of this ion into the cell. Correspondingly, angiotensin-stimulated biosynthetic responses, including steroid and prostaglandin synthesis, also are dependent upon extracellular calcium. Indeed, a calcium requirement would also appear to constitute a common mechanism of action of all peptides. Gill, Ill, and Simonian (1977) have demonstrated in cultures of bovine adrenal zona glomerulosa that angiotensin can increase DNA synthesis and enhance protein synthesis, resulting in marked cell proliferation. These responses were inhibited by [Sar[1], Ile[8]] angiotensin II. This intracellular mode of action was not

Table 6. RESPONSES TO ANGIOTENSIN

<u>Biosynthetic</u>

    Steroidogenesis

    Prostaglandin synthesis

    Activation of tyrosine hydroxylase

    Liver enzymes

    Protein synthesis

    DNA synthesis

<u>Stimulus-contraction (secretion) coupling</u>

    Vascular smooth muscle

    Nonvascular smooth muscle

    Myocardium

    Adrenal medulla

    Neurotransmitter release

---

confined to the adrenal, as the octapeptide also increased DNA synthesis in the heart and increased the activity of tyrosine hydroxylase in the sympathetic nervous system and tryptophan hydroxylase
in the central nervous system, particularly in the region of the
raphe nucleus. Recently Garrison, Borland, Florio, and Twible (1979)
have shown that angiotensin acts in the liver to inhibit glycogen
synthetase and to activate phosphorylase, resulting in marked
glycogenolysis and gluconeogenesis. In tissues such as the adrenal
and liver it is clear that cyclic AMP is the second messenger between
the receptor and the observed response for ACTH and glucagon respectively. In the adrenal zona glomerulosa and in the liver, responses
induced by angiotensin II are not correlated with any changes in the
cyclic AMP levels. In other tissues, such as the intestine, where
angiotensin II stimulates salt and water absorption, the mediation
by cyclic AMP has never been implicated. In the kidney, angiotensin
may act via cyclic GMP to increase salt and water reabsorption.

At this point we wish to suggest an experiment combining the
autoradiographic technique of Robertson and Khairallah (1971) with
the reaction product-microscopic technique of Richardson and Beaulnes
(1971). These studies could be extended readily to cultured adrenal
zona glomerulosa cells, using ^{3}H-angiotensin II coupled to a high
molecular weight enzyme. In the adrenal, angiotensin II induces a
rapid steroidogenesis and a slower increase in DNA and protein synthesis. The marriage of these two techniques could have great utility
in determining whether angiotensin produces these effects by combining
with a receptor on the plasma membrane or whether angiotensin II
actually enters the cell to promote nucleic acid and protein synthesis

The ability of peptide hormones to enter cells and induce responses such as DNA and protein synthesis is at the present time highly speculative. However, recently several investigators have provided direct evidence for the entry of polypeptide hormones into cells (see reviews by Kolata, 1978, and by Goldstein, Anderson, and Brown, 1979). Molecules such as insulin, fibroblastic growth factor, and epidermal growth factor have been labelled with fluorescent probes such as rhodamine and fluorescein, and added to cultured adipocytes or fibroblasts under a phase contrast fluorescent microscope. In these experiments very little illuminating light is used to avoid damaging the cells and therefore an image intensification camera attached to the microscope is used to observe the location and behavior of the probed molecules. When first administered to the cells the fluorescent material is widely distributed. However, in a matter of minutes it aggregates and internalizes within the cells. Once across the plasma membrane and inside the cell, the molecules move with a nonrandom, saltatory motion towards specific organelles, such as lysosomes. Based on the observation that many enzymes are activated by the aggregation of individual subunits, it is suggested that the aggregation of receptors on the plasma membrane may produce an active complex. This could either initiate the cellular response *in situ* or pass into the cell to induce increased DNA and protein synthesis. It is speculative at the present time whether these hormone receptor complexes pass the cell membrane to initiate a response or to be degraded; however, the integrity of the probed molecules can be determined readily up until the time of entry into the cell by displacement with the native hormone. A major criticism of this technique is the impossibility of knowing if the hormone and probe are still joined together once inside the cell.

In spite of these criticisms, studies with probed angiotensins could be intriguing, as this molecule is one of the few peptide hormones with extensively characterized specific antagonists. In fact, it could be postulated that the receptor aggregates forming in a contractile or secretory system after exposure to angiotensin actually may represent the formation of a channel for the entry of calcium ions into the cell (see Figure 3). Angiotensin II analogues with COOH terminal aliphatic residues are antagonists of contractile responses. If aggregation of receptors is the key to an acute response, antagonists should disperse or prevent aggregates formed with angiotensin II and may not induce the formation of receptor aggregates when studied alone as the fluorescent probed peptide.

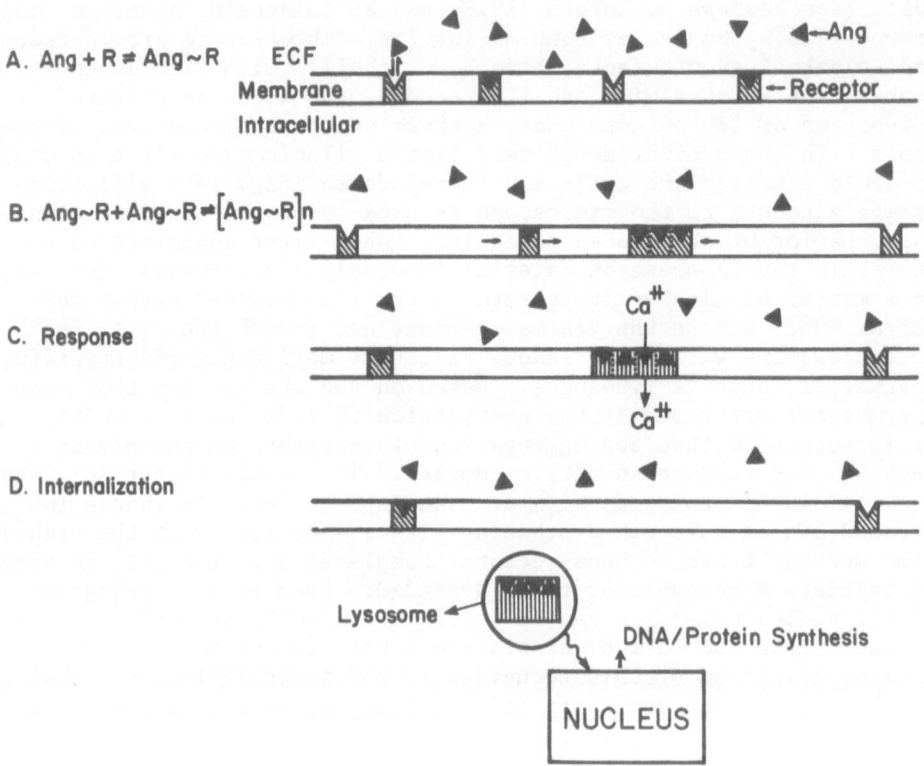

Figure 3. Postulated model for the action of angiotensin II in sensitive tissues.

A. The angiotensin molecule combines with specific receptors on the plasma membrane.

B. and C. These receptors aggregate in a predetermined manner to form channels for the entry of extracellular calcium, which serves to initiate the cellular response.

D. The hormone-receptor aggregates then internalize and become associated with lysosomes. They are then either degraded or pass to the nucleus where they initiate a long-term response involving DNA and protein synthesis.

REFERENCES

Aguilera, G., Hauger, R. L., and Catt, K. J. (1978). Control of aldosterone secretion during sodium restriction: Adrenal receptor regulation and increased adrenal sensitivity to angiotensin II. Proc. Natl. Acad. Sci. 75: 975-979.

Arakawa, K., Smeby, R. R., and Bumpus, F. M. (1962). Synthesis of succinyl-isoleucyl[5]-angiotensin II and N-(poly-o-acetyl-seryl)-isoleucyl[5]-angiotensin II. J. Am. Chem. Soc. 84: 1424-1426.

Beaufils, M., Sraer, J., Lepreux, C., and Ardaillou, R. (1976). Angiotensin II binding to renal glomeruli from sodium-loaded and sodium-depleted rats. Am. J. Physiol. 230: 1187-1193.

Bennett, Jr., J. P. and Snyder, S. H. (1976). Angiotensin II binding to mammalian brain membranes. J. Biol. Chem. 251: 7423-7430.

Bravo, E. L., Khosla, M. C., and Bumpus, F. M. (1976). The role of angiotensins in aldosterone production. Circ. Res. 38 (suppl. 2): 104-107.

Bumpus, F. M., Levens, N. R., Munday, K. A., and Poat, J. A. (1976). Structural activity requirements for the action of angiotensin II on fluid transport by rat jejunum. J. Physiol. (Lond.) 257: 32P.

Bumpus, F. M., Schwartz, H., and Page, I. H. (1957). Synthesis and pharmacology of the octapeptide angiotensin. Science 125: 3253.

Devynck, M. A. and Meyer, P. (1976). Angiotensin receptors in vascular tissue. Am. J. Med. 61: 758-767.

Devynck, M. A. and Meyer, P. (1978). Angiotensin receptors. Biochem. Pharmacol. 27: 1-5.

Devynck, M. A., Rouzaire-Dubois, B., Chevillotte, E., and Meyer, P. (1976). Variations in the number of uterine angiotensin receptors following changes in plasma angiotensin levels. Eur. J. Pharmacol. 40: 27-37.

Douglas, J., Bartley, P., Kondo, T., and Catt, K. (1978). Formation of des-Asp[1]-angiotensin II is not an obligatory step in the steroidogenic action of angiotensin II in the canine adrenal. Endocrinology 102: 1921-1924.

Douglas, J., Saltman, S., Fredlund, P., Kondo, T., and Catt, K. J. (1976). Receptor binding of angiotensin II and antagonists. Correlation with aldosterone production by isolated canine adrenal granulosa cells. Circ. Res. 38 (suppl. 2): 108-112.

Fitzsimons, J. T. (1975). Renin, angiotensin, and drinking. In: Control Mechanisms of Drinking. (Peters, G., Fitzsimons, J. T., and Peters-Haefeli, L., eds.), pp. 97-102, Springer-Verlag, Berlin, Heidelberg.

Freedlender, A. E. and Goodfriend, T. L. (1977). Angiotensin receptors and sodium transport in renal tubules. Fed. Proc. 36: 481.

Fuxe, K., Ganten, D., Hökfelt, T., and Bolme, P. (1976). Immunohistochemical evidence for the existence of angiotensin II-containing nerve terminals in the brain and spinal cord in the rat. Neurosci. Letters 2: 229-234.

Gagnon, D. J., Cousineau, D., and Boucher, P. J. (1973). Release of vasopressin by angiotensin II and prostaglandin E_2 from the rat neurohypophysis *in vitro*. Life Sci. 12: 487-492.

Garrison, J. C., Borland, M. K., Florio, V. A., and Twible, D. A. (1979). The role of calcium ion as a mediator of the effects of angiotensin II, catecholamines, and vasopressin on the phosphorylation and activity of enzymes in isolated hepatocytes. J. Biol. Chem. (in press).

Gill, G. N., Ill, C. R., and Simonian, M. H. (1977). Angiotensin stimulation of bovine adrenocortical cell growth. Proc. Natl. Acad. Sci. 74: 5569-5573.

Glossman, H., Baukal, A. J., and Catt, K. J. (1974). Properties of angiotensin II receptors in the bovine and rat adrenal cortex. J. Biol. Chem. 249: 825-834.

Goldstein, J. L., Anderson, R. G. W., and Brown, M. S. (1979). Coated pits, coated vesicles, and receptor-mediated endocytosis. Nature 279: 679-684.

Goodfriend, T. L., Fyhrquist, F., Gutmann, F., Knych, E., Hollemans, H., Allmann, D., Kent, K., and Cooper, T. (1972). Clinical and conceptual uses of angiotensin receptors. In: *Hypertension '72.* (Genest, J. and Koiw, E., eds.), pp. 549-563, Springer-Verlag, Berlin.

Gurchinoff, S., Khairallah, P. A., Devynck, M. A., and Meyer, P. (1976). Angiotensin II binding to zona glomerulosa cells from rabbit adrenal glands. Biochem. Pharmacol. 25: 1031-1034.

Kalsner, S. and Nickerson, M. (1968). A method for the study of mechanisms of drug disposition in smooth muscle. Can. J. Physiol. Pharmacol. 46: 719-730.

Khairallah, P. A., Robertson, A. L., and Davila, D. (1972). Effects of angiotensin II on DNA, RNA, and protein synthesis. In: *Hypertension '72.* (Genest, J. and Koiw, E., eds.), pp. 218-220, Springer-Verlag, Berlin.

Khosla, M. C., Smeby, R. R., and Bumpus, F. M. (1974). Structure-activity relationship in angiotensin II analogs. In: *Handbook of Experimental Pharmacology XXXVII. Angiotensin.* (Page, I. H. and Bumpus, F. M., eds.), pp. 126-161, Springer-Verlag, Berlin.

Kolata, G. B. (1978). Polypeptide hormones: What are they doing in cells? Science 201: 895-897.

LeMorvan, P. and Palaic, D. (1975). Characterization of the angiotensin receptor in guinea pig aorta. J. Pharmacol. Exp. Ther. 195: 167-175.

Peach, M. J. (1972). Physiological roles of angiotensin. In: *Chemistry and Biology of Peptides.* (Meinhofer, J., ed.), pp. 471-493, Ann Arbor Science Publishers, Inc., Ann Arbor, Mich.

Peach, M. J., Bumpus, F. M., and Khairallah, P. A. (1969). Inhibition of norepinephrine uptake in hearts by angiotensin II and analogs. J. Pharmacol. Exp. Ther. 167: 291-299.

Peach, M. J. and Ober, M. (1974). Inhibition of angiotensin-induced catecholamine release by 8-substituted analogs of angiotensin II. J. Pharmacol. Exp. Ther. 190: 49-58.

Pernollet, M-G., Devynck, M. A., Matthews, P. G. and Meyer, P. (1977). Post-nephrectomy changes in adrenal angiotensin II receptors in the rat; influence of exogenous angiotensin and a competitive inhibitor. Eur. J. Pharmacol. 43: 361-372.

Richardson, J. B. and Beaulnes, A. (1971). The cellular site of action of angiotensin. J. Cell Biol. 51: 419-432.

Robertson, A. L. and Khairallah, P. A. (1971). Angiotensin II: Rapid localization in nuclei of smooth and cardiac muscle. Science 172: 1138-1139.

Sirett, N. E., Mclean, A. S., Bray, J. J., and Hubbard, J. I. (1977). Distribution of angiotensin II receptors in rat brain. Brain Res. 122: 299-312.

Srauer, J., Baud, L., Cosyns, J-P., Verroust, P., Nivez, M-P., and Ardaillou, R. (1977). High affinity binding of ^{125}I-angiotensin II to rat glomerular membranes. J. Clin. Invest. 59: 69-81.

Wideman, C. H., Khosla, M. C., and Smeby, R. R. (1972). Effects of analogs of angiotensin II on isolated frog skin. Fed. Proc. 31: 228.

DISCUSSION AFTER DR. PEACH'S PAPER

Dr. Davis

I have just one specific question. You mentioned the isoleucine angiotensin III blocker. I would like to know what is your opinion about the evidence that it is specific for angiotensin III.

Dr. Peach

It is not specific, but is perhaps selective, under the right experimental conditions. And by selective, you really don't have the break in dose that is enjoyed with the beta-1, beta-2 adrenergic receptor game where you can use a cardio-selective antagonist, like metoprolol which has just come on the market. With the Ile[7]-angiotensin III you really don't have a very large dosage range to play with. The other curious thing we have run into with the so-called hepta-blocker, [Ile[7]] angiotensin III, is its effectiveness against exogenous vs endogenous angiotensin. Historically, exogenous systems put angiotensin or norepinephrine into a system from the outside. Antagonists enter the system in the same way, from the outside. So things will work against exogenous systems that won't work against endogenous systems. Endogenous systems are notoriously more difficult to block with alpha blockers or angiotensin blockers, or whatever type of blocker you use. In fact, electrophysiologists who work in the brain are not deterred at all if they can't block a synapse. They know what the transmitter is when they electrically stimulate neurons, but that synapse is so well protected they have no idea what the real barriers are to getting a blocker into that

synapse, so they don't even flinch if they don't have that type of
confirmation of the transmitter of the synapse. The wild thing we
ran into with [Ile^7] angiotensin III was that it had absolutely no
selectivity in our hands except perhaps in adrenal cells that had
been handled and washed and pelleted and all sorts of things repeatedly; that was the only time we have seen selectivity against exogenous angiotensin. The times we've been most impressed with its
selectivity have been under circumstances where we have activated
the endogenous system. That's wrong as far as everything I was
taught. Endogenous systems are rough to get to, but that is the
time we have been most impressed with the selectivity of [Ile^7]
angiotensin III...when we've activated the angiotensin system with
low salt diets or when we've produced Goldblatt hypertension that
was angiotensin dependent. It impresses me every time I look at
the data, but I am convinced that it is real. So I say that under
the right conditions it is selective at best, and I think you really
will have to work hard to find it if you're in the wrong tissue at
the wrong time. We can reproduce what we've published, but it is
selective.

Dr. Nishimura
      If you treat the tissue with angiotensin II antagonists which
bind to receptors, does this inhibit radioactive angiotensin from
entering the cell or binding to the nucleus?

Dr. Peach
      That study has been done partially with the techniques I showed
you, by the people I showed you. You can compete with those materials entering the eclls. For example, if you take horseradish
peroxidase-angiotensin you can prevent it from going wherever it is
going by adding it in the presence of angiotensin. You can do the
same thing with [poly-o-acetyl-seryl] angiotensin. That just tells
you that the material is going to a receptor site for angiotensin II.
The only person who has looked carefully at the blockers, and that
was very early, was Khairallah. They could prevent perinuclear
graining by autoradiographic techniques by using 8-substituted
analogues of angiotensin. Angiotensin III also was very effective.
There were a couple of other analogues that were good but which
didn't make any sense. If you accept classic structure-activity
relationship studies, some analogues worked that shouldn't have
worked. I more or less disregard all historic structure-activity
studies until I do them myself. Our biggest problem right now is
the purity of the angiotensin II preparations. I suppose I might
as well open that can of worms. Most angiotensin II preparations
that we obtained have been contaminated with one of two things:
either [β-Aspartyl] angiotensin II or angiotensin III. If what
you want to do is look for a mechanism of action, you are up the
creek. You are studying the very peptides that perhaps you want
to study separately, but they are combined in the same little
bottle that comes from Joe Schmuck Pharmaceuticals or somewhere!

It's tough! It's difficult to separate angiotensin III from angiotensin II. It's even more difficult to separate the [β-Aspartyl]
angiotensin. The only way you can pick up [β-Aspartyl] angiotensins
is to incubate them exhaustively with leucine aminopeptidase, which
will not hydrolyze that bond, or to have access to high pressure
liquid chromatography, which will separate the [β-Aspartyl] from the
[α-Aspartly] angiotensins. We have angiotensin II preparations in
our laboratory that have no dependency on extracellular calcium to
contract the rabbit aorta, just as angiotensin III does not. We
have preparations that have some dependency and we have preparations
that are completely dependent upon extracellular calcium. They all
say "angiotensin II" on the label and when you assay them by ninhydrin or fluorescamine assay or by tyrosine , mole to mole comparison with the peptide, they all come out at the same level of tyrosine. Angiotensin III has tyrosine, [β-Aspartyl] angiotensin II has
tyrosine, angiotensin II has tyrosine. They all say mole to mole
the same purity and that they are the only peptides in there.
Uh-huh. But there's angiotensin II, angiotensin III, and [β-Aspartyl]
angiotensin II. And if you go to the literature you will see the
same thing: Angiotensin II doesn't always require calcium; angiotensin II always requires calcium. They don't know what angiotensin II they were working with.

Dr. Nishimura
     When angiotensin enters the cells, is it still angiotensin?
Is it possible to extract the angiotensin from a tissue and check
the biological activity?

Dr. Peach
     Yes, this has been done by three or four people now. The prob-
lem in most studies people have done of that nature has been proving
that what they extracted was not angiotensin on the surface of the
cells. You don't know from whence you extracted it. There is some
angiotensin on the surface and there may be some inside the cells.
I think what could probably be done, and done rather easily, is to
expose the tissue to angiotensin under conditions where if it is
going to internalize, it will; then you compete off the surface
material by using antagonists like Saralasin or [Sar[1], Ile[8]] angiotensin II. You should compete it off even aggregated receptors on
the surface. Once you have that scrubby-dubbed off, then homogenize
the tissue under stabilizing conditions for peptides. What you have
to do is to get all of the surface material off, and then you can
identify the label which has internalized and then you can make a
positive identification of angiotensin II.

Dr. Moore
     Mike, one fascinating thing you mentioned was about the aggre-
gation of receptors. The thing that struck me straightaway was
tachyphylaxis. Are you working along those lines?

Dr. Peach

Oh, absolutely! I can go one step more than that. I don't
know how many of you know it, but angiotensin II causes tachyphylaxis
to angiotensin III, but angiotensin III doesn't cause tachyphylaxis
to angiotensin II. That is a mind boggler. If those peptides are
working on the same receptor, then why shouldn't they have complete,
full cross-tachyphylaxis? Well, all you've got to do is play with
the aggregated states and say that angiotensin II causes a tetramer
and angiotensin III causes a trimer, and the angiotensin III can't
interact with the tetramer. You can just dream until the cows come
home, but you need to come up with a testable model. No idea is any
good unless you can put it in the laboratory and test it...unless
you can come up with proof! Our problem with receptors is that we
keep coming down on the fence. We can say the data are consistent
with whichever model we want to believe, and so I haven't gone anywhere. So I can come up with an hypothesis based upon aggregation,
which I am convinced occurs, and I can test that hypothesis, and I
can go forward. That is what I want to do.

Dr. Bauer

I want to thank Dr. Peach for that most enthusiastic discussion.

DEVELOPMENT OF ANGIOTENSIN II RECEPTORS

Alan Moore[1]

Department of Pharmacology
Institute for Cardiovascular Studies
University of Houston
Houston, TX 77004

Many investigators have described the positive inotropic action of angiotensin II on isolated heart preparations (for a review, see Peach, 1977). During a brief sabbatical spent with Drs. Peach and Ackerely at the University of Virginia, the development of angiotensin II receptors in the heart was studied. We chose the embryonic chicken heart because this provided easily available material of a known embryonic age, and also because Dr. Peach and his colleagues previously had demonstrated the similarity of the mechanism of action of angiotensin II on isolated heart preparations of chickens and mammals (Freer, Pappano, Peach, *et al.*, 1976).

Initially, isolated perfused hearts were used that were taken from embryos 19 days and older, and these showed clear inotropic responses to angiotensin II at a threshold value of 10^{-10} to 10^{-9} M (Fig. 1a), which was in agreement with previously reported values (Freer, Pappano, Peach, *et al.*, 1976). The threshold value for angiotensin I in these preparations was 10^{-6} M. When younger hearts were used, from 10 to 15 day old embryos, it was apparent that the sensitivities to angiotensin I and angiotensin II were similar; 10^{-6} M was the approximate threshold value for both compounds (Fig. 1b and 1c).

It appears that in the period between 15 to 18 days the chicken embryo heart becomes selectively 1000-fold more sensitive to the inotropic action of angiotensin II. The two most likely explanations for this are: 1) Angiotensin II receptor differentiation, or 2) development of post-receptor mechanisms. It is known that

---

[1]Present address: Norwich-Eaton Pharmaceuticals, P. O. Box 191, Norwich, NY 13815

(a)   19 DAY OLD CHICKEN EMBRYO HEART INOTROPIC RESPONSES TO AII

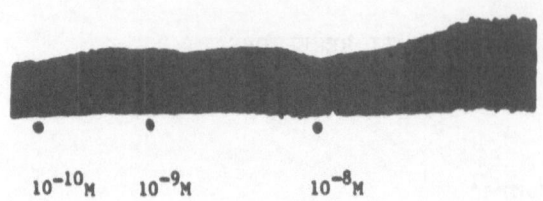

10^{-10}M 10^{-9}M 10^{-8}M

(b)   15 DAY OLD CHICKEN EMBRYO HEART INOTROPIC RESPONSES TO AI

1.5 x 10^{-7}M 10^{-6}M

(c)   15 DAY OLD CHICKEN EMBRYO HEART INOTROPIC RESPONSES TO AII

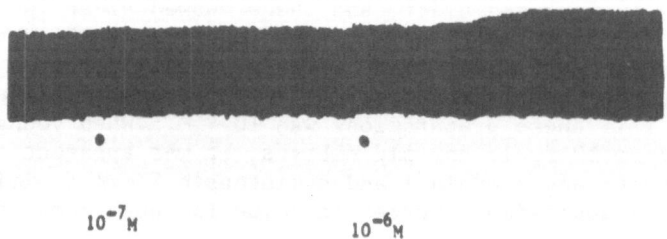

10^{-7}M 10^{-6}M

*Figure 1.   Inotropic response of isolated perfused chicken heart
            paced at 2 beats/sec.   (a) Response of 19-day old
            chicken embryo heart to AII at 10^{-10}, 10^{-9} and 10^{-8} M.
            (b) Response of 15-day old chicken embryo heart to AI,
            with a threshold of approximately 10^{-6} M.   (c) Response
            of 15-day old chicken embryo heart to AII, with a thres-
            hold of approximately 10^{-6} M.*

Table 1.   *125I-ANGIOTENSIN II BINDING TO 19 DAY OLD CHICKEN EMBRYO HEART (COLLAGENASE DISPERSED)*

High affinity group: K_D = 6.8 x 10^{-9} M
No. of sites = 4.2 x 10^{-10} Moles/gm. protein

Low affinity group: K_D = 8.0 x 10^{-7} M
No. of sites = > 10^{-8} Moles/gm. protein

---

angiotensin II and β-adrenoreceptor stimulants appear to act by a final common pathway in this preparation: i.e., by opening of "slow" calcium channels in the membrane (Freer, Pappano, Peach, *et al.*, 1976)   and we found that in the younger hearts that were less sensitive to angiotensin II, there was a clear response to isoprenaline. This suggested that the receptor itself was involved rather than a post-receptor mechanism, although it did not exclude the role of a mechanism coupling receptor occupancy to calcium channels. To study this further, binding studies were performed. Nineteen day old chicken embryo hearts were minced, collagenase dispersed, and were studied by standard ligand-displacement with ^{125}I-angiotensin II. Two populations of angiotensin II receptors were observed: (1) a high affinity group, with a dissociation constant corresponding to the ED_{50} (dose required to produce a 50% of maximum response) of angiotensin II in the older hearts, and (2) a low affinity group with a dissociation constant corresponding approximately to the ED_{50} of angiotensin II in the younger hearts (Table 1).

It appears that the difference in sensitivity to angiotensin II between the younger and older chicken embryo hearts reflects a difference in receptor affinity, and studies are now being conducted to relate endogenous angiotensin II levels to receptor differentiation in this preparation.

REFERENCES

Freer, R. J., Pappano, A. J., Peach, M. J., Bing, K. T., McLean, M. J., Vogel, S., and Speralakis, N. (1976). Mechanism for the positive inotropic effect of angiotensin II on isolated cardiac muscle. Circ. Res. 39: 178-183.
Peach, M. J. (1977). Renin-angiotensin system: Biochemistry and mechanism of action. Physiol. Rev. 57: 313-370.

DISCUSSION AFTER DR. MOORE'S PAPER

Dr. Nishimura
    I didn't catch exactly what angiotensins you used. Were these
fowl angiotensins I and II?

Dr. Moore
    No, these were the standard mammalian angiotensins I and II.

Dr. Nishimura
    I think it might be interesting to use the fowl angiotensin;
that is [Asp^1, Val^5] angiotensin II. Also, although I don't know
about angiotensin, neurohypophyseal hormones change during the
fetal period, almost as if they repeat the phylogenetic history,
changing from vasotocin to vasopressin. So differences of the
receptor properties might reflect the differences of the hormones.

Dr. Moore
    Exactly. That is a very good point. I think what we have to
do now is to go back and look at hormone levels, because we haven't
compared the levels of angiotensin. As we know, the angiotensin
receptors are modulated by the levels of the hormones in the blood,
and we have to go back and do that. Actually, these experiments
are what led to the chicken experiment I talked about yesterday,
because after working with Mike Peach on this, when I went back to
Cleveland I thought I would switch to vascular smooth muscle because
these heart preparations are very difficult to set up. I tried the
chicken aorta and found that it didn't respond to angiotensin. So
then the question became: Why doesn't the chicken aorta respond to
angiotensin?

INHIBITORS OF ANGIOTENSIN-CONVERTING ENZYME

D. W. Cushman, M. A. Ondetti, H. S. Cheung,
M. J. Antonaccio, V. S. Murthy, and B. Rubin

The Squibb Institute for Medical Research
Princeton, NJ   08540

OUTLINE

I.   Introduction

II. Development of potent specific inhibitors
     A. Snake venom peptides
     B. Active-site directed inhibitors

III. Specificity of action
     A. *In vitro* studies
     B. *In vivo* studies

IV. Antihypertensive activity
     A. Normotensive animals
     B. Renal hypertensive animals
     C. Genetic hypertensive rats
     D. DOCA-salt hypertensive rats
     E. Human hypertensives

V.   Mechanism and specificity of antihypertensive action

I.   INTRODUCTION

     Angiotensin-converting enzyme is the historically appropriate
trivial name for a widely distributed peptidyldipeptide hydrolase
(EC 3.4.15.1) that cleaves dipeptide residues from the carboxyl-
terminal end of polypeptides (Erdös, 1976a). Two reactions of this
enzyme (Figure 1) are of potential importance for regulation of
blood pressure under normophysiological or pathophysiological
conditions: removal of the terminal histidylleucine dipeptide from

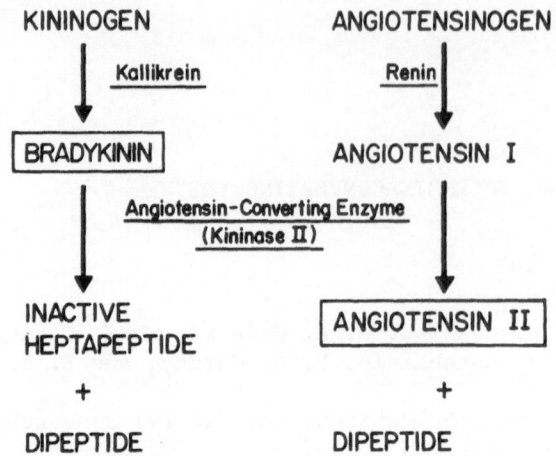

*Figure 1. Physiologically and pathologically important reactions
of angiotensin-converting enzyme. The inactive decapeptide angiotensin I is hydrolyzed to yield the vasopressor
antinatriuretic octapeptide angiotensin II; the vasodepressor natriuretic nonapeptide bradykinin is inactivated by hydrolytic removal of its carboxyl-terminal
dipeptide residue.*

the inactive decapeptide angiotensin I to form the potent vasopressor octapeptide angiotensin II (Skeggs, Kahn, and Shumway, 1956),
and inactivation of the vasodepressor nonapeptide bradykinin by
hydrolytic removal of its carboxyl-terminal phenylalaninylarginine
dipeptide (Igic, Erdös, Yeh, *et al.*, 1972). Angiotensin II is
formed in various vascular beds, the most important being lung and
kidney (Vane, 1972); it may act locally as a vasoconstrictor and
also may escape into the general circulation. In addition to its
direct vasoconstrictor action, angiotensin II causes sodium retention and plasma volume expansion that may be due in part to a direct
intrarenal action of the peptide, but certainly over a long period
of time is due to its stimulation of aldosterone secretion by the
adrenal cortex (Peach, 1977). Bradykinin is efficiently inactivated
in most tissues (Erdös, 1976b), allowing its vasodilatory or renal
natriuretic actions to be exerted only at the site of production.
Inhibitors of angiotensin-converting enzyme (a.k.a. kininase II) are
capable of producing a lowered blood pressure, natriuresis, and
diuresis either by inhibiting angiotensin II production or by pre-
venting the destruction of locally formed bradykinin, and perhaps
by allowing escape of the latter into the arterial circulation.
The relative contribution of these two fundamental actions of con-

verting enzyme inhibitors to their antihypertensive actions is difficult to assess at the present time.

II. DEVELOPMENT OF POTENT SPECIFIC INHIBITORS

A. Snake Venom Peptides

The first inhibitors of angiotensin-converting enzyme with sufficient potency and specificity of action for study as potential antihypertensive drugs were a series of nontoxic peptides found in the venom of the Brazilian arrowhead viper, *Bothrops jararaca*. A mixture of these peptides possessing bradykinin-potentiating activity was first described by Ferreira (1965), who referred to the crude mixture as bradykinin-potentiating factor (BPF). A great stimulus for the fractionation of BPF into its individual peptide components came in 1968 with the observation that this mixture was also a potent inhibitor of angiotensin-converting enzyme (Bakhle, 1968). It was not obvious at this time that the two activities were due to the same components of the venom. Ferreira, Bartelt, and Greene (1970) isolated nine bradykinin-potentiating peptides from the venom and determined the amino acid sequence of one, a pentapeptide that they later named bradykinin-potentiating peptide 5a (BPP$_{5a}$; see Figure 2). Synthetic BPP$_{5a}$ and the other pure or nearly-pure peptide fractions isolated by Ferreira *et al.* were all found to inhibit angiotensin-converting enzyme (Stewart, Ferreira, and Greene, 1971). Ondetti, Williams, Sabo, *et al.* (1971) purified six similar peptides from *B. jararaca* venom using their activity as inhibitors of angiotensin-converting enzyme (Cushman and Cheung, 1971; Cheung and Cushman, 1973) as a guide. They determined the sequences of all six of these venom peptides, which were of similar structure but ranged in size from nonapeptide to tridecapeptide; five of the six probably were identical to peptides isolated by Ferreira's group. The most thoroughly studied of these longer venom peptides is the nonapeptide SQ 20,881, which is used clinically under the generic name teprotide (Figure 2). Like BPP$_{5a}$, teprotide and the other longer peptides from the venom of *B. jararaca* all augment biological activities of bradykinin (Engel, Schaeffer, Gold, and Rubin, 1972). Similar but less thoroughly studied inhibitors of angiotensin-converting enzyme have been isolated from the venom of the Asian pit viper *Agkistrodon halys blomhoffii* (Kato and Suzuki, 1971).

The pentapeptide BPP$_{5a}$ is a potent inhibitor of angiotensin-converting enzyme *in vitro*, but is itself rapidly hydrolyzed by the converting enzyme under some assay conditions (Cheung and Cushman, 1973) and probably by other peptidases as well. It has a short duration of inhibitory activity *in vivo* (Krieger, Salgado, Assan, *et al.*, 1971; Engel, Schaeffer, Waugh, and Rubin, 1973).

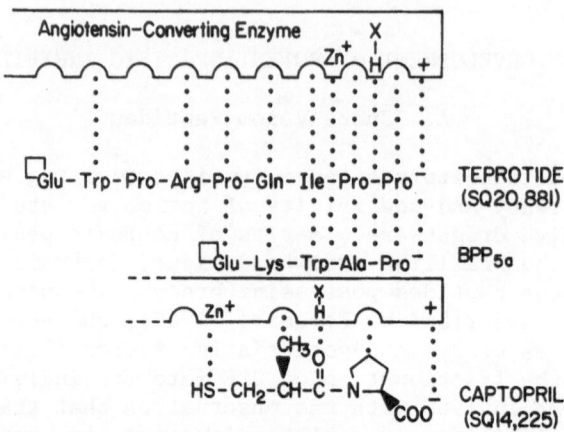

Figure 2.   *Potent competitive inhibitors of angiotensin-converting
             enzyme and their postulated interactions with the active
             site of the enzyme. The snake venom peptides teprotide
             (SQ 20,881) and BPP$_{5q}$ bind to the enzyme like typical
             peptide substrates via their three carboxyl-terminal
             amino acid residues, but they also interact strongly
             with other subsites (circular indentations) on the
             enzyme that are more removed from the catalytic center
             (zinc ion). Captopril (SQ 14,225) interacts with the
             enzyme in much the same way as the terminal dipeptide
             residue of a peptide substrate or competitive inhibitor,
             but it has a much stronger interaction, via its sulfhydryl
             group, with the zinc ion of the enzyme, and its structure
             has been optimized for maximal interaction with the enzyme
             of each of the groups shown.*

Teprotide, as discussed below, has a much longer duration of action
in vivo, and is the only one of the venom peptides to be studied
extensively as an antihypertensive agent. Clinical trials have
suggested that teprotide is a safe and effective antihypertensive
drug in most renovascular hypertensive patients and in a high
percentage of patients with essential hypertension (Gavras, Brunner,
Laragh, and Vukovich, 1974; Johnson, Black, Vukovich, *et al.*, 1975;
Case, Wallace, Keim, *et al.*, 1977); the only major limitation for
its use is its lack of oral activity.

B. Active-Site Directed Inhibitors

Recently, a new class of specific inhibitors of angiotensin-converting enzyme has been developed, the most potent of which is captopril, or SQ 14,225 (Figure 2). This nonpeptide inhibitor is unique in several respects. It is an extremely tight-binding competitive inhibitor of angiotensin-converting enzyme, but has a much simpler structure than the peptide inhibitor, teprotide. It has evolved from a rational program of chemical design that utilized a hypothetical model of the active site of angiotensin-converting enzyme as the basis for synthesis of a series of compounds with increasingly greater affinities for the enzyme (Ondetti, Rubin, and Cushman, 1977; Ondetti, Sabo, Losee, *et al.*, 1977; Cushman, Cheung, Sabo, and Ondetti, 1977). The hypothetical active site, in turn, is based on the assumption that substrate binding and peptide bond cleavage by angiotensin-converting enzyme occur in much the same way as with the well-characterized enzyme, carboxypeptidase A of bovine pancreas, the only major difference being the position of the peptide bond that is cleaved.

Captopril is visualized as binding to the active site of angiotensin-converting enzyme in a manner that is quite similar to the binding of the two most terminal amino acid residues of a typical substrate of this enzyme, such as angiotensin I (Figure 2). The terminal negatively-charged carboxyl group interacts ionically with a positively-charged residue of the enzyme; the amide carbonyl forms a hydrogen bond with a donor group on the enzyme; and the proline ring and methyl side-chains interact with the enzyme in the same, but unspecified, manner as do the side-chains of the last two amino acid residues of a peptide substrate. In addition, however, captopril has a sulfhydryl group that can interact strongly with the zinc ion at the active site of the enzyme, an interaction that contributes greatly to the tight binding of this inhibitor with the enzyme. The nonapeptide teprotide (Figure 2) lacks such a strong interaction with the zinc ion of the enzyme; it owes its potency to several additional interactions of amino acid residues with sites on the enzyme that are beyond the catalytic center (Cushman, Pluscec, Williams, *et al.*, 1973; Cheung and Cushman, 1973).

The most important property of captopril, however, is not directly related to the logical basis of its design. Unlike teprotide, captopril is orally active as an inhibitor of the converting enzyme, a property that is of the utmost importance for the development of this compound as a drug for the treatment of chronic hypertension.

III. SPECIFICITY OF ACTION

A. *In Vitro* Studies

Teprotide (SQ 20,881) and captopril (SQ 14,225) both are potent competitive inhibitors of purified angiotensin–converting enzyme of rabbit lung, with K_i values (enzyme–inhibitor dissociation constants) of 1.0×10^{-7} M and 1.7×10^{-9} M, respectively (Table 1). Both are remarkably specific for inhibition of this peptidyldipeptide hydrolase, inasmuch as this can be determined by testing these compounds for inhibition of five other common peptidases (Table 1). Teprotide was 600 to 3000 times more potent as an inhibitor of the converting enzyme than as an inhibitor of carboxypeptidases A and B, leucine aminopeptidase, trypsin, and chymotrypsin. The potency (I_{50} value) of captopril as a converting enzyme inhibitor was 40,000 to 70,000 times greater than its potency as an inhibitor of the two carboxypeptidases or the two endopeptidases, but only 230 times greater than its inhibitory activity *vs*. leucine aminopeptidase. Carboxypeptidases A and B, and leucine aminopeptidase are all zinc–containing enzymes; the carboxypeptidases, as described above, have mechanisms of action thought to be similar to that of angiotensin–converting enzyme.

Inhibition of angiotensin–converting enzyme (kininase II) in isolated strips of guinea pig ileum or other smooth muscles has two consequences: contraction of the muscle by angiotensin I is inhibited, and contraction by bradykinin is augmented and prolonged in duration (Rubin, Laffan, Kotler, *et al.*, 1978). Specific inhibitors should be completely free of other activities such as effects on resting muscle tone or on agonistic activities of other myotropic agents. Both teprotide and captopril at low concentrations inhibit the contractile action of angiotensin I and augment the contractile action of bradykinin. Neither drug at 10,000 to 100,000 times higher concentrations has any effect on smooth muscle tone or on contractions induced by a wide variety of agonists, including angiotensin II, acetylcholine, histamine, prostaglandins, or alpha and beta adrenergic receptor agonists (Table 1). Augmentation of bradykinin action is the most sensitive test for inhibitors of angiotensin-converting enzyme; it is also a quite specific test, since nonspecific agents most often inhibit the actions of bradykinin along with those of other agonists. However, since 50% augmentation of the effect of bradykinin is only a small fraction of the maximum augmentation obtainable, the AC_{50} normally used to report bradykinin augmentation is not directly comparable with the IC_{50} used to describe angiotensin I inhibition. The AC_{50} for bradykinin is always a lower and more variable value than the IC_{50} for angiotensin I.

Table 1.   SPECIFICITY OF SQ 20,881 AND SQ 14,225 AS INHIBITORS OF
           ANGIOTENSIN-CONVERTING ENZYME

Action	SQ 20,881	SQ 14,225
Inhibition of Rabbit Lung Angiotensin-Converting Enzyme		
I_{50} (μM)*	0.56	0.023
K_i (μM)	0.10	0.0017
Type of Inhibition	competitive	competitive
Inhibition of Other Peptidases		
I_{50} (μM)		
Carboxypeptidase A	1800	1500
Carboxypeptidase B	520	800
Leucine Aminopeptidase	>100	5.4
Trypsin	1000	>1000
Chymotrypsin	380	>1000
Effect on Smooth Muscle Agonists		
AC_{50} (μM)[†]		
Bradykinin	0.0015	0.0032
IC_{50} (μM)[†]		
Angiotensin I	0.060	0.023
Angiotensin II	>30	>500
Acetylcholine	>30	>500
Histamine	>30	>500
Prostaglandin E_2	>30	>500
Norepinephrine	>30	>500
Isoproterenol	>30	>500

*pH 8.3, 0.3 M NaCl, 5 mM hippuryl-L-histidyl-L-leucine.

[†]Values represent 50% inhibition or augmentation of the smooth muscle response at a single agonist concentration; guinea pig ileum was used with all agonists except norepinephrine (rabbit aorta) and isoproterenol (rat portal vein).

B.   *In Vivo* Studies

Most of the inhibitory and many of the antihypertensive actions
described below for captopril have also been demonstrated with teprotide administered by intravenous, intramuscular, or subcutaneous
routes (Engel, Schaeffer, Gold, and Rubin, 1972; Engel, Schaeffer,
Waugh, and Rubin, 1973). Indeed, as described above, the antihypertensive potential of inhibitors of angiotensin-converting enzyme
was first demonstrated in clinical studies with the parenterally
active drug. Studies with captopril, however, are both more extensive and of greater interest, since this orally active compound is
now undergoing clinical trial as an antihypertensive drug for long-
term treatment of all forms of hypertension.

As shown in Figures 3 and 4, captopril produces a dose-dependent
inhibition of the vasopressor action of angiotensin I and an increase
in the magnitude and duration of the vasodepressor action of bradykinin in unanesthetized rats; maximal inhibition required oral doses
of 1 mg/kg or higher, and the inhibition persisted for 3 hours or
more (Rubin, Laffan, Kotler, *et al.*, 1978). Captopril at these
doses had no effect on the vasopressor actions of angiotensin II or
norepinephrine, or the vasodepressor activity of acetylcholine. A
similar spectrum of activities *in vivo* has been obtained in cats,
dogs, rabbits, and humans (Vollmer and Boccagno, 1977; Murthy,
Waldron, Goldberg, and Vollmer, 1977; Murthy, Waldron, and Goldberg,
1978a and 1978b; Ferguson, Turini, Brunner, *et al.*, 1977). In conscious rabbits (Murthy, Waldron, Goldberg, and Vollmer, 1977) the
drug had no effect on the vasodepressor actions of isoproterenol or
prostaglandin E_2; a slight increase in the pressor activity of angiotensin II was probably due to decreased concentration of endogenous
angiotensin II and a resulting decreased occupancy of the angiotensin
receptors. In rabbits, the increased duration of vasodepressor
action of bradykinin produced by captopril was shown to be due not
primarily to increased circulating levels of bradykinin, but to a
greater degree to an augmentation of the intrarenal action of bradykinin as an activator of phospholipase, and the consequent increase
in circulating levels of arachidonic acid and other precursors of
vasodilatory prostaglandins or prostacyclin (Murthy, Waldron, and
Goldberg, 1978b).

Captopril perfused through the cerebral ventricles of anesthetized cats inhibited the blood pressure and heart rate increases
produced by centrally injected angiotensin I (Vollmer and Boccagno,
1977); the related central action of angiotensin II was unaffected.
An intravenous dose of 3.1 mg/kg, ten times higher than that required
for inhibition of the peripheral angiotensin-converting enzyme activity, did not affect activities of centrally-injected angiotensin I.
Autoradiographic experiments with ^{35}S-labeled captopril also failed
to show any accumulation of this drug within the brain (Heald and
Ita, 1977). The specific central inhibition of angiotensin-

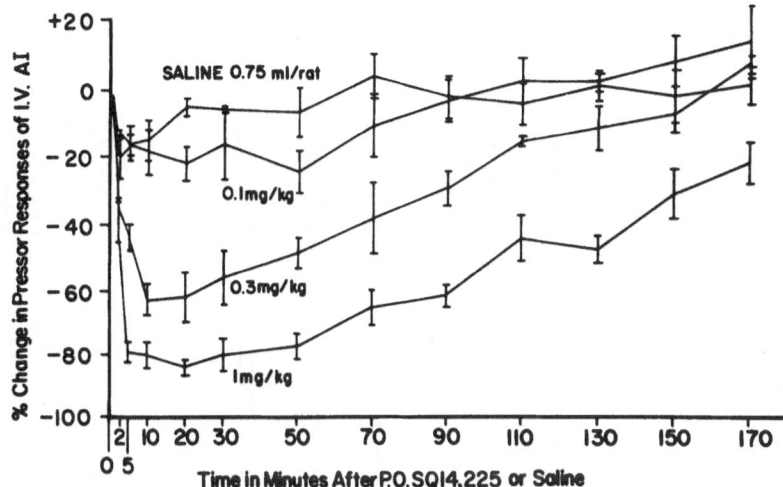

Figure 3. *Inhibition of the vasopressor action of angiotensin I in unanesthetized rats by orally administered captopril (SQ 14,225). Four rats per dose were injected with 310 ng/kg of angiotensin I at the indicated times following oral dosing with captopril; results are expressed as percent change in the pressor response ± standard error. (Reproduced with permission from the Journal of Pharmacology and Experimental Therapeutics (1978), 204:275. Copyright by the Williams and Wilkins Co., Baltimore, MD).*

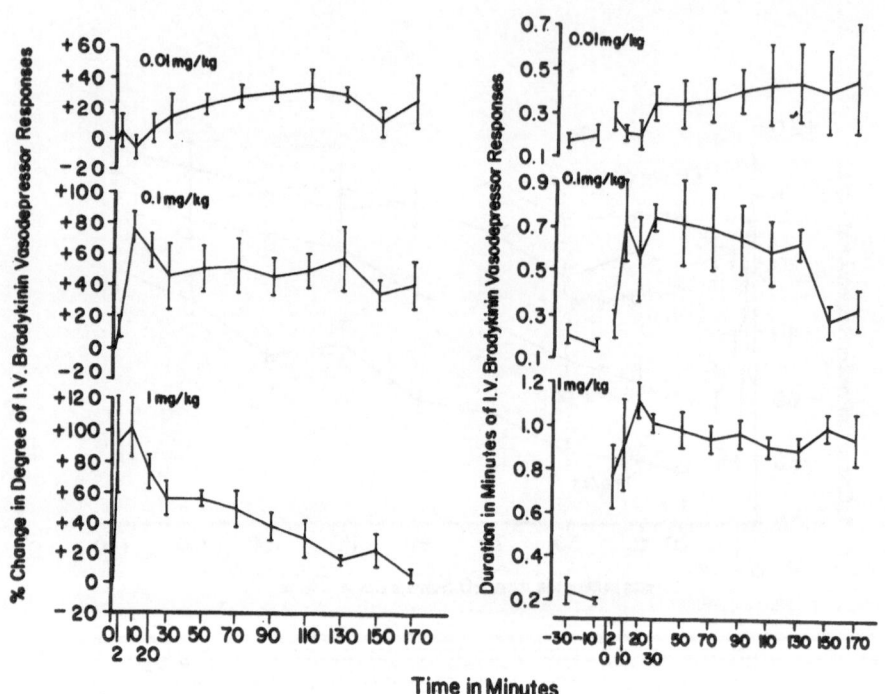

Time in Minutes

Figure 4.   Augmentation and prolongation of the vasodepressor action of bradykinin in unanesthetized rats by oral doses of captopril (SQ 14,225).   Four rats per dose were injected with 10 µg/kg bradykinin at the indicated times following oral dosing with captopril; results are expressed as percent change in the depressor response ± standard error (left) and as absolute duration of the depressor response ± standard error (right).   (Reproduced with permission from the Journal of Pharmacology and Experimental Therapeutics (1978), 204:278.   Copyright by the Williams and Wilkins Co., Baltimore, MD).

converting enzyme by captopril contrasts with an earlier report (Solomon, Cavero, and Buckley, 1974) that teprotide inhibited the central responses to both angiotensins I and II. Teprotide has also been suggested to inhibit another bradykinin-degrading enzyme (LeDuc, Marshall, and Needleman, 1978; Ondetti and Engel, 1975); such results may indicate the peptidic inhibitor, in addition to lacking oral activity, may not be as specific in its actions *in vivo* as the nonpeptidic inhibitor captopril.

IV. ANTIHYPERTENSIVE ACTIONS

A. Normotensive Animals

The renin-angiotensin system does not appear to be essential for day-to-day maintenance of blood pressure in normotensive animals or man except under conditions of lowered "effective blood volume" such as those produced by hemorrhage or sodium depletion (Gavras, Brunner, Vaughn, and Laragh, 1973). Maximally inhibitory doses of captopril produced no more than a 5 to 10 mm Hg drop in blood pressure in unanesthetized rats, rabbits, and man, or in chloralose anesthetized cats (Laffan, Goldberg, High, *et al.*, 1978; Ondetti, Rubin, and Cushman, 1977; Murthy, Waldron, Goldberg, and Vollmer, 1977; Vollmer, and Baccagno, 1977; Bengis, Coleman, Young, and McCaa, 1978; Ferguson, Turini, Brunner, *et al.*, 1977). A greater decrease in blood pressure was obtained in conscious or pentobarbital anesthetized normotensive dogs (Murthy, Waldron, and Goldberg, 1978a; Harris, Heran, Goldenberg, *et al.*, 1978). In sodium deficient normotensive rats and dogs (McCaa, Hall, and McCaa, 1978; Bengis, Coleman, Young, and McCaa, 1978) oral administration of captopril at 20-40 mg/kg for 1-3 weeks produced a dramatic hypotensive response of about 30 mm Hg. In the sodium depleted dogs, this hypotensive action was accompanied by a 3.8-fold increase in plasma renin activity, a 2.7-fold decrease in plasma aldosterone concentration, and a 2.4-fold increase in blood kinins. Similar results in rats and dogs have been obtained with the peptidic inhibitor teprotide (Thurston and Laragh, 1975; Stephens, Davis, Freeman, *et al.*, 1977; Samuels, Miller, Fray, *et al.*, 1976; McCaa, 1977).

B. Renal Hypertensive Animals

The anesthetized aortic-ligated rat is a model of acute high-renin hypertension. In these animals, an intravenous infusion of 3 mg/kg of captopril produced a marked sustained decrease in diastolic blood pressure (Laffan, Goldberg, High, *et al.*, 1978).

The one-kidney renal hypertensive rat (one renal artery partially occluded by a silver clip, the contralateral kidney removed) has a high blood pressure that is associated with high plasma renin

activity for only the first few days after clipping, during the
development of the hypertensive state. Thus, the high blood pressure in these animals probably is maintained beyond this developmental period by a nonrenin-dependent mechanism, perhaps by increased sodium retention (Doyle, Duffy, and MacDonald, 1976; Brunner,
Kirshman, Sealey, and Laragh, 1971). Six weeks after clipping, such
rats had no significant lowering of blood pressure after 2 days of
oral dosing with captopril at 30 mg/kg (Laffan, Goldberg, High, et
al., 1978). However, a significant lowering of blood pressure was
obtained in this model after 7 days of dosing with captopril at an
average daily dose of 46 mg/kg (Bengis, Coleman, Young, and McCaa,
1978). In one-kidney renal hypertensive dogs, captopril given
orally at 35 mg/kg before and after renal artery clipping delayed
but did not prevent the onset of hypertension (Watkins, Davis,
Freeman, et al., 1978).

The two-kidney renal hypertensive rat (one renal artery clipped,
the unclipped kidney left intact) has high blood pressure that is
associated with high levels of plasma renin for at least the first
few weeks (Doyle, Duffy, and MacDonald, 1976). As shown in Figure 5,
captopril given at oral doses of 3 mg/kg to 30 mg/kg rapidly lowered
blood pressure by 50-60 mm Hg in such rats six weeks after clipping
of the renal artery (Laffan, Goldberg, High, et al., 1978; Ondetti,
Rubin, and Cushman, 1977); the total duration of this antihypertensive
effect was greater than 24 hours. In this model, oral captopril was
effective at a dose that was 10 times lower than the effective dose
of subcutaneously administered teprotide. Similar antihypertensive
activity of captopril in this model was obtained by Bengis, Coleman,
Young, and McCaa (1978), who administered the drug for a period of
seven days.

Two-kidney renal hypertensive rats have now been treated for
several months with captopril alone and in combination with the
diuretic hydrochlorothiazide (Rubin, Antonaccio, Goldberg, et al.,
1978); in these studies, systolic blood pressures were measured
indirectly in conscious animals. As shown in Table 2, captopril
administered orally at 30 mg/kg maintained systolic blood pressure
for at least 4 months at a level of 40-50 mm Hg lower than that of
control animals given only water. After 4 months of treatment,
poor survival of the control animals with the highest blood pressures makes direct comparison of control and treated animals less
meaningful, but blood pressures of the treated animals had not increased greatly after the 10th month of drug administration (see
Table 2). Hydrochlorothiazide alone at 6 mg/kg had only a slight
effect on the blood pressure of these two-kidney renal hypertensive
rats, but the combination of captopril with hydrochlorothiazide
produced a sustained lowering of blood pressure for at least 10
months to a level that was 20 mm Hg lower than that achieved with
captopril alone. The direct vasodilator hydralazine produced a
greater hypotensive response than captopril during the first few

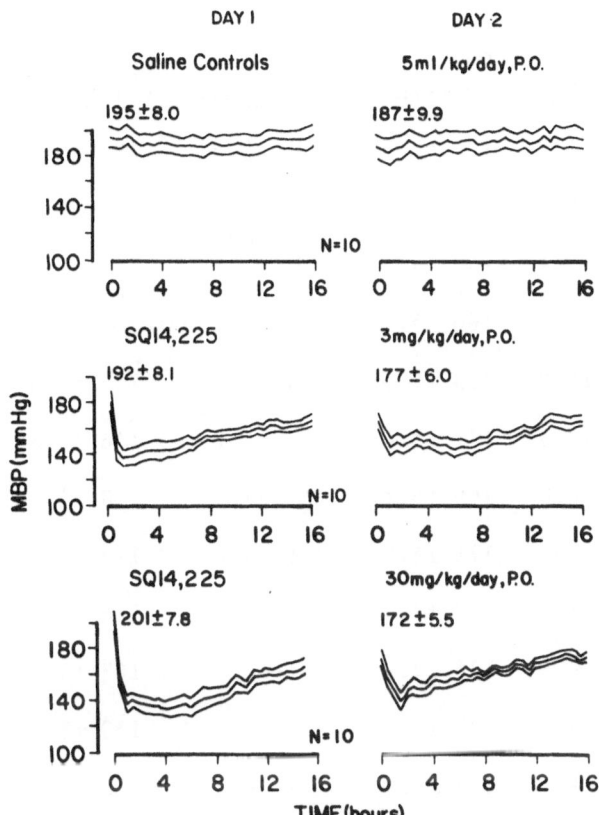

Figure 5. *Antihypertensive action of orally administered captopril (SQ 14,225) in unanesthetized two-kidney renal hypertensive rats. For each experiment, groups of 10 hypertensive rats received saline, captopril at 3 mg/kg, or captopril at 30 mg/kg on two successive days; results are plotted as mean blood pressure ± standard error. (Reproduced with permission from the Journal of Pharmacology and Experimental Therapeutics (1978), 204: 283. Copyright by the Williams and Wilkins Co., Baltimore, MD).*

TABLE 2.   EFFECT OF CHRONIC TREATMENT OF RENAL HYPERTENSIVE RATS
WITH SQ 14,225 AND OTHER ANTIHYPERTENSIVE DRUGS

Time (mo.)	Systolic Blood Pressure ±SE (mm Hg)				
	H_2O	SQ 14,225 (30 mg/kg)	Hydrochloro- thiazide (6 mg/kg)	SQ 14,225 + Hydrochloro- thiazide *	Hydralazine (6 mg/kg)
0	198 ±4.9	197 ±5.3	197 ±5.8	198 ±5.1	201 ±5.5
0.5	202 ±5.3	162 ±5.7	192 ±7.6	----	174 ±4.5[†]
1	208 ±5.4	160 ±4.4	191 ±5.5	147 ±6.2	182 ±6.0
2	215 ±5.7	166 ±5.0	197 ±8.2	----	194 ±4.9
3	211 ±5.9	169 ±5.6	197 ±7.1	148 ±4.8	187 ±5.7
4	209 ±8.3	171 ±5.4	199 ±9.2	146 ±5.8	190 ±5.4
5	201 ±8.8	169 ±6.1	198 ±10	158 ±4.6	190 ±3.5
6	191 ±13	171 ±5.5	199 ±7.6	153 ±4.0	196 ±10
7	194 ±14	177 ±7.4	190 ±10	156 ±2.6	198 ±4.5
8	----	176 ±3.9	----	162 ±3.5	----
9	----	177 ±4.8	----	153 ±3.7	----
10	----	173 ±4.9	----	156 ±3.6	----

Groups of 15 animals, 6 weeks after clipping of their left renal
arteries, were dosed orally once a day with water or the indicated
drugs. Systolic blood pressures were determined indirectly 4 hours
after dosing. Standard errors are based on a maximum of 15 animals
per group and a minimum of 5 animals in groups where survival rates
were low.

*Animals in this group were treated continuously with SQ 14,225, but
were given hydrochlorothiazide only at 5 day intervals each month
until the third month, after which time they were treated continuously with both drugs.

†Hydralazine lowered blood pressure dramatically during the first
few days of administration: day 1, 127 ± 6.9 mm Hg; day 2, 130 ± 5.3
mm Hg; day 5, 148 ± 6.2 mm Hg.

days of its administration, but only a very slight antihypertensive action was observed after one month of treatment with this drug (Table 2).

In addition to the blood pressure reduction, the incidence of its pathological sequelae also was reduced in two-kidney renal hypertensive rats treated chronically with captopril or captopril plus a diuretic. At nine months, survival rates among the 15 rats in each group shown in Table 2 were as follows: water-treated, 1/15; captopril-treated, 9/15; hydrochlorothiazide-treated, 3/15; captopril + hydrochlorothiazide-treated, 13/15; and hydralazine-treated, 3/15. The heart weight to body weight ratios of surviving untreated two-kidney renal hypertensive rats were much higher than those of normotensive control animals of the same age. After about one month of treatment of the renal hypertensive rats with captopril, this ratio had decreased to a value that was indistinguishable from that of normotensive controls (Rubin, Antonaccio, Goldberg, *et al.*, 1978).

C. Genetic Hypertensive Rats

Mature spontaneously hypertensive rats of the Wistar-Kyoto Okamoto-Aoki strain do not have elevated plasma renin activity (Sen, Smeby, and Bumpus, 1972), and have not been considered to have renin-dependent hypertension. Nevertheless, as shown in Figure 6, orally administered captopril produces a significant dose-related fall in blood pressure in these animals (Laffan, Goldberg, High, *et al.*, 1978). Subcutaneously administered teprotide (30 mg/kg) produced a similar lowering of blood pressure. The acute antihypertensive effect of captopril in these rats is abolished by total nephrectomy. The blood pressure lowering produced by captopril in spontaneously hypertensive rats has been shown to be brought about solely by a decrease in total peripheral vascular resistance (Muirhead, Prewitt, Brooks, and Brosius, 1978), as would be expected for a drug that only inhibits angiotensin production or augments bradykinin action.

Chronic treatment of spontaneously hypertensive rats with captopril (100 mg/kg, p.o.) produced an even more profound change in the blood pressure (Antonaccio, Rubin, Horovitz, *et al.*, 1978). After 6 or 12 months, animals treated with this drug had mean blood pressures that were indistinguishable from those of normotensive controls (Table 3), and 70 mm Hg lower than those of untreated hypertensive rats. Hydralazine (3 mg/kg) lowered blood pressure to a lesser degree than did captopril, but without the rapidly developing tolerance that was seen in the renal hypertensive rats. A complete normalization of the heart weight to body weight ratio was achieved in rats treated with captopril; hydralazine at 6 months had produced a partial reversal of cardiac hypertrophy.

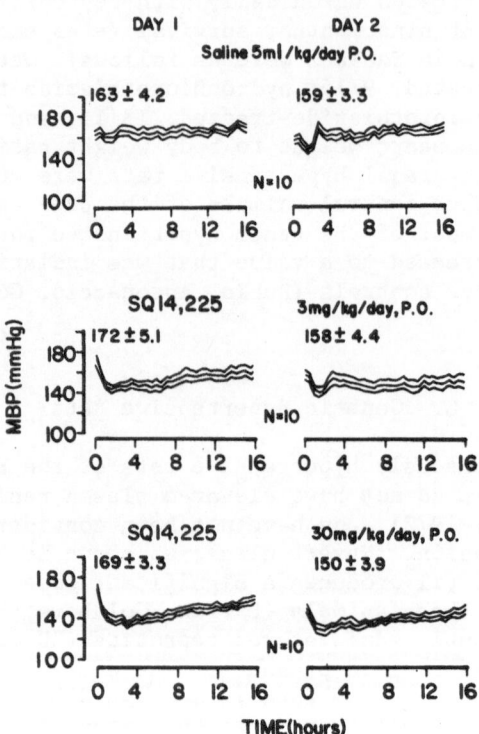

Figure 6. *Antihypertensive action of orally administered captopril
(SQ 14,225) in unanesthetized spontaneously hypertensive
rats. For each experiment, groups of 10 hypertensive
rats received saline, captopril at 3 mg/kg, or captopril
at 30 mg/kg; results are plotted as mean blood pressure
± standard error. (Reproduced with permission from the
Journal of Pharmacology and Experimental Therapeutics
(1978), 204:284. Copyright by the Williams and Wilkins
Co., Baltimore, MD).*

*TABLE 3.   EFFECT OF CHRONIC TREATMENT OF SPONTANEOUSLY
HYPERTENSIVE RATS WITH SQ 14,225 AND HYDRALAZINE*

Time (mo.)	Normotensive Wistar-Kyoto	Mean Blood Pressure ±SE (mm Hg)		
		Wistar-Kyoto	Spontaneously Hypertensive Rats	
	H_2O	H_2O	SQ 14,225 (100 mg/kg)	Hydralazine (3 mg/kg)
0.5	123 ±1.7	193 ±2.4	148 ±2.7	167 ±2.3
3	126 ±3.6	201 ±2.3	141 ±2.8	159 ±3.2
6	121 ±2.7	198 ±1.4	128 ±2.6	160 ±3.2
12	130 ±1.0	202 ±2.1	126 ±2.3	143 ±3.7

*Normotensive or spontaneously hypertensive rats at 10 to 14 weeks
of age were given water or drug once a day by the oral route.
Eighteen days before measurement of blood pressure, 10-12 rats
from each of the four groups were cannulated for direct determination of blood pressure.*

D.   DOCA-Salt Hypertensive Rats

Hypertension induced by the mineralocorticoid deoxycorticosterone acetate (DOCA) is associated with low renin activity and, among
other factors, with sodium retention. In this model, captopril did
not affect the development or the final magnitude of hypertension
(Douglas, Langford, and McCaa, 1978).

E.   Human Hypertension

The first inhibitor of angiotensin-converting enzyme to be
studied in hypertensive patients was the nonapeptide teprotide
(Gavras, Brunner, Laragh, and Vukovich, 1974; Johnson, Black,
Vukovich, *et al.*, 1975; Case, Wallace, Keim, *et al.*, 1977). This
inhibitor, administered intravenously at doses of 1-4 mg/kg,
appeared to normalize blood pressures of renovascular hypertensive
patients, it produced dramatic lowering of blood pressure in patients
with malignant hypertension, and significantly lowered blood pressure

in a high percentage of those patients diagnosed as essential hypertensives. The efficacy of this drug in essential hypertension was
related to the level of plasma renin. A blood pressure lowering
was obtained in almost all patients with high plasma renin activity,
in the majority of patients with "normal" plasma renin activity
(normal for a normotensive individual), and in almost none of the
patients with low plasma renin activity. The antihypertensive
action of teprotide was potentiated by plasma volume depletion
achieved by low sodium diet or the use of diuretics.

Captopril administered orally in doses of about 6 mg/kg to
15 mg/kg had a similar antihypertensive activity to that observed
earlier with teprotide (Gavras, Brunner, Turini, *et al.*, 1978).
Perhaps because of the high doses employed over a longer period of
time (3 to 24 weeks), captopril appeared to be even more effective
as an antihypertensive drug than teprotide. It lowered blood pressure in some patients with low-renin essential hypertension. In
fact, in this first reported clinical study with captopril the maximal blood pressure lowering obtained correlated only poorly with
the measured plasma renin activities of the patients; however, these
maximal effects were obtained in various patients with different
doses of the drug. Interestingly, captopril lowered blood pressure
significantly in some patients who had hitherto been resistant to
various combinations of commonly employed antihypertensive drugs.

V. MECHANISM AND SPECIFICITY OF ANTIHYPERTENSIVE ACTION

Both captopril (SQ 14,224) and teprotide (SQ 20,881) are remarkably specific antihypertensive drugs with a well understood primary
mechanism of action, *i. e.*, inhibition of angiotensin-converting
enzyme. Nevertheless, a certain ambiguity exists regarding the
exact mechanism of their antihypertensive actions in various forms
of hypertensive disease. Such inhibitors prevent formation of
angiotensin II, and should lower blood pressure when it is supported by circulating or locally-produced excesses of this peptide.
The decrease in circulating angiotensin II, however, can lead to a
decrease in aldosterone secretion by the adrenal cortex, and to a
more slowly developing hypotension caused by increased sodium
excretion. A third possible hypotensive mechanism resulting from
inhibition of the converting enzyme results from inhibition of its
action as a bradykinin-inactivating enzyme, which may lead to
increased local production of this vasodepressor polypeptide, or
to increased blood levels due to decreased pulmonary inactivation
of circulating bradykinin.

Both teprotide and captopril cause large increases in plasma
renin activity in normotensive or hypertensive animals and man
(Miller, Samuels, Haber, and Barger, 1972; Bing and Poulsen, 1975;
Antonaccio, Rubin, Horovitz, *et al.*, 1978; Harris, Heran, Goldenberg,

et al., 1978; Bengis, Coleman, Young, and McCaa, 1978; Stephens, Davis, Freeman, *et al.*, 1977; Gavras, Brunner, Laragh, and Vukovich, 1974; Gavras, Brunner, Turini, *et al.*, 1978; Ferguson, Turini, Brunner, *et al.*, 1977). This increase occurs even in the absence of significant blood pressure reduction, and is thought to be due to decreased blood concentration of angiotensin II and a consequent reversal of the feedback inhibition of renin release normally exerted by angiotensin II. Angiotensin II itself is difficult to measure at low levels, but it has been reported to be lowered significantly in essential hypertensive patients treated with teprotide (Williams and Hollenberg, 1977). Plasma aldosterone concentration has been shown to be significantly decreased by captopril or teprotide in sodium-depleted animals and in hypertensive patients (McCaa, 1977; McCaa, Hall, and McCaa, 1978; Bengis, Coleman, Young, and McCaa, 1978; Gavras, Brunner, Laragh, and Vukovich, 1974; Gavras, Brunner, Turini, *et al.*, 1978). Teprotide did not increase plasma bradykinin levels in normal human volunteers or in sodium-depleted normotensive humans who responded to this drug with a dramatic lowering of blood pressure (Sancho, Re, Burton, *et al.*, 1976; Williams and Hollenberg, 1977); sodium depleted essential hypertensive patients, however, responded with a 2.3-fold increase in plasma bradykinin concentration (Williams and Hollenberg, 1977). Studies in rabbits, however, have shown that an increase in the hypotensive action of locally produced bradykinin need not involve increases in circulating bradykinin, but may be mediated by increased intrarenal release of prostaglandin precursors such as arachidonic acid (Murthy, Waldron, and Goldberg, 1978b). Thus, just as it is difficult to determine the role of the renin-angiotensin system in hypertensive disease by merely measuring renin activity in the general circulation, it is equally difficult to elucidate the mechanism of antihypertensive action of angiotensin-converting enzyme inhibitors by measuring changes in the circulating levels of components of the renin-angiotensin system or kallikrein-kinin system.

Although the precise mechanism of the antihypertensive action of converting enzyme inhibitors cannot yet be determined, it is reasonably clear that mechanisms unrelated to inhibition of the enzyme do not operate. These drugs do not have a significant direct effect on the autonomic nervous system or heart, or on a variety of vascular smooth muscle receptors. In anesthetized dogs (Murthy, Waldron, and Goldberg, 1978a), captopril had no effect on the rate or force of contraction of the heart and, unlike most hypotensive drugs, it increased renal blood flow. Marked decreases in blood pressure produced by captopril in hypertensive animals or man have not been accompanied by significant reflex tachycardia (Laffan, Goldberg, High, *et al.*, 1978; Gavras, Brunner, Turini, *et al.*, 1978; Bengis, Coleman, Young, and McCaa, 1978), although the hypotensive effect obtained in sodium depleted rats is associated with an increase in heart rate (Bengis, Coleman, Young, and McCaa, 1978).

Both captopril (SQ 14,225) and teprotide (SQ 20,881) are remarkably free of acute side-effects, as might be expected for drugs that specifically inhibit an enzyme that is not essential for normal homeostatic control of blood pressure or, as far as is known, for any other critical physiological function. The acute oral LD_{50} of SQ 14,225 in rats is about 25,000 times higher than its effective dose for inhibition of the angiotensin I pressor response (Rubin, Laffan, Kotler, *et al.*, 1978). In animal and human studies, no sign of any acute toxicity has been obtained at very high doses. Some toxicological effects have been observed in humans given high doses of captopril for several weeks (Gavras, Brunner, Turini, *et al.*, 1978), but the incidence of such effects upon long term dosing in humans can be evaluated only after study at appropriate dose levels in a large number of patients. At our present state of knowledge, captopril appears to have great potential as a remarkably effective and remarkably well tolerated drug for use in the long term control of most forms of human hypertensive disease.

REFERENCES

Antonaccio, M. J., Rubin, B., Horovitz, Z. P., Laffan, R. J., Goldberg, M. E., High, J. P., Harris, D. N., and Zaidi, I. (1979). Effects of chronic treatment with SQ 14,225 (captopril) an orally active inhibitor of angiotensin I-converting enzyme, in spontaneously hypertensive rats. Jpn. J. Pharmacol. 29: 285-294.

Bakhle, Y. S. (1968). Conversion of angiotensin I to angiotensin II by cell-free extracts of dog lung. Nature 220: 919-921.

Bengis, R. G., Coleman, T. G., Young, D. B., and McCaa, R. E. (1978). Long-term blockade of angiotensin formation in various normo-tensive and hypertensive rat models using converting enzyme inhibitor (SQ 14,225). Circ. Res. 43 (Suppl. 1): 45-53.

Bing, J. and Poulsen, K. (1975). Time course of changes in plasma renin after blockade of the renin system. Acta Path. Microbiol. Scand. 83: 454-466.

Brunner, H. R., Kirshman, J. D., Sealey, J. E., and Laragh, J. H. (1971). Hypertension of renal origin: Evidence of two different mechanisms. Science 174: 1344-1346.

Case, D. B., Wallace, J. M., Keim, H. J., Weber, M. A., Sealey, J. E. and Laragh, J. H. (1977). Possible role of renin in hyperten-sion as suggested by renin-sodium profiling and inhibition of converting enzyme. New Eng. J. Med. 296: 641-646.

Cheung, H. S. and Cushman, D. W. (1973). Inhibition of homogeneous angiotensin-converting enzyme of rabbit lung by synthetic venom peptides of *Bothrops jararaca*. Biochim. Biophys. Acta 293: 451-463.

Cushman, D. W. and Cheung, H. S. (1971). Spectrophotometric assay and properties of the angiotensin-converting enzyme of rabbit lung. Biochim. Pharmacol. 20: 1637-1648.

Cushman, D. W., Cheung, H. S., Sabo, E. F., and Ondetti, M. A. (1977). Design of potent competitive inhibitors of angiotensin-converting enzyme. Carboxyalkanoyl and mercaptoalkanoyl amino acids. Biochemistry 16: 5484-5491.

Cushman, D. W., Pluscec, J., Williams, N. J., Weaver, E. R., Sabo, E. F., Kocy, O., Cheung, H. S., and Ondetti, M. A. (1973). Inhibition of angiotensin-converting enzyme by analogs of peptides from *Bothrops jararaca* venom. Experientia 29: 1032-1035.

Douglas, B. H., Langford, H. G., and McCaa, R. E. (1978). Failure of an angiotensin I converting enzyme inhibitor to alter deoxycorticosterone acetate-sodium chloride (DCA-NaCl) hypertension. Clin. Res. 26: 510 (abstract).

Doyle, A. E., Duffy, S., and MacDonald, G. J. (1976). Exchangable sodium in experimental hypertension in rats. Clin. Sci. Mol. Med. 51 (Suppl. 3): 133s-135s.

Erdös, E. G. (1976a). Conversion of angiotensin I to angiotensin II. Am. J. Med. 60: 749-759.

Erdös, E. G. (1976b). The kinins. Biochem. Pharmacol. 25: 1563-1569.

Engel, S. L., Schaeffer, T. R., Gold, B. I., and Rubin, B. (1972). Inhibition of pressor effects of angiotensin I and augmentation of depressor effects of bradykinin by synthetic peptides. Proc. Soc. Exp. Biol. Med. 140: 240-244.

Engel, S. L., Schaeffer, T. R., Waugh, M. H., and Rubin, B. (1973). Effects of the nonapeptide SQ 20,881 on blood pressure of rats with experimental hypertension. Proc. Soc. Exp. Biol. Med. 143: 483-487.

Ferreira, S. H. (1965). A bradykinin-potentiating factor (BPF) present in the venom of *Bothrops jararaca*. Br. J. Pharmacol. 24: 163-169.

Ferreira, S. H., Bartelt, D. C., and Greene, L. J. (1970). Isolation of bradykinin-potentiating peptides from *Bothrops jararaca* venom. Biochemistry 9: 2583-2593.

Ferguson, R. K., Turini, G. A., Brunner, H. R., Gavras, H., and McKinstry, D. N. (1977). A specific orally active inhibitor of angiotensin-converting enzyme in man. Lancet 1: 775-778.

Gavras, H., Brunner, H. R., Laragh, J. H., and Vukovich, R. A. (1974). An angiotensin-converting enzyme inhibitor to identify and treat vasoconstrictor and volume factors in hypertensive patients. New Eng. J. Med. 291: 817-821.

Gavras, H., Brunner, H. R., Turini, G. A., Kershaw, G. R., Tifft, C. P., Cuttelod, S., Gavras, I., Vukovich, R. A., and McKinstry, D. N. (1978). Antihypertensive effect of the oral angiotensin converting enzyme inhibitor SQ 14,225 in man. New Eng. J. Med. 298: 991-995.

Gavras, H., Brunner, H. R., Vaughan, E. D., Jr., and Laragh, J. H. (1973). Angiotensin-sodium interaction in blood pressure maintenance of renal hypertensive and normotensive rats. Science 180: 1369-1372.

Harris, D. N., Heran, C. L., Goldenberg, H. J., High, J. P., Laffan, R. J., Rubin, B., Antonaccio, M. J., and Goldberg, M. E. (1978). Effects of SQ 14,225, an orally active inhibitor of angiotensin converting enzyme, on blood pressure, heart rate, and plasma renin activity of conscious normotensive dogs. Eur. J. Pharmaco 51: 345-349.

Heald, A. F. and Ita, C. E. (1977). Distribution of an inhibitor of angiotensin-converting enzyme, SQ 14,225, as studied by whole-body autoradiography and liquid scintillation counting. Pharmacologist 19: 129 (abstract).

Igic, R., Erdös, E. G., Yeh, H. S. J., Sorrells, K., and Nakajima, T. (1972). Angiotensin-converting enzyme of the lung. Circ. Res. 31 (Suppl. 2): 51-61.

Johnson, J. G., Black, W. D., Vukovich, R. A., Hatch, F. E., Jr., Friedman, B. I., Blackwell, C. F., Shenouda, A. N., Share, L., Shade, R. E., Acchiardo, S. R., and Muirhead, E. E. (1975). Treatment of patients with severe hypertension by inhibition of angiotensin-converting enzyme. Clin. Sci. Mol. Med. 48: 53s-56s.

Kato, H. and Suzuki, T. (1971). Bradykinin-potentiating peptides from the venom of *Agkistrodon halys blomhoffii*. Isolation of five bradykinin potentiators and the amino acid sequence of two of them, potentiators B and C. Biochemistry 10: 972-987.

Krieger, E. M., Salgado, H. C., Assan, C. J., Greene, L. J., and Ferreira, S. H. (1971). Potential screening test for detection of overactivity of the renin-angiotensin system. Lancet 1: 269-271.

Laffan, R. J., Goldberg, M. E., High, J. P., Schaeffer, T. R., Waugh, M. H., and Rubin, B. (1978). Antihypertensive activity in rats of SQ 14,225, an orally active inhibitor of angiotensin I-converting enzyme. J. Pharmacol. Exp. Ther. 204: 281-288.

LeDuc, L. E., Marshall, G. R., and Needleman, P. (1978). Differentiation of bradykinin receptors and kininases with conformational analogues of bradykinin. Mol. Pharmacol. 14: 413-421.

McCaa, R. E. (1977). Role of the renin-angiotensin system in the regulation of aldosterone biosynthesis and arterial pressure during sodium deficiency. Circ. Res. 40 (Suppl. 1): 157-162.

McCaa, R. E., Hall, J. E., and McCaa, C. S. (1978). The effects of angiotensin I-converting enzyme inhibitors on arterial blood pressure and urinary sodium excretion. Role of the renal renin-angiotensin and kallikrein-kinin systems. Circ. Res. 43 (Suppl. 1): 32-39.

Miller, E. D., Jr., Samuels, A. I., Haber, E., and Barger, A. C. (1972). Inhibition of angiotensin conversion in experimental renovascular hypertension. Science 177: 1108-1109.

Muirhead, E. E., Prewitt, R. L., Brooks, B., and Brosius, W. L. (1978). Antihypertensive action of the orally active converting enzyme inhibitor (SQ 14,225) in spontaneously hypertensive rats. Circ. Res. 43 (Suppl. 1): 53-59.

Murthy, V. S., Waldron, T. L., and Goldberg, M. E. (1978a). Inhibition of angiotensin-converting enzyme by SQ 14,225 in anesthetized dogs: Hemodynamic and renal vascular effects. Proc. Soc. Exp. Biol. Med. 157: 121-124.

Murthy, V. S., Waldron, T. L., and Goldberg, M. E. (1978b). The mechanism of bradykinin potentiation after inhibition of angiotensin-converting enzyme by SQ 14,225 in conscious rabbits. Circ. Res. 43 (Suppl. 1): 40-45.

Murthy, V. S., Waldron, T. L., Goldberg, M. E., and Vollmer, R. R. (1977). Inhibition of angiotensin-converting enzyme by SQ 14,225 in conscious rabbits. Eur. J. Pharmacol. 46: 207-212.

Ondetti, M. A. and Engel, S. L. (1975). Bradykinin analogs containing β-homoamino acids. J. Med. Chem. 18: 761-763.

Ondetti, M. A., Rubin, B., and Cushman, D. W. (1977). Design of specific inhibitors of angiotensin-converting enzyme: A new class of orally active antihypertensive agents. Science 196: 441-444.

Ondetti, M. A., Sabo, E. F., Losee, K. A., Cheung, H. S., Cushman, D. W., and Rubin, B. (1977). The use of an active site model in the design of specific inhibitors of angiotensin-converting enzyme. In: Peptides. Proceedings of the Fifth American Peptide Symposium. (Goodman, M. and Meienhofer, J., eds.), pp. 576-578, John Wiley and Sons, New York.

Ondetti, M. A., Williams, N. J., Sabo, E. F., Pluscec, J., Weaver, E. R., and Kocy, O. (1971). Angiotensin-converting enzyme inhibitors from the venom of Bothrops jararaca. Isolation, elucidation of structure, and synthesis. Biochemistry 10: 4033-4039.

Peach, M. J. (1977). Renin-angiotensin system: Biochemistry and mechanisms of action. Physiol. Rev. 57: 313-370.

Rubin, B., Antonaccio, M. J., Goldberg, M. E., Harris, D. N., Itkin, A. G., Horovitz, Z. P., Panasevich, R. B., and Laffan, R. J. (1978). Chronic antihypertensive effects of captopril (SQ 14,225), an orally active angiotensin I-converting enzyme inhibitor, in conscious 2-kidney renal hypertensive rats. Eur. J. Pharmacol. 51: 377-388.

Rubin, B., Laffan, R. J., Kotler, D. G., O'Keefe, E. H., DeMaio, D. A., and Goldberg, M. E. (1978). SQ 14,225 (D-3-mercapto-2-methylpropanoyl-L-proline), a novel orally active inhibitor of angiotensin-converting enzyme. J. Pharmacol. Exp. Ther. 204: 271-280.

Samuels, A. I., Miller, E. D., Fray, J. C. S., Haber, E., and Barger, A. C. (1976). Renin-angiotensin antagonists and the regulation of blood pressure. Fed. Proc. 35: 2512-2520.

Sancho, J., Re, R., Burton, J., Barger, A. C., and Haber, E. (1976). The role of the renin-angiotensin-aldosterone system in cardiovascular homeostasis in normal human subjects. Circulation 53: 400-405.

Sen, S., Smeby, R. R., and Bumpus, F. M. (1972). Renin in rats with spontaneous hypertension. Circ. Res. 31: 876-880.

Skeggs, L. T., Kahn, J. R., and Shumway, N. P. (1956). Preparation
    and function of the hypertension-converting enzyme. J. Exp.
    Med. 103: 295-299.
Solomon, T. A., Cavero, I., and Buckley, J. P. (1974). Inhibition
    of central pressor effects of angiotensin I and II. J. Pharm.
    Sci. 63: 511-515.
Stephens, G. A., Davis, J. O., Freeman, R. H., Watkins, B. E., and
    Khosla, M. C. (1977). The effects of angiotensin II blockade
    in conscious sodium-depleted dogs. Endocrinology 101: 378-388.
Stewart, J. M., Ferreira, S. H., and Greene, L. J. (1971). Brady-
    kinin potentiating peptide PCA-Lys-Trp-Ala-Pro. An inhibitor
    of the pulmonary inactivation of bradykinin and conversion of
    angiotensin I to II. Biochem. Pharmacol. 20: 1557-1567.
Thurston, H. and Laragh, J. H. (1975). Prior receptor occupancy as
    a determinant of the pressor activity of infused angiotensin II
    in the rat. Circ. Res. 36: 113-117.
Vane, J. R. (1972). Sites of conversion of angiotensin I. In:
    Hypertension '72. (Genest, J. and Koiw, E., eds.), pp. 523-
    532, Springer-Verlag, New York.
Vollmer, R. R. and Boccagno, J. A. (1977). Central cardiovascular
    effects of SQ 14,225, an angiotensin-converting enzyme inhibitor
    in chloralose-anesthetized cats. Eur. J. Pharmacol. 45: 117-
    125.
Watkins, B. E., Davis, J. O., Freeman, R. H., Stephens, G. A., and
    DeForrest, J. M. (1978). Effects of the oral converting enzyme
    inhibitor SQ 14,225 on one-kidney hypertension in the dog.
    Proc. Soc. Exp. Biol. Med. 157: 245-249.
Williams, G. H. and Hollenberg, N. K. (1977). Accentuated vascular
    and endocrine response to SQ 20,881 in hypertension. New Eng.
    J. Med. 297: 184-188.

DISCUSSION AFTER DR. CUSHMAN'S PAPER

Dr. Rowe

There is evidence that two-kidney hypertensive rats escape renin
dependency. In your experiments, did you see any animals that became
unresponsive?

Dr. Cushman

No, I don't believe so, not in the long-term studies. I don't
think our rats were classically renin dependent, even at the start
of our long-term studies, in that they did not have elevated plasma
renin activities. They had renal clips for six weeks before the
experiment started. Of course, the spontaneously hypertensive rats
also remained responsive to captopril and did not have high plasma
renin activities. This result could be interpreted in a number of
ways, which is where the ambiguity of the drug sets in. Does it
mean that we should leave the renin-angiotensin system and concen-

trate on bradykinin? Or, does it mean that dependence on measurements of plasma renin activity may be somewhat naive, and that the
functional importance of the renin-angiotensin system goes beyond
merely an active elevation of angiotensin II in the bloodstream?
I think those kinds of questions are very important. I'm like
Dr. Peach - I would rather raise questions than give answers!

Dr. Peach
        I would like to comment on the last question. We used hyper-
tensive two-kidney one clip Goldblatt rats after sixteen weeks of
hypertension and saw no response to [Sar^1, Ala^8] angiotensin II
(saralasin) and no acute response to SQ 14,225 (Weed, Vaughan, and
Peach, 1979). By day 3 of treatment the pressure started down, and
by day 7 the pressure was normal. You see the same thing in one-
kidney Goldblatt rats if you intervene at any time when they're
supposedly angiotensin independent. People are just in a big hurry;
angiotensin causes an immediate pressor response, so let's be in a
big hurry to reverse it. If you just wait around, they'll respond.
I have a question for Dr. Cushman. Those primary hyperaldosterone
patients that you showed, were those adenomas, or did they have bilateral hyperplasia?

Dr. Cushman
        I don't have the foggiest idea. I don't even know which par-
ticular investigators were studying those patients.

Dr. Peach
        I probably shouldn't say this, but when we administered
SQ 14,225 to patients with bilateral ideopathic adrenal hyperplasia
they did not respond, nor do patients with adenomas. The other
comment is, we have used this drug in patients with end-stage renal
disease, and there it can scare you. The pressures in these patients can fall to about 60 over nothing! These are patients who are
brittle end-stage renals, whose pressures go up when you dialyze
them and who are not controlled by routine or combination antihypertensive therapy.

Dr. Cushman
        These patients have undergone dialysis, haven't they?

Dr. Peach
        They are on routine chronic dialysis. When we administer
SQ 14,225 in the lowest dose, which is 10 mg, their blood pressure
drops to 60 over nothing. In one patient, Dr. Vaughan and I went
to get a cup of coffee, and when we called the Clinical Research
Center they said "She's better now", but they had to give her three
units of saline i. v. to bring her pressure back up. That particular patient had a creatinine excretion of two mg, so she had essentially no renal function. The pressure remained down for five days

in that particular patient, which attests to the importance of the
kidney in getting rid of the drug. That patient also subsequently
underwent a bilateral nephrectomy, and postnephrectomy the pressure
came to exactly where the pressure went with careful titration with
SQ 14,225.

Dr. Cushman

I should have pointed out that this is one potential side
effect of converting enzyme inhibitors. It has already been reported in the literature. Apparently the blood pressures of these
patients, because of dialysis or otherwise, are quite dependent
upon the renin-angiotensin system, and that is something that one
certainly has to watch out for. Extreme sodium depletion is another
situation where if you give this drug you may see some rather dras-
tic drops in blood pressure. This is something one should be able
to look out for, once you know about it.

Dr. Williams

I would like to make two comments. First, in our AV fistula
dogs treated with SQ 14,225 in doses of 10 to 15 mg per kg, one of
our dogs became anuric because the blood pressure dropped so low,
and the animal died. Secondly, another side effect of SQ 14,225
that I find, at least in AV fistula dogs, is that these dogs inevi-
tably develop watery stools, but not diarrhea by the clinical definition. Have you seen these side effects in any other species, and
if not, why in this particular animal model?

Dr. Cushman

I know that the drug has been tested for toxicologic effects
in dogs at very high doses, but not in AV fistula dogs, of course.
This is one of those instances where, even though I think of myself
as being a pharmacologist, I plead to being a biochemist. I really
don't know the answer. There may have been some slight effects upon
the stool even in normal dogs, but I don't think they were considered
to be important or related to the drug's mechanism of action. If
you give an animal that much of any sulphydryl compound you might
produce similar effects. This is an observation that would be
interesting to pursue, but I am not sure that our toxicological
studies with normal dogs would shed much light on it.

Dr. Davis

I think you should add congestive heart failure to your list.
I gather in talking with Dr. Horovitz that there are several studies
being done currently on heart failure. From the standpoint of animal models, Dr. Williams should mention that the AV fistula dog is
a good model for high output heart failure, and he has seen a very
good natriuretic response with SQ 14,225 in this model. Dr. Freeman
has been looking at the low output failure model, the dog with caval
constriction, and he also noticed a very striking natriuresis with
SQ 14,225.

Dr. Cushman

We are certainly very interested in those studies.

Dr. Miller

I thought I might add something to the information on the renin-angiotensin system in the chronic Goldblatt rat. Several years ago we published an article on pepstatin as an inhibitor of renin, and we were able to lower the blood pressure of chronic Goldblatt animals with pepstatin at a very low dosage.

Dr. Cushman.

What is the drawback of pepstatin, if anything?

Dr. Miller

It has a half-life of about one and one-half circulation times ...unless some peptide chemists can make it longer acting.

DISCUSSION REFERENCES

Miller, R. P., Poper, C. J., Wilson, C. W., and DeVito, E. (1972). Renin inhibition by pepstatin. Biochem. Pharmacol. 21: 2941-2944.

Weed, W. C., Vaughan, Jr., E. D., and Peach, M. J. (1979). Prolongation of saralasin responsive state of two-kidney, one clip Goldblatt hypertension in the rat by the orally administered converting enzyme inhibitor captopril (SQ 14,225). Hypertension 1: 8-12.

ROLE OF ANGIOTENSIN II IN THE REGULATION OF ALDOSTERONE BIOSYNTHESIS[1]

R. E. McCaa, A. C. Guyton, D. B. Young, and C. S. McCaa

Department of Physiology and Biophysics
University of Mississippi School of Medicine
Jackson, MS 39216

OUTLINE

I. Introduction

II. Regulation of aldosterone biosynthesis
   A. Role of ACTH
   B. Role of potassium ions
   C. Role of the renin-angiotensin system
   D. Role of sodium ions

III. Regulation of aldosterone biosynthesis during sodium deficiency
   A. Aldosterone response to long-term beta-adrenergic blockade with propranolol in sodium deficient dogs
   B. Aldosterone response to long-term infusion of angiotensin II inhibitory analogues in sodium deficient dogs
   C. Aldosterone response to long-term administration of angiotensin I converting enzyme inhibitors in sodium deficient dogs
   D. Evidence for an important role of both potassium and angiotensin II in the control of aldosterone biosynthesis during dietary sodium restriction

IV. The renin-angiotensin system in experimental renovascular hypertension

V. Conclusions

---

[1]The investigations from the authors' laboratory reported in this review were supported by USPHS Grant HL 09921 from the National Institutes of Health and by a grant from the Mississippi Heart Assn.

I.   INTRODUCTION

Aldosterone plays a primary role in maintaining the overall
adequacy of the circulatory system. A hypodynamic state of the
circulation is usually followed within minutes by increased aldosterone secretion, and a hyperdynamic state of the circulation
results in decreased aldosterone secretion. Despite the vast
importance of the role of aldosterone in overall circulatory regulation, it has been difficult to arrive at conclusions on the
regulation of aldosterone biosynthesis for several reasons. First,
aldosterone biosynthesis is under multifactorial control, and it
has been difficult to maintain several variables constant while
altering only a single factor. Second, measurement of aldosterone
in peripheral plasma has been exceedingly difficult, time consuming,
and expensive. Finally, most of our knowledge of the physiological
control of aldosterone secretion is derived from short-term animal
experiments and clinical studies, while very few research studies
have been long-term, lasting for several weeks. The majority of
these earlier experimental studies indicated that aldosterone
secretion was primarily regulation by the renin-angiotensin system,
while alterations in sodium and potassium metabolism and the
pituitary secretion of adrenocorticotropic hormone (ACTH) were
thought to play important secondary roles.

During the past ten years we have collected considerable
quantitative data in experimental animals and man in an effort to
develop a composite quantitative control systems analysis for the
regulation of aldosterone secretion. Our method of approach to
the investigation of the regulation of aldosterone secretion is
divided into three phases: First, systems analyses of the basic
known regulatory mechanisms, including both control system block
analyses and computer solutions. Second, physiological experimen-
tation to fill in data needed to make the analysis complete and to
validate the concepts upon which the systems were predicted.
Finally, reanalysis of the system after additional experimental data
were added.

This chapter presents a review of the recent experimental research studies performed in our laboratory to differentiate between
acute and chronic stimuli of aldosterone secretion and to determine
the quantitative and temporal relationships of the various stimuli
and aldosterone biosynthesis. Special emphasis is placed on three
phases of our research studies: (1) the aldosterone response to
long-term infusion of ACTH, potassium ions, and angiotensin II in
intact conscious dogs maintained on normal sodium intake, (2) the
use of pharmacologic agents to evaluate quantitatively the role of
the renin-angiotensin system in mediating increased aldosterone
biosynthesis during sodium deficiency, and (3) chronic blockade of
angiotensin II formation with angiotensin I converting enzyme inhibitors to determine the role of the renin-angiotensin-aldosterone system

in mediating the elevated arterial blood pressure in animal models of experimental renovascular hypertension. Since all of our studies were performed in intact conscious animals, the data obtained from this experimental model will be collated with observations of other investigators who have used different experimental approaches to study aldosterone regulation in other animal species and in man.

All of the long-term experiments presented from this laboratory were performed in intact unanesthetized mongrel dogs with chronic indwelling catheters in the right femoral artery and vein. The venous catheter was used to maintain continuous infusion of various pharmacologic agents at a constant rate from a syringe infusion pump. Continuous twenty-four hour arterial blood pressure measurements were obtained from the arterial catheter by a pressure transducer and a recorder. The animals were housed in separate, stainless steel metabolic cages during the control, experimental, and recovery stages of the study. The experimental animal preperation used in these studies and the procedure for collection and analysis of the blood samples by radioimmunoassay have been described in complete detail in previous publications. (McCaa, McCaa and Guyton, 1975; McCaa, McCaa, Read, *et al.*, 1972b).

II. REGULATION OF ALDOSTERONE BIOSYNTHESIS

Though all the details of the regulatory mechanisms controlling aldosterone biosynthesis are not known, it is apparent that at least four different factors, and possibly several others, play important roles in aldosterone regulation. These regulatory mechanisms include the pituitary secretion of ACTH, alterations in sodium and potassium metabolism, and the renal renin-angiotensin system. Figure 1 illustrates the plasma aldosterone responses to long-term infusions of ACTH, angiotensin II, or potassium ions in intact conscious dogs maintained on a normal sodium intake.

A. Role of ACTH

Much of our knowledge of the role of ACTH on aldosterone secretion has been obtained from studies in human beings maintained on long-term administration of ACTH (Newton and Laragh, 1968) or from studies of patients with Cushing's syndrome with chronic excessive secretion of endogenous ACTH. In both instances aldosterone secretion remains at normal or even below normal levels. The normal or decreased production of aldosterone in the face of chronically high levels of ACTH is thought to result from suppression of aldosterone secretion by increased body fluid volume resulting from excessively high levels of circulating cortisol. It is generally believed by most investigators that ACTH, although

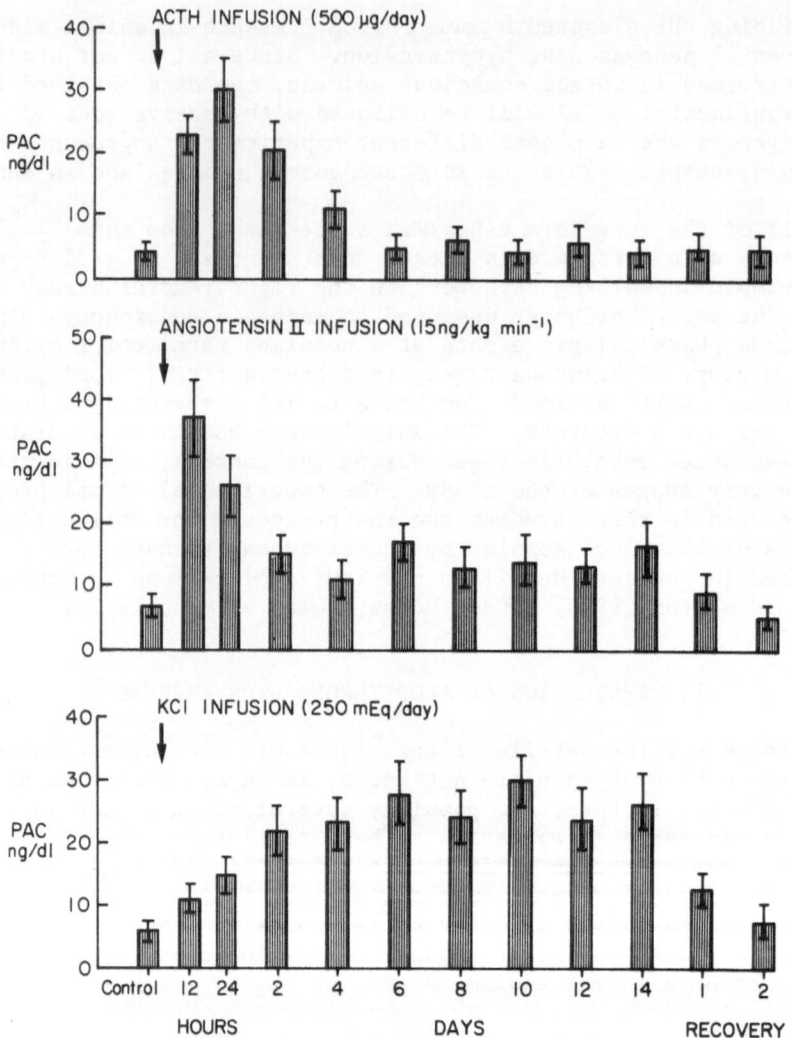

Figure 1. *The response of plasma aldosterone concentration to*
long-term infusion of ACTH (top panel), angiotensin II
(middle panel), and potassium chloride (bottom panel)
in eight sodium-replete dogs. Vertical lines indicate
± SEM.

important in maintaining the steroid precursors necessary for the
synthesis of aldosterone, plays a minor role in the day-to-day
control of aldosterone secretion except for the increases
produced by acute stress such as surgical treatment, anxiety, or
physical trauma.

   The aldosterone response to long-term infusion of ACTH in eight
sodium-replete dogs is illustrated in Figure 1. Within twenty-four
hours after continuous ACTH infusion at a rate of 500 μg/day, plasma
aldosterone concentration increased from 6.7 $\pm$ 1.3 (SEM) to 29.3 $\pm$
7.6 ng/dl and remained significantly elevated above control levels
for the next three days. However, on the fourth day plasma
aldosterone concentration returned to the level that existed during
the control period, despite continuous ACTH infusion that maintained
plasma cortisol concentrations elevated sixteen times greater than
control levels (0.73 $\pm$ 0.25 to 11.6 $\pm$ 2.9 μg/dl). A similar
transient increase in aldosterone secretion in response to continuous
ACTH infusion was observed in conscious dogs during sodium
deficiency. Although aldosterone secretion returned to control
levels after four days of continuous ACTH infusion in sodium-
replete and sodium-deplete dogs, arterial blood pressure increased
by 27 $\pm$ 5 mm Hg in both groups of dogs and the animals remained
hypertensive until ACTH infusion was discontinued (McCaa,
Muirhead, Pitcock, et al., 1978). Since infusion of high levels
of aldosterone and cortisol failed to increase arterial blood
pressure in adrenalectomized dogs, it was concluded that the ACTH-
induced hypertension was due to the production of an unidentified
adrenocortical hormone(s) with mineralocorticoid and/or pressor
activity (Kastner and McCaa, 1978). Other investigators have
demonstrated ACTH-induced hypertension in experimental animals
(Coghlan, Denton, Fan, et al., 1977; Scoggins, Butkus, Coghlan,
et al., 1978) and man (New, Saenger, Peterson and Ulick, 1975;
New, Peterson, Saenger and Levine, 1976).

                    B. Role of Potassium Ions

   Increased serum potassium concentration induced either by
increased dietary intake of potassium or by direct intravenous
infusion of potassium ions resulted in marked increases in
aldosterone secretion in experimental animals and man (Laragh
and Stoerk, 1957). Earlier research studies indicated that
large increases in serum potassium concentration were required to
elicit increased aldosterone secretion. However, more recent
studies have demonstrated marked increases in plasma aldosterone
concentration in response to minor increases in serum potassium
concentration (Boyd, Mulrow, Palmore and Silvo, 1973; McCaa,
Ott and McCaa, 1974), and clinical studies in nephrectomized
human beings indicate that potassium may be the primary regulatory
mechanism controlling aldosterone biosynthesis (McCaa, McCaa, Read
and Bower, 1972a; Bayard, Cooke, Tiller, et al., 1971).

   The aldosterone response to long-term infusion of potassium
ions in eight sodium-replete dogs is illustrated in Figure 1.
In response to continuous infusion of potassium chloride at a rate

of 250 mEq/day, plasma aldosterone concentration increased from
6.2 ±2.4 to 13.6 ±3.4 ng/dl within twenty-four hours and averaged
24.4 ±4.3 ng/dl by forty-eight hours after continuous infusion of
potassium chloride. Serum potassium concentration averaged 4.1 ±
0.5 mEq/L during the control period and increased to 4.8 ±0.5 mEq/L
within forty-eight hours after potassium chloride infusion. During
long-term continuous infusion of potassium chloride in intact
conscious dogs plasma aldosterone concentration and serum potassium
concentration remained significantly elevated above control levels.
These studies demonstrate that minor increases in serum potassium
concentration produce marked increases in aldosterone secretion and
indicate that alterations in potassium metabolism may play a major
role in both short-term and long-term regulation of aldosterone
biosynthesis (McCaa, McCaa, and Guyton, 1975).

C. Role of the Renin-Angiotensin System

Although acute intravenous infusions of angiotensin II increase
aldosterone secretion (Laragh, Angers, Kelly, and Lieberman, 1960),
plasma concentration (McCaa, Read, Cowley, et al., 1973; Fraser,
James, Brown, et al., 1965; Horton, 1969) and urinary excretion
(Genest, Nowaczynski, Koiw, et al., 1960; Biron, Koiw, Nowaczynski,
et al., 1961), the physiological role of the renal renin-angiotensin
system in the long-term regulation of aldosterone secretion is
less certain. In normal man, aldosterone secretion remained elevated
during prolonged infusion of pressor doses of the vasopressor
octapeptide, angiotensin II (Ames, Borkowski, Sicinski, and Laragh,
1965). In contrast, the adrenal glomerulosa cell in nephrectomized
human beings and in patients with hypopituitarism is almost totally
insensitive to acute or prolonged infusion of angiotensin II (McCaa,
Read, Cowley, et al., 1973; Williams, Bailey, Hampers, et al., 1973;
Weidmann, Horton, Maxwell, et al., 1973). In conscious sodium-replete
sheep, long-term infusions of angiotensin II resulted in a transient
increase in aldosterone secretion that lasted only 6 to 12 hours
(Blair-West, Coghlan, Denton, et al., 1972). Although acute intravenous infusion of angiotensin II into intact conscious rats resulted
in a marked increase in aldosterone secretion (Coleman, McCaa, and
McCaa, 1974· Campbell, Brooks, and Pettinger, 1974), long-term infusion of angiotensin II into conscious rats for 7 to 12 days failed to
sustain aldosterone secretion or adrenal aldosterone production above
control levels (Marieb and Mulrow, 1965).

The aldosterone response to the long-term infusion of angiotensin II in eight sodium-replete dogs is illustrated in Figure 1. In
response to acute infusion of angiotensin II at a rate of 15 ng/kg/
min, plasma aldosterone concentration increased from 7.1 ±2.9 to
48.3 ±9.7 ng/dl, plasma cortisol concentration increased from
0.92 ±0.35 to 3.85 ±0.87 µg/dl, and plasma renin activity decreased

from 0.82 ±0.23 to 0.39 ± 0.34 ng/ml/hr. Within twenty-four hours
after beginning the angiotensin II infusion, plasma aldosterone
concentration decreased from the high levels observed during the
acute phase of angiotensin II infusion. During long-term continuous
angiotensin II infusion, plasma aldosterone concentration averaged
14.7 ± 4.6 ng/dl, plasma cortisol concentration averaged 1.03 ±
0.43 µg/dl, plasma renin activity was undetectable by radioimmunoassay, and arterial blood pressure remained elevated above control
levels, averaging 142 ± 5 mm Hg, an increase of 42 mm Hg (McCaa,
1978).

The failure of long-term infusions of pressor doses of
angiotensin II to sustain elevated aldosterone secretion to the
same levels as those observed in response to sodium depletion has
led several investigators to postulate that the heptapeptide
metabolite of angiotensin II, des-asp[1] angiotensin II (angiotensin
III), may be the active component of the renin-angiotensin system
and may play a physiological role in the regulation of aldosterone
biosynthesis. However, recent studies from our laboratory (McCaa,
1978) and other laboratories (Carey, Vaughan, Peach, and Ayers, 1978;
Aguilera, Baukal, Fujita, *et al.*, 1978) indicate that angiotensin
III has less than one-half the aldosterone-stimulating effect of
angiotensin II, has only a slight effect on the feedback suppression
of renin secretion, and little or no effect on arterial blood
pressure.

D. Role of Sodium Ions

Marked alterations in sodium concentration *per se* have little
or no direct effect on adrenal aldosterone biosynthesis in
experimental animals *in vivo* (McCaa, Young, Guyton, and McCaa,
1974) or *in vitro* (Muller, 1965; Saruta, Cook and Kaplan, 1972).
Yet, slight alterations in sodium balance have profound effects on
aldosterone secretion in experimental animals and man. Since
dietary sodium restriction or removal of sodium from the body by
hemodialysis, diuresis, or any of several other means is associated
with parallel increases in plasma renin activity and plasma aldosterone concentration, most investigators believe that the aldosterone response to alterations in sodium balance is mediated by
the activity of the renal renin-angiotensin system.

In our laboratory a technique for studying headless animals
has been utilized that has made it possible to study animals whose
bodies have no secretory substances and no nervous control from the
head. This procedure has been combined with total nephrectomy so
that, in addition to the removal of head factors, the renal renin-
angiotensin system is also removed from the animals. Both of these
procedures have been combined with hemodialysis so that the plasma

concentration of sodium and potassium and other substances, as well
as the total body fluid volume, can be controlled (McCaa, McCaa,
Cowley, *et al.*, 1973). Figure 2 illustrates the aldosterone response
to reductions in sodium concentration by hemodialysis in decapitated-
nephrectomized dogs. These studies demonstrated that acute reduction
in plasma sodium concentration by 25 mEq/L failed to stimulate
aldosterone secretion in decapitated-nephrectomized animals. Similar
results were observed in hypophysectomized-nephrectomized animals.
These observations indicate that sodium concentration *per se* has
little or no direct effect on the zona glomerulosa to stimulate
aldosterone secretion. In conscious dogs, continuous infusion of
antidiuretic·hormone and hypotonic saline for 14 days resulted in
a decrease in plasma sodium concentration from 143.6 ± 0.5 to 125.0 ±
0.5 mEq/L while plasma aldosterone concentration decreased from
9.1 ± 2.8 to 5.7 ± 1.6 ng/dl (Manning, Guyton, Coleman, and McCaa,
1979). Similar results have been observed in human beings maintained
on antidiuretic hormone (Fichman, Michelakis, and Horton, 1974), and
in several clinical studies investigators have observed normal or
decreased aldosterone secretion in patients with inappropriate ADH
syndrome with plasma sodium concentration markedly reduced below
normal levels.

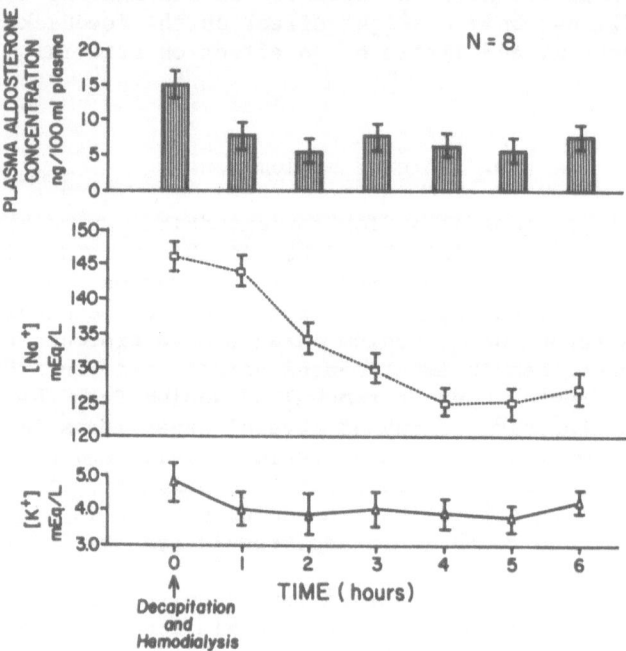

*Figure 2.   The response of plasma aldosterone concentration to acute
             sodium depletion with reduction in serum sodium concen-
             tration by hemodialysis in eight nephrectomized-
             decapitated dogs.   Vertical lines indicate ± SEM.*

III.   REGULATION OF ALDOSTERONE BIOSYNTHESIS DURING SODIUM DEFICIENCY

Despite the controversy over the role of the renin-angiotensin system in the regulation of aldosterone biosynthesis and the control of arterial pressure during sodium deficiency, most investigators have observed parallel increases in activity of the renin-angiotensin system and aldosterone secretion in response to sodium depletion in experimental animals and man. Yet, some studies have indicated that changes in plasma angiotensin II concentration, the active component of the renin-angiotensin system, are not sufficient to explain completely the increased aldosterone secretion associated with sodium deficiency (Blair-West, Coghlan, Cran, *et al.*, 1973; Mendelsohn, Johnston, Doyle, *et al.*, 1972; Boyd, Adamson, Arnold, *et al.*, 1972). Also, several experimental studies have demonstrated that long-term infusion of pressor doses of the octapeptide, angiotensin II, failed to sustain increased aldosterone secretion or plasma aldosterone concentration to the same levels of those observed in untreated sodium deficient animals. In contrast, still other investigators have observed a marked potentiation in adrenal sensitivity to angiotensin II during sodium deficiency (Oelkers, Brown, Fraser, *et al.*, 1974; Hollenberg, Chenitz, Adams and Williams, 1974), indicating that the aldosterone response to angiotensin II may be augmented with decreased sodium intake (Davis, Burwell and Bartter, 1969; Cowley and McCaa, 1976).

Recently we have evaluated the role of the renal renin-angiotensin system in the long-term regulation of aldosterone biosynthesis and the control of arterial blood pressure in intact conscious sodium deficient dogs. Our studies were designed to inhibit renin secretion with the beta-adrenergic blocking agent, propranolol, to block the action of angiotensin II at the vascular smooth muscle and adrenal glomerulosa receptors sites with angiotensin II inhibitory analogues, and to block the conversion of angiotensin I to angiotensin II with angiotensin I converting enzyme inhibitors. It is important to emphasize that these studies were performed in dogs maintained on dietary sodium restriction (5 mEq Na /day) for at least twenty-one days and diuretics were not used at any time in these studies. The reason diuretics were not used is because they stimulate renin secretion to extreme levels and have profound effects on both urinary sodium and potassium excretion.

A.   Aldosterone Response to Long-Term Beta-Adrenergic Blockade
         With Propranolol in Sodium Deficient Dogs

The response of mean arterial pressure, plasma renin activity, serum potassium concentration and plasma aldosterone concentration to long-term infusion of propranolol in eight sodium-depleted dogs is illustrated in Table 1. In sodium deficient dogs, long-term beta-

TABLE 1. THE EFFECTS OF BETA-ADRENERGIC BLOCKADE WITH PROPRANOLOL ON MEAN ARTERIAL BLOOD PRESSURE, PLASMA RENIN ACTIVITY, SERUM POTASSIUM CONCENTRATION AND PLASMA ALDOSTERONE CONCENTRATION IN EIGHT SODIUM-DEPLETED DOGS. VALUES ARE MEANS ± SEM.

Time Days	Dose of Propranolol (mg/day)	Propranolol			
		MAP	PRA	K^+	PAC
0	0	105 ± 5	4.0 ± 0.8	4.3 ± 0.3	35.7 ± 7
1	200	100 ± 3	3.6 ± 0.6	4.6 ± 0.3*	48.3 ± 9*
2	200	97 ± 3	3.4 ± 0.7	4.9 ± 0.3*	54.5 ± 10*
4	200	94 ± 3*	3.1 ± 0.3*	5.1 ± 0.4*	63.5 ± 12*
6	200	90 ± 5*	2.9 ± 0.3*	5.3 ± 0.4*	68.3 ± 9*
8	200	87 ± 2*	2.9 ± 0.4*	5.5 ± 0.5*	60.4 ± 10*
10	200	84 ± 3*	2.1 ± 0.4*	5.3 ± 0.5*	63.4 ± 11*
12	200	86 ± 2*	2.2 ± 0.2*	5.4 ± 0.5*	58.5 ± 7*
14	200	84 ± 3*	1.9 ± 0.2*	5.6 ± 0.5*	64.7 ± 14*
R_2	0	88 ± 4	3.5 ± 0.4	5.1 ± 0.3*	48.4 ± 8*
R_4	0	96 ± 5	3.7 ± 0.5	4.8 ± 0.3*	41.0 ± 7

MAP = Mean arterial pressure (mmHg), PRA = plasma renin activity (ng/ml/hr), $[K^+]$ = serum potassium concentration (mEq/L) and PAC = plasma aldosterone concentration, (ng/100 ml plasma). R_2 and R_4 = 2 and 4 days after stopping propranolol.
*Statistically different from control.

adrenergic blockade with propranolol produced a significant decrease in plasma renin activity and arterial blood pressure. However, plasma aldosterone concentration increased significantly within 24 hours after beginning continuous infusion of propranolol. The increase in aldosterone secretion during propranolol infusion was associated with a significant increase in serum potassium concentration induced by propranolol (McCaa, 1977a). There is a large volume of experimental data indicating that propranolol and other beta-adrenergic blocking agents induce a massive efflux of bulk potassium ions from human red blood cells (Ekman, Manninen, and Salminin, 1969; Minninen, 1970). Despite the decrease in plasma renin activity induced by propranolol, the increase in serum potassium concentration rendered the beta-adrenergic blocker ineffective in defining the role of the renin-angiotensin system in the regulation of aldosterone secretion in sodium deficient dogs. However, future studies with specific inhibitors of renin release, inhibitors that do not have an effect on potassium ion movement, may provide valuable experimental data on the role of the renin-angiotensin system in the regulation of aldosterone biosynthesis and the control of arterial blood pressure during sodium deficiency.

B. Aldosterone Response to Long-Term Infusion of Angiotensin II
       Inhibitory Analogues in Sodium Deficient Dogs

The response of mean arterial pressure, plasma renin activity, and plasma aldosterone concentration to long-term infusion of two angiotensin II inhibitory analogues in eight sodium-depleted dogs is given in Table 2. In sodium deficient dogs the long-term infusion of two potent angiotensin II inhibitory analogues, [Sar^1, Ala^8] angiotensin II and [Sar^1, Ile^8] angiotensin II, reduced arterial blood pressure significantly, and the blood pressure remained below control levels during continuous infusion of the inhibitory analogues of angiotensin II. However, the intrinsic agonistic properties of these inhibitory analogues of angiotensin II on the adrenal glomerulosa cells negated their use for defining the role of the renal renin-angiotensin system in mediating increased aldosterone secretion during sodium deficiency. The agonistic properties of these angiotensin II inhibitory analogues on the adrenal glomerulosa cells have been observed by several other investigators in experimental animals (Williams, McDonnell, Raux, and Hollenberg, 1974; Bravo, Khosla, and Bumpus, 1975; Steele and Lowenstein, 1974; Beckerhoff, Uhlschmid, Furrer, *et al.*, 1975) and in man (Sealey, Wallace, Case, and Laragh, 1976) and have led some investigators to suggest that functional differences exist between the angiotensin II receptors in vascular smooth muscle and in the adrenal glomerulosa cells (Bravo, Khosla, and Bumpus, 1975; Steele and Lowenstein, 1974; Williams, McDonnell, Raux, and Hollenberg, 1974).

TABLE 2. THE EFFECTS OF ANGIOTENSIN II INHIBITORY ANALOGUES [Sar^1, Ala^8] ANGIOTENSIN II AND [Sar^1, Ile^8]ANGIOTENSIN II, ON MEAN ARTERIAL PRESSURE, PLASMA RENIN ACTIVITY AND PLASMA ALDOSTERONE CONCENTRATION IN EIGHT SODIUM DEPLETED DOGS. VALUES ARE MEANS ± SEM.

Time Days	Dose of Analogue µg/kg Min^{-1}	[Sar^1,Ala^8]A II			[Sar^1,Ile^8]A II		
		MAP	PRA	PAC	MAP	PRA	PAC
0	0	105 ± 5	4.2 ± 0.4	36.5 ± 8	107 ± 5	3.9 ± 0.5	38.7 ± 7
1	5	95 ± 3	16.9 ± 1.8*	33.4 ± 7	90 ± 3*	14.8 ± 1.1*	46.4 ± 10
2	5	90 ± 3*	17.3 ± 1.9*	41.3 ± 9	87 ± 2*	17.3 ± 1.3*	51.3 ± 12*
4	5	86 ± 2*	13.4 ± 1.3*	47.3 ± 10*	82 ± 2*	13.8 ± 0.9*	43.4 ± 11
6	5	85 ± 2*	10.5 ± 1.0*	26.4 ± 7*	80 ± 2*	11.5 ± 1.1*	41.0 ± 8
8	5	82 ± 2*	8.3 ± 0.9*	29.5 ± 6*	83 ± 2*	9.6 ± 0.8*	47.5 ± 10*
10	5	80 ± 3*	11.2 ± 1.0*	38.7 ± 9	80 ± 2*	11.4 ± 1.0*	44.6 ± 7
12	5	82 ± 3*	10.6 ± 0.8*	40.3 ± 11	78 ± 3*	10.3 ± 0.9*	51.3 ± 11*
14	5	82 ± 2*	9.8 ± 0.7*	29.3 ± 9*	82 ± 2*	12.7 ± 1.1*	46.5 ± 12*
R$_2$	0	94 ± 4	5.1 ± 0.4	30.7 ± 8	92 ± 4	6.5 ± 0.6	40.6 ± 7
R$_4$	0	100 ± 3	3.3 ± 0.3	34.0 ± 6	100 ± 5	4.4 ± 0.3	41.2 ± 9

MAP = Mean arterial pressure (mmHg), PRA = plasma renin activity (ng/ml/hr) and PAC = plasma aldosterone concentration (ng/100 ml plasma). R$_2$ and R$_4$ = 2 and 4 days after stopping the AII analogues.
*Statistically different from control.

C. Aldosterone Response to Long-Term Administration of
Angiotensin I Converting Enzyme Inhibitors in Sodium Deficient Dogs

The most effective pharmacologic agents used thus far for studying the role of the renin-angiotensin system in the regulation of
aldosterone secretion and the control of arterial blood pressure
during sodium deficiency have been the angiotensin I converting
enzyme inhibitors, teprotide and captopril (McCaa, 1977b; McCaa,
Hall, and McCaa, 1978; Aguilera and Catt, 1978). The response of
mean arterial blood pressure, plasma renin activity, serum potassium
concentration, and plasma aldosterone concentration to long-term
administration of two potent inhibitors of angiotensin I converting
enzyme in eight sodium-depleted dogs is illustrated in Table 3.
Mean arterial blood pressure decreased markedly in sodium deficient
dogs in response to inhibition of angiotensin I converting enzyme
with the nonapeptide, teprotide, and with the orally active synthetic
compound, captopril[2]. Although plasma aldosterone concentration decreased to sodium-replete levels in response to long-term continuous
infusion of teprotide, plasma aldosterone concentration failed to
return to sodium-replete levels during long-term oral administration
of captopril. However, a positive correlation was observed between
changes in serum potassium concentration and plasma aldosterone
concentration during long-term administration of these angiotensin I
converting enzyme inhibitors. The changes in serum potassium concentration during administration of the inhibitors of angiotensin I converting enzyme are shown in Table 3. In response to continuous infusion of teprotide, serum potassium concentration decreased significantly while serum potassium concentration failed to change from
control levels during long-term oral administration of the synthetic
inhibitor, captopril. The mechanism(s) responsible for the changes
in serum potassium concentration during teprotide infusion, and the
lack of changes in serum potassium concentration during long-term
oral administration of captopril, remain to be elucidated. Nevertheless, these data demonstrate the importance of both angiotensin II
and potassium ions in the regulation of aldosterone biosynthesis
during sodium deficiency.

D. Evidence for an Important Role of Both Potassium and
Angiotensin II in the Control of Aldosterone Biosynthesis
During Dietary Sodium Restriction

We have previously described experimental studies in which
beta-adrenergic blockade with propranolol produced a significant
decrease in plasma renin activity and arterial blood pressure in
sodium deficient dogs. Despite the significant decrease in plasma
renin activity, plasma aldosterone concentration increased markedly.

---

[2]Teprotide and captopril were supplied by the Squibb Institute for
Medical Research, Princeton, NJ.

TABLE 3.   THE EFFECTS OF ANGIOTENSIN I CONVERTING ENZYME INHIBITORS, TEPROTIDE AND CAPTOPRIL, ON MEAN ARTERIAL PRESSURE, PLASMA RENIN ACTIVITY, SERUM POTASSIUM CONCENTRATION AND PLASMA ALDOSTERONE CONCENTRATION IN EIGHT SODIUM DEPLETED DOGS.

Time Days	Dose of Teprotide µg/kg min -1	Teprotide			
		MAP	PRA	$[K^+]$	PAC
0	0	100 ± 5	3.9 ± 0.4	4.4 ± 0.5	38.7 ± 8
1	10	90 ± 3*	37.3 ± 3.4*	4.2 ± 0.5	11.2 ± 3*
2	10	80 ± 2*	34.7 ± 4.2*	4.0 ± 0.3*	9.3 ± 2*
4	10	72 ± 2*	32.2 ± 3.9*	3.9 ± 0.4*	10.4 ± 3*
6	10	76 ± 2*	26.7 ± 4.1*	3.7 ± 0.3*	8.9 ± 2*
8	10	72 ± 2*	19.3 ± 2.9*	3.7 ± 0.4*	7.3 ± 1*
10	10	70 ± 2*	21.6 ± 3.0*	3.9 ± 0.5*	5.1 ± 2*
12	10	68 ± 2*	15.9 ± 2.7*	3.7 ± 0.3*	6.8 ± 2*
14	10	70 ± 3*	13.6 ± 2.3*	3.7 ± 0.4*	7.9 ± 3*
R_2	0	95 ± 3	6.3 ± 1.4*	4.0 ± 0.4*	30.7 ± 6*
R_4	0	100 ± 3	4.3 ± 0.9	4.1 ± 0.5	34.5 ± 7

MAP = Mean arterial pressure (mmHg), PRA = plasma renin activity (ng/ml/hr), $[K^+]$ = serum potassium concentration (mEq/L) and PAC = plasma aldosterone concentration, (ng/100 ml plasma). R_2 and R_4 = 2 and 4 days after stopping teprotide.
*Statistically significant from control.

TABLE 3 (con't). THE EFFECTS OF ANGIOTENSIN I CONVERTING ENZYME INHIBITORS, TEPROTIDE AND CAPTOPRIL, ON MEAN ARTERIAL PRESSURE, PLASMA RENIN ACTIVITY, SERUM POTASSIUM CONCENTRATION AND PLASMA ALDOSTERONE CONCENTRATION IN EIGHT SODIUM DEPLETED DOGS.

Time Days	Dose of Captopril (mg/kg/day)	Captopril			
		MAP	PRA	$[K^+]$	PAC
0	0	107 ± 5	5.1 ± 0.6	4.4 ± 0.5	41.2 ± 8
1	20	82 ± 3*	34.2 ± 4.3*	4.5 ± 0.4	32.0 ± 7*
2	20	72 ± 3*	21.7 ± 3.8*	4.3 ± 0.4	21.7 ± 6*
4	20	75 ± 2*	17.3 ± 2.6*	4.5 ± 0.5	16.3 ± 6*
6	20	68 ± 2*	15.8 ± 2.7*	4.6 ± 0.5	22.5 ± 7*
8	20	70 ± 3*	11.6 ± 1.9*	4.5 ± 0.5	17.3 ± 6*
10	20	70 ± 2*	9.3 ± 1.7*	4.6 ± 0.5	14.7 ± 5*
12	20	72 ± 3*	12.4 ± 1.9*	4.3 ± 0.5	18.3 ± 4*
14	20	70 ± 3*	8.9 ± 1.1*	4.5 ± 0.5	20.7 ± 5*
R_2	0	94 ± 4	6.3 ± 0.9	4.4 ± 0.5	38.4 ± 8
R_4	0	105 ± 5	5.7 ± 0.5	4.3 ± 0.5	38.7 ± 8

MAP = Mean arterial pressure (mmHg), PRA = plasma renin activity (ng/ml/hr), $[K^+]$ = serum potassium concentration (mEq/L) and PAC = plasma aldosterone concentration, (ng/100 ml plasma). R_2 and R_4 = 2 and 4 days after stopping captopril.
*Statistically significant from control.

The increase in plasma aldosterone concentration was associated
with a significant increase in serum potassium concentration induced
by propranolol. The response of arterial blood pressure, serum
potassium concentration, and plasma aldosterone concentration in
sodium-depleted dogs maintained on both propranolol and captopril
and then after kayexalate was administered to prevent absorption
of potassium is shown in Figure 3. In response to propranolol infusion for 14 days in sodium deficient dogs, arterial blood pressure decreased from 103 ±4 to 82 ±3 mm Hg, serum potassium concentration increased from 4.3 ±0.5 to 5.5 ±0.5 mEq/L, and plasma aldosterone concentration increased from 36.4 ±8.6 to 63.2 ±12.7 ng/dl.
In the same animals after complete inhibition of angiotensin I converting enzyme with captopril, arterial pressure decreased from 82
±3 to 70 ±2 mm Hg, serum potassium concentration failed to change
significantly, averaging 5.3 ±0.3 mEq/L, and plasma aldosterone
concentration decreased from 63.2 ±12.7 to 31.3 ±7.7 ng/dl. Since
angiotensin II formation was totally blocked by captopril in the
animals maintained on propranolol infusion, it was assumed that the
failure of aldosterone secretion to decrease to sodium-replete
levels was due to the increase in serum potassium concentration.
Additional studies proved this to be true. Administration of
kayexalate, which prevented the absorption of potassium in the
animals maintained on both propranolol and captopril, resulted in
a significant decrease in serum potassium concentration, and plasma
aldosterone concentration decreased to near sodium-replete levels.

IV. THE RENIN-ANGIOTENSIN-ALDOSTERONE SYSTEM IN EXPERIMENTAL RENOVASCULAR HYPERTENSION

The role of the renin-angiotensin-aldosterone system in the
development and maintenance of experimental renovascular hypertension has been studied extensively in animal models (Carpenter,
Davis, and Ayers, 1961; Singer, Losito, and Salmon, 1963; McCaa,
Richardson, McCaa, *et al*., 1965; Blair-West, Coghlan, Denton, *et
al*., 1968; Liard, Cowley, McCaa, *et al*., 1974). In experimental
renovascular benign hypertension, plasma renin activity, blood
angiotensin II concentration, and plasma aldosterone concentration
are elevated during the early developmental phase of hypertension.
However, plasma renin activity, blood angiotensin II concentration,
and plasma aldosterone concentration return to near-normal levels
after three to five days, while arterial blood pressure remains
elevated. In contrast, in experimental renovascular malignant
hypertension, plasma renin activity, blood angiotensin II concentration, and plasma aldosterone concentration remain elevated
throughout the development and maintenance of the hypertension.
Clinical studies support these observations (Laragh, Ulick,
Januszewicz, *et al*., 1960). Most investigators agree that the
elevated arterial blood pressure in malignant hypertensive models

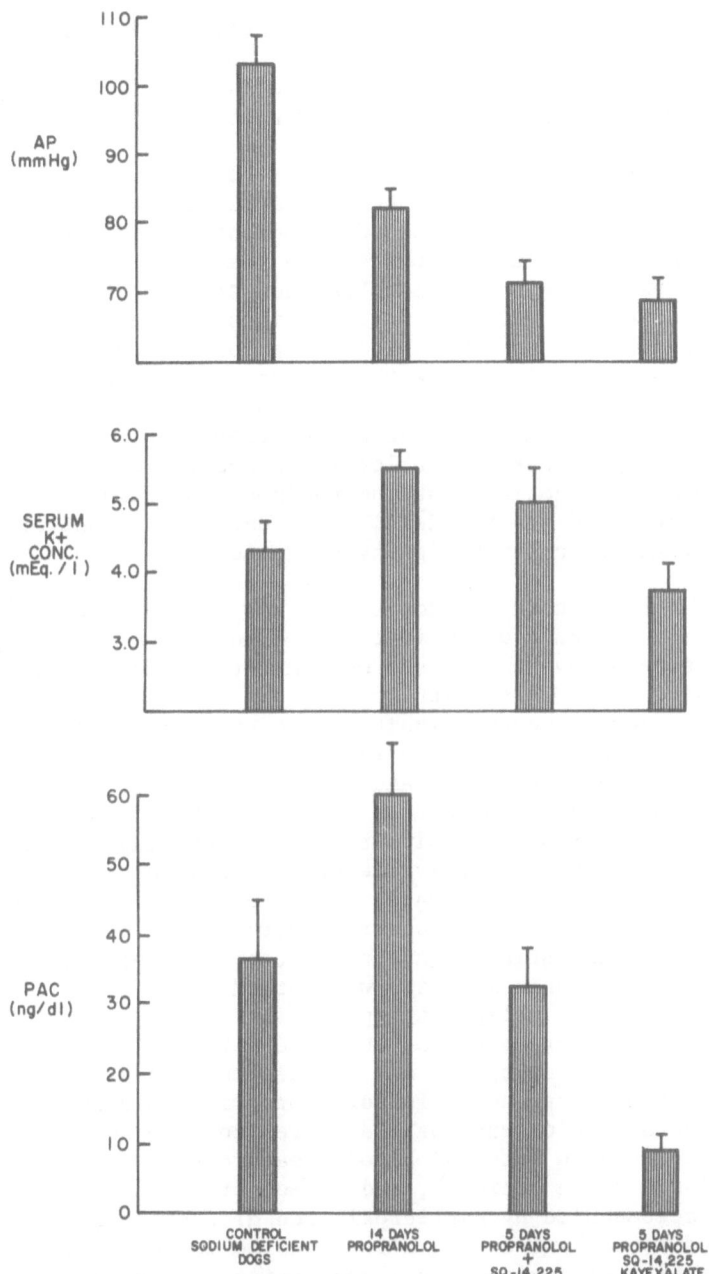

Figure 3. The response of arterial blood pressure, serum potassium
concentration, and plasma aldosterone concentration to
kayexalate administration in sodium deficient dogs
maintained on long-term administration of propranolol and
captopril. Vertical lines indicate ± SEM.

is mediated by the powerful vasoconstrictive action of the octapeptide, angiotensin II, on the vascular smooth muscle cells, while
the elevated aldosterone secretion rate is produced by the action
of angiotensin II on the adrenal glomerulosa cells.

Recently, the potent angiotensin I converting enzyme inhibitors
teprotide and captopril, have been used to evaluate the role of the
renin-angiotensin system in the development and maintenance of
experimental renovascular hypertension (Watkins, Davis, Freeman,
et al., 1978a; Watkins, Davis, Freeman, *et al.*, 1978b; Bengis,
Coleman, Young, and McCaa, 1978). Administration of the angiotensin I converting enzyme inhibitors prior to, and for several
days after unilateral renal artery constriction and contralateral
nephrectomy in dogs caused a delay in the development of hypertension. However, one week later the arterial blood pressure
reached the same hypertensive levels as control one-kidney hypertensive dogs, indicating that the renin-angiotensin system need
never be activated for the development and maintenance of chronic
one-kidney renovascular benign hypertension.

In our laboratory Dr. Roy Bengis has evaluated the effects
of long-term blockade of angiotensin II formation in normotensive,
one- and two-kidney benign, and one- and two-kidney malignant
hypertensive rat models, with the use of the orally active angiotensin I converting enzyme inhibitor, captopril. A decrease in
arterial blood pressure and an increase in urinary sodium excretion
were observed in normal rats and in sodium-depleted rats during
long-term angiotensin converting enzyme inhibition with captopril.
In those groups of hypertensive rats in which plasma renin activity
was normal or only moderately elevated, i.e., in one- and two-
kidney benign hypertensive rats, a progressive but slow decrease in
arterial blood pressure was observed during a seven day period of
captopril administration. In those groups of hypertensive rats in
which the plasma renin activity was markedly elevated, i.e., in
one- and two-kidney malignant hypertensive rats, a precipitous fall
in arterial blood pressure was observed within 24 hours after the
administration of captopril, and the decrease in arterial pressure
persisted throughout the period of captopril administration. The
hypotensive action of captopril appeared to have two components:
a rapid decrease in arterial blood pressure that was proportional
to the plasma renin activity, and a slow progressive component
that was accompanied by natriuresis and diuresis. Since circulating and renal kinins have been shown to increase during the
administration of angiotensin I converting enzyme inhibitors
(McCaa, Hall, and McCaa, 1978), the hypotensive and natriuretic
effects of captopril may be due in part to decreased circulating
and renal levels of angiotensin II, and in part to increased
circulating and renal levels of kinins.

Previous studies (Liard, Cowley, McCaa, *et al.*, 1974) have demonstrated that plasma renin activity and plasma aldosterone concentration return to near control levels within 3 days after renal artery constriction in unilaterally nephrectomized dogs despite arterial blood pressure remaining markedly elevated (one-kidney benign Goldblatt hypertension). However, plasma renin activity and plasma aldosterone concentration remain markedly elevated in man and experimental animals with malignant hypertension. The plasma aldosterone concentration in normal, in sodium-depleted, in benign hypertensive, and in malignant hypertensive rats before and 14 days after captopril administration is illustrated in Figure 4. Studies in renovascular hypertensive animals and in man with moderate or marked elevations in plasma renin activity and plasma aldosterone concentrations indicate that plasma aldosterone concentrations return to near control levels during inhibition of angiotensin I converting enzyme with captopril. These observations support the concept that elevated aldosterone secretion in malignant hypertensive animals and man is mediated by increased activity of the renin-angiotensin system. However, it remains to be determined whether hypertension would persist with elevated aldosterone secretion in malignant hypertensive models during angiotensin converting enzyme inhibition with captopril.

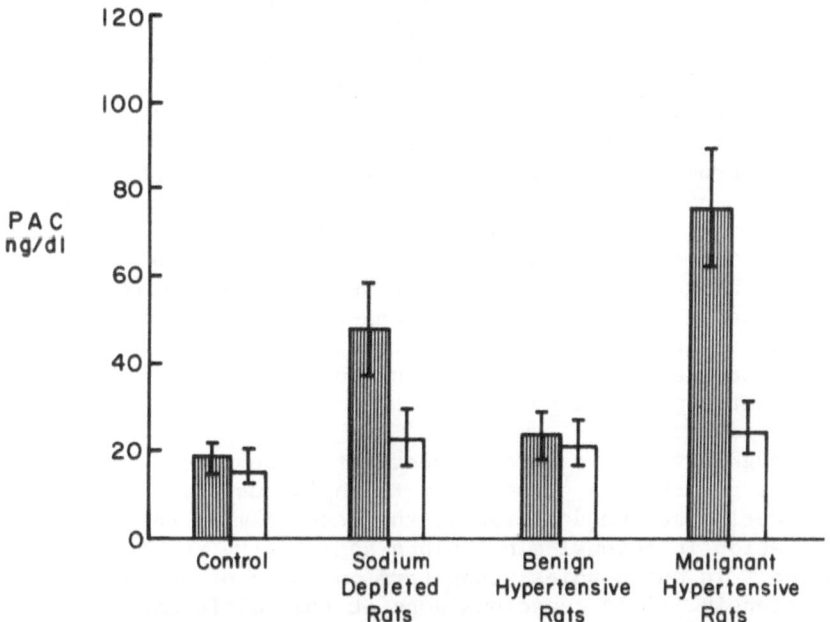

Figure 4. Plasma aldosterone concentration in control, sodium-depleted, benign hypertensive, and malignant hypertensive rats before and 14 days after administration of captopril. Vertical lines indicate ±SEM.

V. CONCLUSIONS

During the past twelve years we have collected considerable
quantitative data in animals and man under a variety of different
experimental conditions in an effort to develop a composite control
systems analysis for the regulation of aldosterone biosynthesis.
Though all the details of the regulatory mechanisms controlling
aldosterone biosynthesis have not been evaluated, our studies
demonstrate several important facts that we believe will be
significant in finally understanding the regulation of aldosterone
biosynthesis.

Dietary sodium restriction or removal of sodium from the body
by any of several means results in marked increases in aldosterone
biosynthesis in experimental animals and man. Since marked changes
in sodium concentration *per se* have little or no direct effect on the
adrenal biosynthesis of aldosterone, the aldosterone response to
alterations in sodium balance must be mediated through some other
mechanism. Many investigators believe that the aldosterone response
to alterations in sodium balance is mediated by the activity of the
renal renin-angiotensin system. Yet, still other investigators
believe some additional unidentified factor(s) or undefined
mechanism(s) may be involved in the regulation of aldosterone
biosynthesis during sodium deficiency. Indeed, aldosterone
secretion fails to increase in hypophysectomized animals or man in
response to sodium deficiency, despite a normal increase in plasma
renin activity and blood angiotensin II concentration, suggesting
a permissive role for some unknown pituitary factor(s). Our
studies demonstrate that pressor doses of angiotensin II are
required to produce a significant increase in aldosterone secretion
in conscious animals maintained on normal sodium intake. Long-term
infusion of angiotensin II at a rate of 15 ng/kg/min, a rate that
increased blood angiotensin II concentration five hundred per cent,
caused only a one hundred per cent increase in plasma aldosterone
concentration. In sharp contrast, long-term infusion of potassium
chloride at a rate that increased serum potassium concentration
only seventeen per cent caused a four hundred per cent increase in
plasma aldosterone concentration.

Although several research investigators have postulated that
the adrenal glomerulosa sensitivity to angiotensin II increases
markedly during sodium deficiency, the mechanism(s) responsible for
the alteration in adrenal glomerulosa sensitivity remains to be
elucidated. In our studies, long-term infusion of angiotensin II
and angiotensin III in conscious dogs at four different rates
produced almost the same percentage change in plasma aldosterone
concentration before and after dietary sodium restriction. Although
the dose-response curve was shifted upwards, there was very little
change in the slope of the curve. It is noteworthy that our studies

were performed during long-term steady state conditions while the earlier studies were acute studies lasting at most only a few hours.

Most of our knowledge of the role of the renin-angiotensin system in the regulation of aldosterone secretion during sodium deficiency is based on acute studies performed in animals or man in which sodium deficiency was induced by low sodium intake and the use of diuretics. However, diuretics have profound effects on the activity of the renin-angiotensin system and urinary excretion of sodium and potassium. In our studies, sodium deficiency was produced entirely by dietary sodium restriction, and diuretics were not used at any time. The importance of the role of the renin-angiotensin system in mediating increased aldosterone biosynthesis in our experimental model was confirmed with the use of the angiotensin I converting enzyme inhibitors, teprotide and captopril. In sodium deficient dogs maintained on long-term infusion of teprotide, aldosterone secretion decreased to sodium-replete levels; however, teprotide increased urinary potassium excretion and decreased serum potassium concentration. In contrast, in sodium deficient dogs maintained on long-term administration of captopril, aldosterone secretion decreased by fifty per cent but remained significantly elevated above sodium-replete levels; however, serum potassium concentration failed to decrease in response to captopril administration. These observations suggest that both angiotensin II and potassium ions play important roles in the regulation of aldosterone biosynthesis during sodium deficiency induced by dietary sodium restriction alone. Additional studies using kayexalate to block potassium absorption in sodium deficient animals maintained on long-term administration of propranolol and captopril proved that potassium also played an important role in the control of aldosterone secretion during sodium deficiency induced by dietary sodium restriction.

Despite the controversy over the role of the renin-angiotensin system in the long-tern regulation of aldosterone biosynthesis or the control of aldosterone secretion during sodium deficiency, most investigators agree that the markedly elevated aldosterone secretory rate observed in human beings and experimental animals with malignant hypertension is mediated by increased activity of the renal renin-angiotensin system. Studies in our laboratory indicate that aldosterone secretion decreases to near control levels during long-term blockade of angiotensin II formation with captopril in animals with benign and malignant hypertension in which plasma renin activity and blood angiotensin II concentrations are moderately or markedly increased.

REFERENCES

Aguilera, G., Baukal, A., Fujita, K., Hauger, R. and Catt, K. J. (1978). Metabolism and biological activities of angiotensin peptides in isolated rat glomerulosa cells. Abstracts--The Endocrine Soc. p. 80 (Abstract).

Aguilera, G. and Catt, K. J. (1978). Regulation of aldosterone secretion by the renin-angiotensin system during sodium restriction in rats. Physiol. Sci. 75:4057-4061.

Ames, R. P., Borkowski, A. J., Sicinski, A. M. and Laragh, J. H. (1965). Prolonged infusions of angiotensin II and norepinephrine on blood pressure, electrolyte balance, and aldosterone and cortisol secretion in normal man and in cirrhosis with ascites. J. Clin. Invest. 44:1171-1186.

Bayard, R., Cooke, C. R., Tiller, D. J., Beitins, I. Z., Kowarski, A., Walker, W. G. and Migeon, C. J. (1971). Regulation of aldosterone secretion in anephric man. J. Clin. Invest. 50:1585-1595.

Beckerhoff, R., Uhlschmid, G., Furrer, J., Nussberger, J., Schmied, U., Vetter, W. J. and Siegenthaler, W. (1975). *In vivo* effects of angiotensin antagonists on plasma aldosterone in the dog. Eur. J. Pharmacol. 34:363-367.

Bengis, R. G., Coleman, T. G., Young, D. B., and McCaa, R. E. (1978). Long-term blockade of angiotensin formation in various normotensive and hypertensive rat models using converting enzyme inhibitor (SQ 14,225). Circ. Res. 43(Suppl. 1):45-53.

Biron, P., Koiw, E., Nowaczynski, W., Brouillet, J. and Genest, J. (1961). Effects of intravenous infusions of valine-5 angiotensin II and other pressor agents on urinary electrolytes and corticosteroids, including aldosterone. J. Clin. Invest. 40:338-347.

Blair-West, J. R., Coghlan, J. P., Cran, E., Denton, D. A., Funder, J. W. and Scoggins, B. A. (1973). Increased aldosterone secretion during sodium depletion with inhibition of renin release. Am. J. Physiol. 224:1409-1414.

Blair-West, J. R., Coghlan, J. P., Denton, D. A., Funder, J. W. and Scoggins, B. A. (1972). Role of the renin-angiotensin system in control of aldosterone secretion. Adv. Exp. Med. Biol. 17:167-181.

Blair-West, J. R., Coghlan, J. P., Denton, D. A., Orchard, E., Scoggins, B. A. and Wright, R. D. (1968). Renin-angiotensin-aldosterone system and sodium balance in experimental renal hypertension. Endocrinology 83:1199-1209.

Boyd, G. W., Adamson, A. R., Arnold, M., James, V. H. T. and Peart, W. S. (1972). Role of angiotensin II in the control of aldosterone in man. Clin. Sci. 42:91-104.

Boyd, J., Mulrow, P. J., Palmore, W. P., and Silvo, P. (1973). Importance of potassium in the regulation of aldosterone production. Circ. Res. 32-33(Suppl. 1):39-45.

Bravo, E. L., Khosla, M. C. and Bumpus, F. M. (1975). Vascular and adrenocortical responses to a specific antagonist of angiotensin II. Am. J. Physiol. 228:110-114.

Campbell, W. B., Brooks, S. N. and Pettinger, W. A. (1974). Angiotensin II- and angiotensin III induced aldosterone release *in vivo* in the rat. Science 184:994-996.

Carey, R. M., Vaughan, D., Jr., Peach, M. J., and Ayers, C. (1978). Activity of [des-Aspartyl[1]]-angiotensin II and angiotensin II in man--Differences in blood pressure and adrenocortical responses during normal and low sodium intake. J. Clin. Invest. 61:20-31.

Carpenter, C. C. J., Davis, J. O. and Ayers, C. R. (1961). Relation of renin angiotensin II and experimental renal hypertension to aldosterone secretion. J. Clin. Invest. 40:2026-2042.

Coghlan, J. P., Denton, D. A., Fan, J. S. K., McDougall, J. G. and Scoggins, B. A. (1977). Further studies on the ACTH induced hypertension in sheep--Involvement of new hypertensinogenic steroid hormones. In: *Juvenile Hypertension*. (New, M. I. and Levine, L. S., eds.), pp. 69-77, Raven Press, New York.

Coleman, T. G., McCaa, R. E., McCaa, C. S. (1974). Effect of angiotensin II on aldosterone secretion in the conscious rat. J. Endocrinol. 60:421-427.

Cowley, A. W., Jr. and McCaa, R. E. (1976). Acute and chronic dose response relationships of angiotensin, aldosterone and arterial pressure at varying levels of sodium intake. Circ. Res. 39: 788-797.

Davis, W. W., Burwell, L. and Bartter, F. C. (1969). Inhibition of the effects of angiotensin II on adrenal steroid production by dietary sodium. Proc. Natl. Acad. Sci. USA 63:718-723.

Ekman, A., Manninen, V. and Salminin, S. (1969). Ion movements in red cells treated with propranolol. Acta Physiol. Scand. 75:333-334.

Fichman, M. P., Michelakis, A. M., and Horton, R. (1974) Regulation of aldosteorne in the syndrome of inappropriate antidiuretic hormone secretion (SIADH). J. Clin. Endocrinol. Metab. 39:136-144.

Fraser, R., James, V. H., Brown, J. J., Isaac, P., Lever, A. F. and Robertson, J. I. S. (1965). Effects of angiotensin and of furosemide on plasma aldosterone, corticosterone, cortisol and renin in man. Lancet 2:989-991.

Genest, J., Nowaczynski, W., Koiw, E., Sandor, T. and Biron, P. (1960). Adrenocortical function in essential hypertension. In: *Essential Hypertension* (Bock, K. D. and Cottier, P. T., eds.), pp. 126-146, Springer-Verlag, Berlin.

Hollenberg, N. K., Chenitz, W. R., Adams, D. F. and Williams, G. H. (1974). Reciprocal influence of salt intake on adrenal glomerulosa and renal vascular responses to angiotensin II in normal man. J. Clin. Invest. 54:34-42.

Horton, R. (1969). Stimulation and suppression of aldosterone in
    plasma of normal man and primary aldosteronism. J. Clin.
    Invest. 48:1230-1236.
Kastner, P. R. and McCaa, R. E. (1978). Blood pressure response to
    chronic infusion of ACTH, cortisol and aldosterone in adrenal-
    ectomized dogs. Physiologist 21:62 (Abstract).
Laragh, J. H., Angers, M., Kelly, W. G. and Lieberman, S. (1960).
    Hypotensive agents and pressor substances: Effects of
    epinephrine, norepinephrine, angiotensin II, and others on the
    secretory rate of aldosterone in man. JAMA 174:234-240.
Laragh, J. H. and Stoerk, H. C. (1957). Study of the mechanism of
    secretion of the sodium-retaining hormone (aldosterone).
    J. Clin. Invest. 36:383-392.
Laragh, J. H., Ulick, S., Januszewicz, S., Deming, Q. B., Kelly,
    W. G., and Lieberman, S. (1960). Aldosterone secretion and
    primary and malignant hypertension. J. Clin. Invest. 39:1091-
    1106.
Liard, J. F., Cowley, A. W., Jr., McCaa, R. E., McCaa, C. S., and
    Guyton, A. C. (1974). Renin, aldosterone, body fluid volumes,
    and the baroreceptor reflex in the development and reversal
    of Goldblatt hypertension in conscious dogs. Circ. Res.
    34:549-559.
Manninen, V. (1970). Movements of sodium and potassium ions and
    their tracers in propranolol-treated red cells and diaphragm
    muscle. Acta Physiol. Scand. 355(Suppl. 1):1-76.
Manning, R. D., Jr., Guyton, A. C., Coleman, T. G., and McCaa, R. E.
    (1979). Hypertension in dogs during antidiuretic hormone and
    hypotonic saline infusion. Am. J. Physiol. 236:H314-H322.
Marieb, N. J. and Mulrow, P. J. (1965). Role of renin-angiotensin
    system in the regulation of aldosterone secretion in the rat.
    Endocrinology 76:657-664.
McCaa, C. S., Richardson, T. Q., McCaa, R. E., Sulya, L. L. and
    Guyton, A. C. (1965). Aldosterone secretion by dogs during
    the developmental phase of Goldblatt hypertension. J.
    Endocrinol. 33:97-102.
McCaa, R. E. (1977a). Response of arterial pressure and aldosterone
    biosynthesis to continuous infusion of propranolol in intact
    conscious sodium deficient dogs. Physiologist 20:62
    (Abstract).
McCaa, R. E. (1977b). Role of the renin-angiotensin system in the
    regulation of aldosterone biosynthesis and arterial pressure
    during sodium deficiency. Circ. Res. 40(Suppl. 1):157-162.
McCaa, R. E. (1978). Aldosterone response to long-term infusion
    of angiotensin II and angiotensin III in conscious dogs before
    and after dietary sodium restriction. Endocrinology 103:458-
    464.
McCaa, R. E., Hall, J. E., and McCaa, C. S. (1978). The effects of
    angiotensin I-converting enzyme inhibitors on arterial blood
    pressure and urinary sodium excretion--Role of the renal renin-
    angiotensin and kallikrein-kinin systems. Circ. Res.
    43(Suppl. 1):32-39.

McCaa, R. E., McCaa, C. S., Cowley, A. W., Jr., Ott, C. E., and
    Guyton, A. C. (1973). Stimulation of aldosterone secretion
    by hemorrhage in dogs after nephrectomy and decapitation.
    Circ. Res. 22: 356-362.
McCaa, R. E., McCaa, C. S., and Guyton, A. C. (1975). Role of
    angiotensin II and potassium in the long-term regulation of
    aldosterone secretion in intact conscious dogs. Circ. Res.
    36-37 (Suppl. 1): 57-67.
McCaa, R. E., McCaa, C. S., Read, V. H., and Bower, J. D. (1972a).
    Influence of hemodialysis on plasma aldosterone concentration
    in nephrectomized patients. Trans. Am. Soc. Artif. Intern.
    Organs 18: 239-243.
McCaa, R. E., McCaa, C. S., Read, D. G., Bower, J. D., and Guyton,
    A. C. (1972b). Increased plasma aldosterone concentration
    in response to hemodialysis in nephrectomized man. Circ.
    Res. 31: 473-480.
McCaa, R. E., Muirhead, E. E., Pitcock, J. A., Kastner, P. R., and
    McCaa, C. S. (1978). The response of plasma aldosterone
    concentration and arterial blood pressure to long-term infusion
    of adrenocorticotropic hormone (ACTH) in conscious dogs during
    sodium repletion and sodium depletion. Abstracts - The Endo-
    crine Society, p. 401.
McCaa, R. E., Ott, C. E., and McCaa, C. S. (1974). Relation
    between plasma potassium concentration and aldosterone sec-
    retion in nephrectomized dogs. IRCS 2: 1263.
McCaa, R. E., Read, V. H., Cowley, A. W., Jr., Bower, J. D., Smith,
    G. V., and McCaa, C. S. (1973). Influence of acute stimuli on
    plasma aldosterone concentration in anephric man and kidney
    allograft recipients. Circ. Res. 33: 313-322.
McCaa, R. E., Young, D. B., Guyton, A. C., and McCaa, C. S. (1974).
    Evidence for a role of an unidentified pituitary factor in
    regulating aldosterone secretion during altered sodium balance.
    Circ. Res. 34-35 (Suppl. 1): 15-25.
Mendelsohn, F. A. O., Johnston, C. I., Doyle, A. E., Scoggins,
    B. A., Denton, D. A., and Coghlan, J. P. (1972). Renin, angio-
    tensin II, and adrenal corticosteroid relationships during
    sodium deprivation and angiotensin infusion in normotensive
    and hypertensive man. Circ. Res. 31: 728-739.
Muller, J. (1965). Aldosterone stimulation *in vitro*. 1. Evalu-
    ation of assay procedure and determination of aldosterone-
    stimulating activity in a human urine extract. Acta Endocrinol.
    (Kbh). 48: 283-296.
New, M. I., Peterson, R. E., Saenger, P., and Levine, L. S. (1976).
    Evidence for an unidentified ACTH-induced steroid hormone
    causing hypertension. J. Clin. Endocrinol. Metab. 43: 1283-
    1293.
New, M. I., Saenger, P. H., Peterson, R. E., and Ulick, S. (1975).
    Evidence for an ACTH stimulable hormone causing hypertension.
    Bull. N. Y. Acad. Med. 51: 1179.

Newton, M. A. and Laragh, J. H. (1968). Effect of corticotropin on aldosterone excretion and plasma renin in normal subjects in essential hypertension and in primary aldosteronism. J. Clin. Endocrinol. Metab. 28: 1006-1013.

Oelkers, W., Brown, J. J., Fraser, R., Lever, A. R., Morton, J. J., and Robertson, J. I. S. (1974). Sensitization of the adrenal cortex to angiotensin II in sodium-deplete man. Circ. Res. 34: 69-77.

Saruta, T., Cook, R., and Kaplan, N. M. (1972). Adrenocortical steroidogenesis. Studies on the mechanisms of action of angiotensin and electrolytes. J. Clin. Invest. 51: 2239-2245.

Scoggins, B. A., Butkus, A., Coghlan, J. P., Denton, D. A., Fan, J. S., Humphrey, T. J., and Whitworth, J. A. (1978). Adrenocorticotropic hormone-induced hypertension in sheep. A model for the study of the effect of steroid hormones on blood pressure. Circ. Res. 43 (Suppl. 1): 76-81.

Sealey, J. E., Wallace, J. M., Case, D. B., and Laragh, J. H. (1976). Inhibition of aldosterone secretion by converting enzyme blockade contrasted with the agonist/antagonist effect of an angiotensin II analogue. Abstracts - The Endocrine Society, p. 160.

Singer, B., Losito, C., and Salmon, S. (1963). Aldosterone and corticosterone secretion rates in rats with experimental renal hypertension. Acta Endocrinol. (Kbh) 44: 505-518.

Steele, J. M., Jr. and Lowenstein, J. (1974). Differential effects of an angiotensin II analogue on pressor and adrenal receptors in the rabbit. Circ. Res. 35: 592-600.

Watkins, B. E., Davis, J. O., Freeman, R. H., DeForrest, J. M., and Stephens, G. A. (1978a). Continuous angiotensin II blockade throughout the acute phase of one-kidney hypertension in the dog. Circ. Res. 42: 813-821.

Watkins, B. E., Davis, J. O. Freeman, R. H., Stephens, G. A., and DeForrest, J. M. (1978b). Effects of the oral converting enzyme inhibitor (SQ 14,225) on one-kidney hypertension in the dog. Proc. Soc. Exptl. Biol. Med. 157: 245-249.

Weidmann, P., Horton, R., Maxwell, M. H., Franklin, S. S., and Fichman, M. (1973). Dynamic studies of aldosterone in anephric man. Kidney Internat. 4: 280-288.

Williams, G. H., Bailey, G. L., Hampers, C. L., Lauler, D. P., Merrill, J. P., Underwood, R. H., Blair-West, J. R., Coghlan, J. P., Denton, D. A., Scoggins, B. A., and Wright, D. R. (1973). Studies on the metabolism of aldosterone in chronic renal failure and anephric man. Kidney Internat. 4: 280-288.

Williams, G. H., McDonnell, L. M., Raux, M. C., and Hollenberg, N. K. (1974). Evidence for different angiotensin II receptors in rat adrenal glomerulosa and rabbit vascular smooth muscle cells. Circ. Res. 34: 384-390.

DISCUSSION AFTER DR. McCAA'S PAPER

Dr. Jawadi
   I have a question about the pH regulation for aldosterone secretion. Does acidosis have any influence on the secretion of aldosterone?

Dr. McCaa
   Earlier we performed studies on the influence of hemorrhage on
aldosterone secretion in decapitated, nephrectomized dogs. This
preparation, which we refer to as an isolated adrenal preparation,
was maintained on artificial respiration while total body fluid
volume and electrolyte concentrations were controlled by hemodialysis. Removal of 100 ml. of blood resulted in a decrease in arterial
blood pressure to 70 mm Hg, acidosis, and the efflux of potassium
ions from the cells into the plasma. Plasma potassium concentration
and plasma aldosterone concentration increased markedly after hemorrhage. However, aldosterone secretion failed to increase when we
prevented plasma potassium concentration from increasing by hemodialysis during hemorrhage. Although the preparation became acid-
otic, we concluded from these studies that the aldosterone response
to hemorrhage in the decapitated, nephrectomized preparation was due
to the marked increase in plasma potassium concentration. The effect
of acidosis *per se* on aldosterone secretion has never been studied.

Dr. Jawadi
   I think I asked this same question last night, but could some-
one comment on ADH secretion in rats who have malignant hypertension?
Someone in Europe has shown that they have a low responsiveness to
ADH. They also measured ADH in these rats and found it to be high.
Has anyone seen this effect?

Dr. McCaa
   We have performed a number of different research studies in the
decapitated, nephrectomized or isolated adrenal preparation. This
preparation is extremely volume sensitive. We have used several
vasoactive substances to maintain arterial blood pressure at 100 mm
Hg, including norepinephrine, angiotensin II, and ADH. Angiotensin II stimulates aldosterone secretion markedly in this preparation
while norepinephrine and ADH have no effect on aldosterone secretion.
On the other hand, I am aware of several studies by different investigators who are measuring ADH concentration in hypertensive animals
and human beings. In experimental renovascular hypertensive animals,
in particular malignant hypertensive animals, blood ADH levels are
extremely high. Dr. David Young also has recently observed marked
elevations in blood ADH levels in malignant hypertensive dogs, while
blood ADH levels were observed to be normal in benign, high-renin
hypertensive dogs (unpublished). Recently, Mohring reported that
plasma ADH levels were elevated 4 to 5 times normal in Sprague-Dawley
rats with two-kidney malignant hypertension. In some of the malig-

nant hypertensive rats, injection of an antiserum specific for
arginine vasopressin caused the blood pressure to return towards
normal, indicating that ADH may cause significant systemic vasoconstriction and may contribute to the development of malignant
renal hypertension. However, Bengis observed that captopril,
which blocks the formation of angiotensin II, lowers the arterial
blood pressure in one- and two-kidney benign and one- and two-
kidney malignant hypertensive rats. It is obvious that further
studies are needed to quantitate the role of ADH in the development
and maintenance of experimental hypertension.

Dr. Freeman
     Bob, I have a question about your earlier studies with the
angiotensin analogues, where you saw a transient decrease in plasma
aldosterone but you were unable to keep it suppressed. In two of
the slides you showed, two of your animals also had increases in
plasma cortisol, and in those animals you had a nice decrease in
arterial pressure. I was wondering if they could have been stressed
enough to where ACTH levels were increased in your animals, and this
might have been the reason you saw the rise in plasma cortisol and
no fall in aldosterone?

Dr. McCaa
     All of our long-term studies were performed in intact, con-
scious, sodium deficient dogs in which control samples were collected
for several weeks for the determination of plasma aldosterone and
cortisol concentrations, and plasma renin activity. After control
values were established, continuous infusion of angiotensin II,
angiotensin III, [Sar^1,Ala^8] angiotensin II, or [Sar^1, Ile^8] angiotensin II was begun. Cortisol secretion increased during the acute
phase (first 6 hours) of infusion of the octapeptide, the heptapeptide, and both inhibitory analogues. During the chronic phase of
these studies, cortisol secretion was not elevated above control
levels, indicating that the failure of aldosterone secretion to
decrease was not due to increased ACTH secretion produced by stress.
Many other investigators have made similar observations. McKenna
observed an increase in cortisol secretion in human adrenal cells
incubated with high concentrations of angiotensin II. Bravo observed
a ten-fold increase in cortisol secretion during infusion of angiotensin II inhibitory analogues in experimental animals. Also, these
investigators, and others, have failed to observe a significant
decrease in aldosterone secretion during infusion of angiotensin II
inhibitory analogues. In fact, Bravo reported marked increases in
aldosterone secretion in trained conscious dogs in response both to
[Sar^1, Ala^8] angiotensin II and [Sar^1, Ile^8] angiotensin II. Therefore, we have concluded from our studies with the angiotensin II
inhibitory analogues that the intrinsic agonistic properties of the
analogues on the adrenal glomerulosa cells negate their usefulness
for defining the role of the renin-angiotensin system in mediating
increased aldosterone secretion during sodium deficiency.

DISCUSSION REFERENCES

Bengis, R. G., Coleman, T. G., Young, D. B., and McCaa, R. E. (1978).
    Circ. Res. 43 (suppl. 1): 45-53.
Bravo, E. L. (1976). Prog. Biochem. Pharmacol. 12: 33-40.
Bravo, E. L., Khosla, M. C., and Bumpus, F. M. (1975). Am. J.
    Physiol. 228: 110-114.
McCaa, R. E., McCaa, C. S., Cowley, A. W., Jr., Ott, C. E., and
    Guyton, A. C. (1973). Circ. Res. 32: 356-362.
McKenna, T. J., Island, D. P., and Nicholson, W. E. (1977). Clin.
    Res. 25: 14A (Abstract).
Mohring, J., Mohring, B., Petri, M., and Haack, D. (1978). Circ.
    Res. 42: 17-22.

INTERACTIONS BETWEEN THE RENIN-ANGIOTENSIN SYSTEM AND THE BRAIN[1]

Ian A. Reid[2]

Department of Physiology
University of California-San Francisco
San Francisco, CA 94143

OUTLINE

I. Introduction

II. Role of the central nervous system in the control of renin secretion
   A. Effects of stimulation of the central nervous system on renin secretion
   B. Efferent pathways by which the brain influences renin secretion
      1. Role of the sympathetic nervous system
      2. Role of vasopressin

III. Actions of angiotensin on the central nervous system
   A. Blood pressure
   B. Drinking
   C. Vasopressin secretion
   D. ACTH secretion
   E. Plasma renin activity

IV. Physiological significance of the central effects of angiotensin II
   A. The brain renin-angiotensin system
      1. Nature of brain "renin"
      2. Effects of central administration of renin substrate
      3. Measurement of angiotensin in brain and cerebrospinal fluid
   B. Effects of circulating angiotensin on the brain

[1]Contains previously unpublished work supported by USPHS Grant AM06704 and by the L. J. and Mary C. Skaggs Foundation.

[2]Recipient of Research Career Development Award HL 00104.

I. INTRODUCTION

The renin-angiotensin system and the central nervous system interact in two major ways: 1. The central nervous system plays an important role in the control of renin secretion by the kidneys and thereby helps to determine the rate at which angiotensin II is generated. 2. Angiotensin II, the biologically active component of the renin-angiotensin system, acts on the brain to produce a variety of effects, including elevation of blood pressure, stimulation of drinking, and increased secretion of vasopressin and corticotropin (ACTH). This second interaction primarily involves circulating angiotensin II formed by the renal renin-angiotensin system, although there is some evidence for local formation of angiotensin within the brain which could also play a role. In this chapter, current concepts concerning these interactions are reviewed; in addition, the results of recent experiments performed in this laboratory are presented.

II. ROLE OF THE CENTRAL NERVOUS SYSTEM IN THE CONTROL OF RENIN SECRETION

A. Effects of Stimulation of the Central Nervous System on Renin Secretion

Electrical stimulation of a number of brain areas, including the mesencephalon (Ueda, Yasuda, Takabatake, *et al.*, 1967), pons (Richardson, Stella, Leonetti, *et al.*, 1974), medulla oblongata (Passo, Assaykeen, Otsuka, *et al.*, 1971) and hypothalamus (Zanchetti and Stella, 1975; Natcheff, Logofetov, and Tzaneva, 1977) increases the rate of renin secretion. These increases appear to result from activation of the sympathetic nervous system because they are accompanied by increases in arterial pressure and are abolished by renal denervation. Also, renin secretion may be decreased by stimulating certain areas of the hypothalamus, and this response is apparently mediated via a decrease in renal sympathetic neural activity (Zehr and Feigl, 1973).

Alterations in the sodium chloride concentration in cerebrospinal fluid have been reported to cause reciprocal changes in the rate of renin secretion. For example, plasma renin levels increase in dogs (Mouw and Vander, 1970) and sheep (Mouw, Abraham, Blair-West, *et al.*, 1974) when the cerebral ventricles are perfused with artificial cerebrospinal fluid containing a subnormal concentration of NaCl. Plasma renin activity also increases in goats when the concentration of sodium in cerebrospinal fluid is decreased by intraventricular infusion of isotonic fructose; conversely, plasma renin activity decreases in response to intraventricular infusion of hypertonic NaCl (Eriksson and Fyhrquist, 1976). The efferent pathway mediating these responses has not been identified; one possibility is that they are mediated via changes in vasopressin secretion, since it is known that this peptide inhibits renin secretion (see below).

Renin secretion is also altered by a variety of centrally-acting pharmacological agents. These include the general anesthetics, which increase the rate of renin secretion (Pettinger, Tanaka, Keeton, *et al.*, 1975). The mechanism responsible for this effect has not been identified, but there is evidence that in some cases increased sympathetic tone plays a role. In addition, the centrally-acting antihypertensive drug clonidine inhibits renin secretion when it is administered centrally in a low dose which is ineffective when administered intravenously (Reid, MacDonald, Pachnis, and Ganong, 1975). This central effect appears to be responsible for the suppression of renin secretion produced by larger, systemically administered doses of clonidine, since the suppression is blocked by ganglionic blockade (Nolan and Reid, 1978), spinal cord transection (Ganong, Wise, Reid, Holland, *et al.*, 1978), or renal denervation (Reid, MacDonald, Pachnis, and Ganong, 1975). Furthermore, oxymetazoline, which is closely related to clonidine but does not cross the blood-brain barrier, increases rather than decreases the rate of renin secretion (Nolan and Reid, 1978).

Various types of psychological stimuli increase renin secretion. For example, renin secretion increases in baboons during a three-hour Sidman avoidance schedule (Blair, Feigl, and Smith, 1976). In rats, plasma renin levels increase when the animals are exposed to a novel environment or become aware of the presence of a hungry cat (Clamage, Sanford, Vander, and Mouw, 1976). Similarly, plasma renin levels increase in mice when they are subjected to psychological stress induced by manipulation of their housing patterns (Vander, Henry, Stephens, *et al.*, 1978).

B. Efferent Pathways by which the Brain Influences Renin Secretion

There are at least two efferent pathways by which the brain influences renin secretion. One, the sympathetic nervous system, is excitatory and is by far the more important pathway. The other pathway involves vasopressin, which exerts an inhibitory control over renin secretion.

1. Role of the Sympathetic Nervous System. It is now clear that renin secretion is increased in situations in which sympathetic neural tone is increased. Examples of such situations include, in addition to those mentioned above, nonhypotensive hemorrhage (Bunag, Page, and McCubbin, 1966), carotid sinus hypotension (Cunningham, Feigl, and Sher, 1978; Reid and Jones, 1976), exercise (Bozovic and Casterfors, 1967), postural changes (Tobert, Slater, Fogelman, *et al.*,

1973), hypoglycemia (Otsuka, Assaykeen, Goldfien, and Ganong, 1970), administration of vasodilators (Pettinger and Keeton, 1975), and vagotomy (Hodge, Lowe, Ng, and Vane, 1969). Conversely, the rate of renin secretion is reduced in response to distention of the left atrium (Zehr, Hasbargen, and Kurz, 1976).

How do alterations in the level of sympathetic activity lead to changes in renin secretion? It is known that renin secretion is increased when the renal nerves are stimulated electrically (Taher, McLain, McDonald, and Schrier, 1976) and decreased when the renal nerves are cut (Bencsáth, Szalay, Debreczeni, *et al.*, 1972). It is also known that administration of catecholamines increases renin secretion (Johnson, Davis, and Witty, 1971). Thus, the changes in renin secretion listed above could result from alterations in renal sympathetic neural activity or from changes in the concentration of catecholamines in the circulation. It is now known that both mechanisms are important. For example, the renin secretory responses to hemorrhage (Tanigawa, Dua, and Assaykeen, 1974), vagotomy (Mancia, Romero, and Shepherd, 1975), postural changes (Zanchetti and Stella, 1975), and distention of the left atrium (Zehr, Hasbargen, and Kurz, 1976) are blocked by renal denervation or local anesthesia of the renal nerves. On the other hand, the response to hypoglycemia, which is associated with an increase in the rate of secretion of epinephrine, is abolished by adrenalectomy but not by renal denervation (Otsuka, Assaykeen, Goldfien, and Ganong, 1970).

During recent years, considerable attention has been focused on the mechanisms by which catecholamines, either circulating in the blood or released locally from renal sympathetic nerve endings, increase renin secretion. There is now evidence that catecholamines can stimulate renin secretion by acting directly on the juxtaglomerular cells (Ganong and Lopez, 1977). This action appears to be mediated by way of β-adrenoceptors and may involve the activation of adenylate cyclase and the formation of cyclic AMP. Examples of stimuli to renin secretion which are mediated via β-adrenoceptors include electrical stimulation of the brain (Passo, Assaykeen, Goldfien, and Ganong, 1971), stimulation of the renal nerves (Taher, McLain, McDonald, and Schrier, 1976), and administration of vasodilators (Pettinger, Tanaka, Keeton, *et al.*, 1975).

Alpha adrenoceptors also appear to play a role in the neural regulation of renin secretion, but their role is less well defined. Stimulation of α-adrenoceptors could increase renin secretion by constricting the afferent arteriole with resultant activation of the renal vascular receptor (Davis and Freeman, 1976). Alpha adrenoceptor stimulation also would decrease the delivery of sodium and chloride to the macula densa by decreasing glomerular filtration rate and by increasing proximal tubular sodium chloride reabsorption. These α-adrenoceptor-mediated effects might explain the reports that

α-adrenoceptor antagonists block the increase in renin secretion
produced by hemorrhage (Birbari, 1971) and electrical stimulation
of the renal nerves (Coote, Johns, MacLeod, and Singer, 1972).

Finally, it should be noted that in some situations stimulation
of α adrenoceptors inhibits renin secretion (Capponi and Vallotton,
1976). Such inhibition might result from a direct effect on the
juxtaglomerular cells; in addition, it could be due to inhibition of
the release of norepinephrine from renal sympathetic nerve endings
(Starke and Endo, 1976) with a resultant decrease in β-mediated
stimulation of renin secretion. The significance of the inhibitory
effect of α-adrenoceptor stimulation on renin secretion remains to
be determined.

2. Role of Vasopressin. Another pathway by which the brain
influences renin secretion involves the neurohypophyseal peptide,
vasopressin. It has been known for several years that administration
of vasopressin decreases renin secretion (Vander, 1968). The mechanism of this inhibitory action has not been established. It has
been proposed that the inhibition results from a direct action of the
peptide on the renin-secreting cells since vasopressin inhibits renin
secretion when infused into nonfiltering kidneys in doses which do
not affect renal blood flow or arterial pressure (Shade, Davis,
Johnson, et al., 1973). On the other hand, it has been reported
that vasopressin fails to decrease the rate of renin release by
kidney slices in vitro (Rosset and Veyrat, 1971).

The extent to which vasopressin participates in the physiological regulation of renin secretion is still being investigated, but
there are situations in which the peptide does appear to play a significant role. For example, stimulation of vasopressin secretion by
bilateral vagotomy in dogs undergoing a water diuresis decreases
renin secretion (Schrier, Reid, Berl, and Earley, 1975). In addition, renin concentration in the plasma or kidneys of rats with
hereditary diabetes insipidus is higher than in normal animals
(Gutman and Benzakein, 1974). This difference may be due to the
absence of vasopressin in the rats with diabetes insipidus, although
hypovolemia may also be a factor.

Recent studies in this laboratory provide further evidence that
vasopressin may play a significant role in the control of renin secretion (Malayan, Ramsay, Keil, and Reid, 1978). In these experiments, vasopressin was administered intravenously to conscious dogs
in doses ranging from 0.01 to 1.0 ng/kg/min. These infusions, which
produced increments in plasma vasopressin concentration ranging from
1 to 30 pg/ml, suppressed plasma renin activity in a dose-related
manner. The lowest plasma vasopressin concentration at which suppression of renin secretion was observed was approximately 4 pg/ml.
Plasma vasopressin concentrations well in excess of this were observed during water deprivation and during hemorrhage; it is likely,

therefore, that vasopressin blunts the increase in renin secretion which occurs in these situations. Studies with the recently synthesized antagonists of vasopressin should facilitate a more precise definition of the role of vasopressin in the control of renin secretion.

In summary, the central nervous system plays an important role in the control of renin secretion. The major efferent pathway from the brain to the kidneys is the sympathetic nervous system, which increases renin secretion via the renal nerves and via circulating catecholamines. In some situations, the brain also exerts an inhibitory effect on renin secretion via the secretion of vasopressin, but the contribution of this pathway appears to be small compared to that of the sympathetic nervous system.

III. ACTIONS OF ANGIOTENSIN II ON THE CENTRAL NERVOUS SYSTEM

Since the original demonstration by Bickerton and Buckley (1961) that angiotensin II can act on the central nervous system to increase arterial pressure, it has become clear that the peptide has several central actions. These include stimulation of drinking, increased secretion of vasopressin and corticotropin (ACTH), and inhibition of renin secretion by the kidneys. In addition, there is evidence that angiotensin II may inhibit norepinephrine uptake by central adrenergic neurons and may increase the release of acetylcholine at central cholinergic nerve terminals. The purpose of this section is to review some of the current concepts concerning these central actions.

A. Blood Pressure

The central pressor effect of angiotensin II has been demonstrated by injecting the polypeptide into the blood supply to the brain, into the cerebral ventricles, or into specific brain regions (Severs and Daniels-Severs, 1973). Administration of angiotensin II into the blood supply to the brain produces a pressor response which is rapid in onset and offset, and which may or may not be associated with an increase in heart rate or cardiac output. The blood pressure response to intraventricular administration of angiotensin is slower in onset than the response to intra-arterial injection, but is much more prolonged and may be maintained for more than 60 minutes after a single injection. In general, the pressor response to intraventricular angiotensin is not accompanied by a change in heart rate.

Considerable information concerning the site(s) of the central pressor effect of angiotensin is now available. The receptor which mediates the increase in blood pressure produced by intravertebral infusion of angiotensin appears to be located in the area postrema, a circumventricular organ which is located in the caudal medulla and which is devoid of a blood-brain barrier. Ablation of this area abolishes the pressor response to intravertebral angiotensin II (Joy and Lowe, 1970) and reduces the blood pressure response to intravenous angiotensin (Scroop, Katic, Joy, *et al.*, 1971). In addition, microinjection of angiotensin into the area postrema but not into adjacent areas results in increases in blood pressure (Ueda, Katayama, and Kato, 1972).

Although the area postrema appears to be the site of action of blood-borne angiotensin on blood pressure, it does not appear to mediate the pressor effect of angiotensin administered into the cerebral ventricles. For example, Gildenberg, Ferrario, and McCubbin (1973) demonstrated that the pressor response to injection of angiotensin into a lateral ventricle was abolished by midbrain transection, whereas the response to intravertebral angiotensin was unaltered. Destruction of the area postrema, on the other hand, abolished the pressor response to intravertebral angiotensin but did not alter the response to intraventricular angiotensin. Earlier studies by Severs, Daniels, Smookler, *et al.* (1966) indicated that the site of action of intraventricular angiotensin on blood pressure is in the periaqueductal region of the mesencephalon. Subsequently, Deuben and Buckley (1970) localized this site more specifically to the subnucleus medialis. They showed that the pressor response to administration of angiotensin into the cerebral aqueduct was much greater when the injection was made anterior to the subnucleus medialis than when it was made posterior to this nucleus. Furthermore, bilateral lesions placed in the periaqueductal gray at the level of the subnucleus medialis markedly reduced the pressor response to intraventricular angiotensin.

More recently, evidence has been presented for other central sites of action of angiotensin on blood pressure. Areas that have received attention include an area in the anteroventral region of the third ventricle, possibly the organum vasculosum of the lamina terminalis (OVLT) (Buggy, Fink, Johnson, and Brody, 1977; Phillips, Phipps, and Knowles, 1978) and the subfornical organ (SFO) (Simpson and Mangiapane, 1978). However, the extent to which these areas mediate central pressor responses to angiotensin remains to be determined.

Information concerning the efferent pathways which mediate the central pressor effect of angiotensin is also available. In mongrel dogs, a large component of the response appears to be due to an increase in total peripheral resistance, resulting from an increase in sympathetic outflow. For example, the pressor response to intravertebral administration of angiotensin is accompanied by an increase in splanchnic nerve activity (Fukiyama, 1972) and is abolished by ganglionic blockade (Figure 1) and by guanethidine (Fukiyama, 1972).

In addition, the response to intraventricular injection of angiotensin is blocked by α-adrenergic blockade (Severs, Daniels, Smookler
et al., 1966) and by spinal cord section (Buckley, 1972).

On the other hand, the pressor response in the greyhound appears
to be due largely to an increase in cardiac output that is dependent
on withdrawal of parasympathetic activity. Scroop and Lowe (1969)
reported that the pressor response to intravertebral angiotensin in
dogs was reduced by bilateral vagotomy or by administration of atropine. However, there was a residual angiotensin-induced pressor
response which was due to increased total peripheral resistance and
which was blocked by sympathetic nerve blockade with bethanidine.

A third mechanism by which angiotensin may increase arterial
pressure is via stimulation of vasopressin secretion. It is known
that angiotensin is a stimulus to vasopressin secretion (see below)
and it has been reported that the blood pressure response to intraventricular angiotensin in the rat is reduced by hypophysectomy
(Severs, Summy-Long, Taylor, and Connor, 1970). Furthermore, rats
with hereditary hypothalamic diabetes insipidus fail to show a
normal blood pressure response to intraventricular angiotensin
(Hutchinson, Schelling, Möhring, and Ganten, 1976; Haack and Möhring,
1978). On the other hand, the pressor response to centrally administered angiotensin in the dog is not mediated via increased vasopressin secretion. In anesthetized dogs, the increase in blood pressure produced by intraventricular administration of angiotensin is
not significantly reduced by hypophysectomy (Malayan, Keil, Ramsay,
and Reid, 1978). In addition, the increase in blood pressure produce
by infusion of angiotensin into the vertebral artery of conscious dog
is not accompanied by an increase in plasma vasopressin concentration
(see below). Finally, as noted above, centrally-mediated pressor
responses to angiotensin in the dog can be accounted for on the basis
of increased sympathetic or decreased parasympathetic activity.

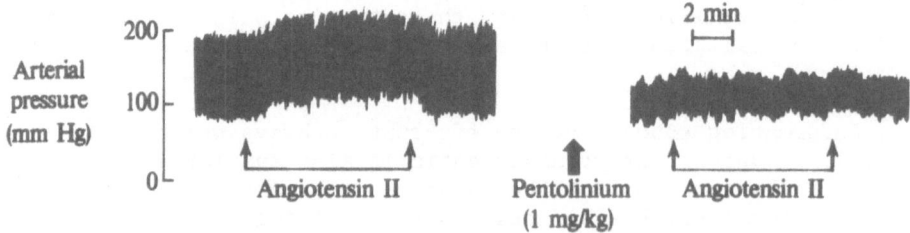

*Figure 1.   Blockade by pentolinium of the increase in blood pressure
produced by bilateral vertebral arterial infusion of
angiotensin II (1.0 ng/kg/min) in a conscious dog.*

B. Drinking

One of the most recently discovered actions of angiotensin II is stimulation of drinking (Severs and Summy-Long, 1975). Administration of the peptide either systemically or directly into the central nervous system elicits drinking in a wide variety of animal species. Furthermore, water intake is increased in a number of situations in which renin secretion and hence circulating angiotensin II levels are elevated; in some of these situations the increase in water intake can be reduced or abolished by administration of agents which block the formation or actions of angiotensin II (Severs and Summy-Long, 1975).

During recent years, considerable attention has been focused on the question of where the receptors which mediate the dipsogenic action of angiotensin are located. Several sites have been proposed but agreement concerning the relative importance of each has not been reached. Much attention has been focused on two circumventricular organs in the third ventricle, the SFO and the OVLT. The evidence supporting a role for the SFO has been reviewed recently (Simpson, Epstein, and Camardo, 1978; Simpson, Mangiapane, and Dellmann, 1978). Their evidence can be summarized as follows: (1) Direct application of angiotensin to the SFO elicits drinking in a dose-related manner. (2) The threshold dose for angiotensin-induced drinking in the SFO is lower than for any other locus tested by these investigators. (3) Selective destruction of the SFO abolishes the drinking response to intravenously administered angiotensin. (4) Direct application of saralasin, a competitive antagonist of angiotensin, to the SFO reduces or abolishes the drinking produced by intravenous angiotensin. Saralasin is less effective when injected into adjacent tissue or into cerebrospinal fluid. Other evidence supporting a role for the SFO in the dipsogenic action of angiotensin includes the observation that iontophoretic application of angiotensin to individual neurons of the SFO increases their firing rate (Felix and Akert, 1974). This effect can be antagonized by saralasin (Phillips and Felix, 1976).

Although most investigators accept that the SFO is a receptor site for the dipsogenic action of angiotensin, other sites have been implicated. One of these is the OVLT which, like the SFO, is devoid of a blood-brain barrier and therefore is accessible to blood-borne angiotensin. Phillips, Phipps, and Knowles (1978) have reported that injection of small amounts of angiotensin into the OVLT region of rats elicits drinking, while destruction of the area abolishes the dipsogenic action of intravenous or intraventricular angiotensin.

Thus, there is evidence that both the SFO and the OVLT are receptor sites for the dipsogenic action of angiotensin, but further investigation is required to determine the relative importance of these and other areas in the control of water intake.

C.   Vasopressin Secretion

Angiotensin has been reported to increase vasopressin secretion when injected intravenously (Ramsay, Keil, Sharpe, and Shinsako, 1978) or directly into the cerebral ventricles (Keil, Summy-Long, and Severs, 1975; Malayan, Keil, Ramsay, and Reid, 1978) (Figure 2). The most impressive responses are produced when angiotensin is administered by the intraventricular route; the responses to intravenous angiotensin are much smaller and some investigators have not observed increases in vasopressin secretion when angiotensin is administered via this route (Cadnapaphornchai, Boykin, Harbottle, *et al.*, 1975; Claybaugh and Share, 1972).   Recently, Claybaugh (1977) reported that intravenous infusion of angiotensin or renin did not change plasma vasopressin concentration in normally hydrated dogs; on the other hand, infusion of similar doses in dehydrated dogs did increase plasma vasopressin levels.

The site at which angiotensin acts to increase vasopressin secretion has not been definitely established.   Evidence for actions at the supraoptic nucleus (Nicoll and Barker, 1971) and posterior pituitary (Gagnon, Cousineau, and Boucher, 1973) has been presented, but further studies are required to settle this question.

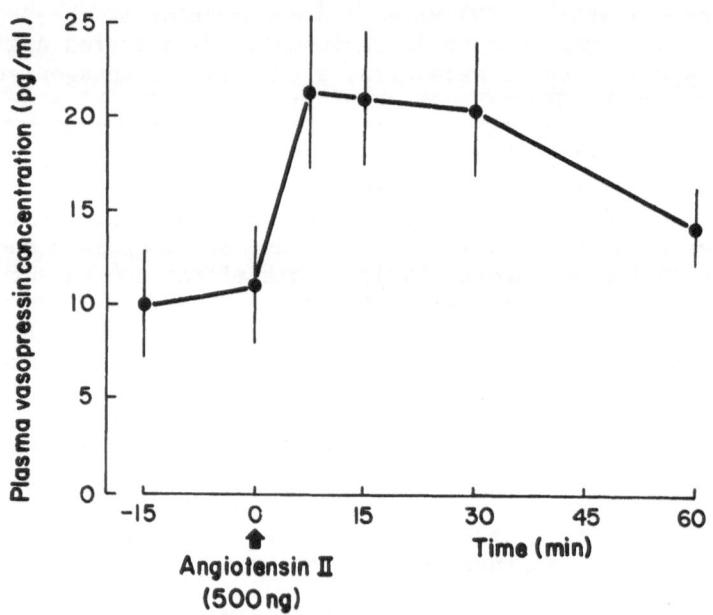

Figure 2.   Effect of intraventricular administration of angiotensin 1 on plasma vasopressin concentration in anesthetized dogs. Data from Malayan, Keil, Ramsay, and Reid (1978).

D. ACTH Secretion

There have several reports that ACTH secretion is increased by central or systemic administration of angiotensin II. In most cases, changes in the concentration of corticosteroids in the blood have been used as an index of changes in ACTH secretion (Maran and Yates, 1977; Reid, 1977a); in others, however, plasma ACTH concentration has been measured directly (Ramsay, Keil, Sharpe, and Shinsako, 1978; Rayyis and Horton, 1971). As in the case of vasopressin, the site of action of angiotensin on ACTH secretion has not been established; sites that have been implicated include the median eminence (Gann, 1969) and the anterior pituitary (Maran and Yates, 1977). It is also possible that angiotensin increases ACTH secretion indirectly by increasing vasopressin release, since it is known that vasopressin is a corticotropin releasing factor.

E. Plasma Renin Activity

Central administration of angiotensin II or renin has been reported to suppress plasma renin activity in dogs (Malayan, Keil, Ramsay, and Reid, 1978) and goats (Eriksson and Fyhrquist, 1976). The suppression of plasma renin occurs without a concurrent increase in plasma angiotensin II concentration, so a direct effect of angiotensin II on the kidney can be excluded (Eriksson and Fyhrquist, 1976).

As noted above, centrally administered angiotensin II increases arterial pressure and vasopressin secretion; either of these changes could mediate the suppression of plasma renin activity. To distinguish between these two possibilities, we recently studied the effect of hypophysectomy on the decrease in plasma renin activity produced by intraventricular angiotensin II in anesthetized dogs (Malayan, Keil, Ramsay, and Reid, 1978). Hypophysectomy completely abolished the changes in plasma renin activity and plasma vasopressin concentration produced by angiotensin; the change in blood pressure, however, was not significantly altered. These results indicate that the suppression of plasma renin activity produced by centrally administered angiotensin is mediated via vasopressin and not by changes in arterial pressure.

IV. PHYSIOLOGICAL SIGNIFICANCE OF THE CENTRAL EFFECTS OF ANGIOTENSIN II

The remainder of this chapter is concerned with the question of the physiological significance of the actions of angiotensin II on the central nervous system. This question will be considered from two standpoints: firstly, the possibility that angiotensin II is formed in the brain by a brain renin—angiotensin system; secondly, the role of circulating angiotensin formed by the renal renin—angiotensin system.

A. The Brain Renin-Angiotensin System

The concept of an intricate brain renin-angiotensin system
originated with the finding that the components required for the
formation of angiotensin, viz., renin substrate, an enzyme with
renin-like activity, and converting enzyme are present in the central nervous system. Much of the information concerning the properties of these components has been reviewed elsewhere (Reid, 1977b;
Ganten, Hutchinson, Schelling, *et al.*, 1976) and will not be discussed here. Instead, this section will focus on the question of
whether or not brain "renin" interacts with the other components
in vivo to form a functional renin-angiotensin system.

1. Nature of Brain "Renin". In the initial studies of brain
"renin", it was clearly shown that the enzyme differs from the renal
enzyme (Ganten, Marquez-Julio, Granger, *et al.* 1971; Daul, Heath,
and Garey, 1975). Although the pH optimum (4.5-5.0) is only
slightly lower than that of renal renin, the activity of the brain
enzyme decreases markedly above pH 5.0 so that at pH 7.4 there is
little or no measurable activity. Both the brain and renal enzymes
hydrolyze the synthetic tetradecapeptide renin substrate (TDP), but
the affinity of the brain enzyme for this substrate is greater than
that of the renal enzyme.

There is now considerable evidence that the renin-like activity
in brain is due to the lysosomal acid protease, cathepsin D. This
was first suggested by Day and Reid (1976) who partially purified
the renin-like enzyme in dog brain by ammonium sulfate fractioni-
zation, Sephadex G-100 chromatography, and concentration by dialysis
at pH 3.3. With these procedures, a 100-fold purification of the
enzyme was achieved. Cathepsin D activity accompanied the renin
activity throughout the purification and showed the same increase in
specific activity. Sephadex gel chromatography and isoelectric
focusing failed to separate the renin activity from the cathepsin
activity. Both enzyme activities were undetectable above pH 6.0
and were irreversibly inhibited by pepstatin.

Recently these findings have been confirmed and extended by
Hackenthal, Hackenthal, and Hilgenfeldt (1978a). These investigators
purified the renin-like enzyme in rat brain to homogeneity by a three
step procedure involving pepstatin affinity chromatography. Renin-
like activity and cathepsin D activity purified in parallel, a 2,000-
fold increase in the specific activity of both enzymes being achieved
Isoelectric focusing again failed to separate the two enzyme activities. In a further study, Hackenthal, Hackenthal, and Hilgenfeldt
(1978b) compared the properties of the purified rat brain enzyme with
those of bovine spleen cathepsin D and hog spleen pseudorenin. Close
similarities were observed with respect to substrate specificity,
inhibition of angiotensin formation from TDP by pepstatin, and the

pH dependence of angiotensin formation. It was therefore concluded
that the brain enzyme and pseudorenin are identical to cathepsin D.
These investigators also pointed out that this enzyme is not an iso-
enzyme of renin so that the term "isorenin" should no longer be used
to designate the brain enzyme.

Further evidence that the renin-like activity in brain is due
to cathepsin D was obtained recently in cell fractionation studies
in this laboratory (Morris and Reid, 1978). The subcellular distribution of the renin-like activity closely paralleled that of cathepsin D, and these in turn paralleled the distribution of the lysosomal
marker, acid phosphatase.

On the other hand, Hirose, Yokosawa, and Inagami (1978) recently
reported the separation of the angiotensin I-generating activity in
brain extracts from nephrectomized rats into two peaks. One peak
apparently represented cathepsin D; the other, however, did not have
general protease activity and was neutralized by an antirenin antiserum. This constitutes the first convincing evidence for the existence of renin in the brain. However, it should be noted that the
concentration of renin measured by Hirose *et al*. was very low, approximately 250 pg/g tissue/hour; this is less than one-tenth the concentration of renin normally present in rat plasma. In addition, the
distribution of the enzyme was not determined, so the possibility
remains that the activity was due to renin contained in blood vessel
walls.

In summary, most reports of the presence of renin-like activity
in brain can be explained on the basis of a nonspecific action of
the lysosomal acid protease, cathepsin D. As we have pointed out
previously, it is unlikely that this enzyme would function as an
angiotensin-forming enzyme *in vivo* (Day and Reid, 1976). On the
other hand, recent evidence suggests that a small amount of authen-
tic renin may also be present in the brain; further investigation
is required to determine if this enzyme is capable of generating
significant amounts of angiotensin II under physiological conditions.

2. Effects of Central Administration of Renin Substrate. One
approach used to determine if there is a functional brain renin-
angiotensin system has been to study the effects of injecting various
components of the renin-angiotensin system into the central nervous
system. It is now clear that renin has a variety of actions when
administered by this route; these include stimulation of drinking and
elevation of arterial pressure (Reid and Ramsay, 1975), and increased
secretion of vasopressin and ACTH (Malayan and Reid, 1976; Reid and
Day, 1977). All of these effects are blocked by saralasin, indicating that they are mediated via the formation of angiotensin II; this
conclusion is supported by the finding that angiotensin II concentration in cerebrospinal fluid increases markedly when renin is

injected via the central route (Reid and Moffat, 1978). These findings indicate that there is an *in vivo* reaction of injected renin with brain renin substrate and converting enzyme, which results in the formation of physiologically active amounts of angiotensin II.

Injecting renin into the central nervous system does not, however, demonstrate endogenous brain renin activity *in vivo*. To address this question, the effects of central administration of renin substrate have been investigated. The first experiments of this type utilized TDP, and it was shown that this synthetic substrate elicits drinking in rats (Epstein, Fitzsimons, and Johnson, 1974). However, subsequent studies showed that brain converting enzyme can form angiotensin II from TDP and that this enzyme, rather than renin, is responsible for the dipsogenic action of TDP (Simpson, Reid, Ramsay, and Kipen, 1978).

The realization that TDP is not the appropriate substrate to use for the detection of brain renin activity (Dorer, Kahn, Lentz, *et al.*, 1975) led to further studies in which the naturally occurring renin substrate was used. Hoffman, Schelling, Phillips, and Ganten (1976) reported that partially purified natural substrate stimulated drinking when administered centrally to rats. However, the responses that they observed were small and inconsistent. Furthermore, a highly purified substrate preparation was less effective in eliciting drinking than were less pure preparations, suggesting that the drinking was caused by a nonspecific factor. In this laboratory, natural renin substrate failed to elicit drinking when administered centrally in rats (Simpson, Reid, Ramsay, and Kipen, 1978). In addition, no evidence for angiotensin II formation was found when purified plasma renin substrate was injected into the third cerebral ventricle of dogs (Reid and Moffat, 1978). Renin substrate concentration in cerebrospinal fluid increased 3-fold but, despite this, no angiotensin II could be detected in spinal fluid; in addition, arterial blood pressure did not change. Similarly, Fitzsimons and Kucharczyk (1978) recently reported that intracranial injection of dog renin substrate failed to elicit drinking in 3 of 4 dogs. Taken together, these observations fail to provide convincing evidence for renin activity in the brain *in vivo*.

3. Measurement of Angiotensin in Brain and Cerebrospinal Fluid. An essential test of the hypothesis that angiotensin is generated in the central nervous system is to determine whether or not angiotensin is present in the brain. The detection and assay of angiotensin I and II in cerebrospinal fluid and brain extracts has been attempted using bioassay, radioimmunoassay, and immunohistochemical techniques, but extremely variable results have been obtained.

Measurements of angiotensin II concentration in cerebrospinal
fluid have been made in a number of species, including the dog, rat,
sheep, and human. Early estimates for the rat ranged from 90-170
fmol/ml (Ganten, Hutchinson, and Schelling, 1975; Simpson, Saad,
and Epstein, 1976) but recently these estimates have been revised
downward to 0-15 fmol/ml (Epstein and Ganten, 1977). In this laboratory, angiotensin II has not been detected in rat spinal fluid
(Simpson and Reid, unpublished observations). Angiotensin II has
not been detected in dog cerebrospinal fluid by either bioassay
(Ganten, Marquez-Julio, Granger, *et al.*, 1971) or radioimmunoassay
(Reid and Moffat, 1978), although a recent report suggests that the
heptapeptide fragment of angiotensin II may be present in the spinal
fluid of some dogs (Hutchinson, Csicmann, Korner, and Johnston, 1978).
Other values reported for cerebrospinal fluid angiotensin II content
include 37 fmol/ml in the human (Severs, Changaris, Kapsha, *et al.*,
1977) and 30-120 fmol/ml in the sheep (Abraham, Baker, Blaine, *et
al.*, 1975). It should be noted that in most of these studies the
identity of the material being measured was not established beyond
the fact that it cross-reacted with angiotensin II antibodies;
further measurements and characterization are clearly required to
determine the true concentration of angiotensin II in cerebrospinal
fluid.

Biological and immunological activity resembling angiotensin
has been found in extracts of brains from various species; however,
there is serious doubt that either of these activities is due to
angiotensin. For example, the pressor activity extracted from rat,
rabbit, and dog brain is not neutralized by saralasin or by antibodies to angiotensin I and II (Horvath, Baxter, Furby, and Tiller,
1977). It is possible that the pressor activity is due to vasopressin. Furthermore, studies in this laboratory (Reid, Day, Moffat,
and Hughes, 1977) indicate that the apparent angiotensin immunoreactivity in crude brain extracts is an artifact caused by angiotensinase. It appears that the angiotensinase in the extracts destroys the ^{125}I-labelled angiotensin used in the angiotensin radioimmunoassay and thus reduces the amount of labelled angiotensin
available for binding to the antibody; the reduced binding could be
erroneously interpreted as displacement of labelled angiotensin.
When more elaborate extraction procedures which eliminate angiotensinase activity have been employed, neither angiotensin I nor angiotensin II immunoreactivity has been detected in rat, rabbit, or dog
brain (Horvath, Baxter, Furby, and Tiller, 1977).

Immunofluorescence and immunohistochemical techniques, which
are also subject to problems of specificity, have been used for the
detection of angiotensin in the brain (Fuxe, Ganten, Hokfelt, and
Bolme, 1976; Changaris, Keil, and Severs, 1978). Positive results
have been obtained by some investigators, but there is not good
agreement as to the distribution of the apparent immunoreactivity.
Using the same techniques in this laboratory, we have not found

evidence for the presence of angiotensin I or II in the brain
(Goldsmith and Iwamoto, unpublished observations). Thus, although
the positive results that have been obtained in some laboratories
are encouraging, additional studies using different antibodies are
required.

In summary, experiments involving the biochemical characterization of brain "renin", the central administration of renin substrate and the measurement of angiotensin I and II in the brain
have not provided convincing evidence for the existence of a functional brain renin-angiotensin system. Of course, the experiments
do not exclude the possibility that such a system exists, and future
research may well prove this to be the case. In the meantime, however, it would seem more fruitful to investigate the effects of
blood-borne angiotensin II, formed by the renal renin-angiotensin
system, on the brain. These effects are the subject of the next
section.

B.   Effect of Circulating Angiotensin II on the Brain

This section summarizes the results of a recent investigation
in this laboratory which was designed to study the central effects
of angiotensin II on blood pressure, heart rate, water intake, and
the secretion of ADH, ACTH, and renin in conscious dogs. In these
experiments, angiotensin was administered either via the vertebral
arteries or via the carotid arteries. This approach was chosen so
that the systemic effects of the peptide would be minimized; in
addition, it was anticipated that comparison of the effects of
intravertebral administration with those of intracarotid administration would help localize the various central sites of action of
angiotensin. Doses of angiotensin estimated to produce physiologically meaningful concentrations of the peptide in the cerebral circulation were used. This is an important feature of these experiments
because in many of the earlier studies, extremely large, unphysio-
logical doses of angiotensin were injected. In additional experiments, the cardiovascular and endocrine effects of hemorrhage were
studied.

The experiments were performed in mongrel dogs of either sex,
and weighed approximately 30 kg. Under pentobarbital anesthesia,
small catheters (0.15 to 0.30 mm internal diameter) were placed in
both vertebral and both carotid arteries using an approach that does
not interfere significantly with blood flow. Cannulas were also
placed in a femoral artery and vein. All cannulas were led subcutaneously to the back of the neck where they were exteriorized and protected by a jacket. The cannulas were flushed daily with saline
and were filled with heparin (1000 units/ml). At least three days
elapsed between the completion of surgery and the first experiment.

On the experimental day, the dogs were brought to the laboratory where they were allowed to stand, loosely restrained by a
sling. Water was available to the dogs at all times, and the volume consumed at any time was recorded. Blood pressure was recorded
continuously from the femoral artery with a Statham strain gauge
and a Grass polygraph. Blood samples for analysis (volume = 12 ml)
were collected from the femoral artery and were replaced with an
equal volume of 0.9% NaCl. After control measurements had been
made, angiotensin II (Schwarz-Mann) was infused either into the left
and right vertebral arteries or into the left and right carotid
arteries. The doses tested were 0.1, 0.33, and 1.0 ng/kg/minute,
infused into each artery. All doses were infused at a rate of 0.5
ml/minute. Assuming vertebral and carotid arterial blood flows of
100-300 ml/minute (unpublished observations), these doses of angiotensin would have increased angiotensin II concentration in the
cerebral circulation by 10 to 300 pg/ml, thus covering the range
encountered under most physiological and experimental conditions.
The duration of the infusion was 15 minutes, and this was followed
by a 15 minute recovery period. At the end of this time, the same
dose of angiotensin was infused into the second pair of arteries.
The other doses of angiotensin II were tested on different days.

The effects of hemorrhage were studied in five dogs. Following
control measurements, blood was pumped from the femoral artery into
a blood bag at the rate of 1.0 ml/kg/min. for 15 minutes. Measurements were made at the end of this period and 15 minutes later; the
blood was then reinfused, and final control measurements were made
15 minutes later.

Plasma vasopressin concentration was measured by radioimmunoassay and was expressed as pg/ml of plasma (Keil and Severs, 1977).
Plasma ACTH was not measured directly but instead, changes in the
concentration of 11-hydroxycorticosteroids in plasma, measured by a
competitive binding technique (Murphy, 1967), were used as an index
of changes in ACTH secretion. Plasma renin activity was measured
as described previously and was expressed as ng angiotensin I generated per ml. of plasma during a 3 hour incubation (ng/ml/3h) (Reid,
Stockigt, Goldfien, and Ganong, 1972). Plasma angiotensin II concentration was measured by radioimmunoassay (Reid and Moffat, 1978).

The effects of intravertebral and intracarotid infusion of
angiotensin II are summarized in Figures 3-5. Intravertebral infusion increased arterial pressure in a dose-related manner, the highest dose increasing mean arterial pressure from 114 ±2 to 129 ±2
mm Hg (P<0.01). Intracarotid angiotensin also increased blood pressure, but to a lesser extent, the largest increase being from
111 ±4 to 120 ±3 mm Hg (P<0.01). The blood pressure responses to
intracarotid angiotensin were slower in onset than the responses to
intravertebral angiotensin (Figure 4). Heart rate increased significantly when angiotensin was infused into the vertebral arteries,

but was unchanged by intracarotid infusion. None of the doses tested elevated the blood pressure or heart rate when infused intravenously. In contrast, water intake was increased in a dose-related manner by the intracarotid infusions but was unaffected by intravertebral infusions. The stimulation of drinking produced by intracarotid angiotensin was usually accompanied by increases in blood pressure ranging from 5 to 25 mm Hg (Figure 5). There was a tendency for plasma vasopressin and 11-hydroxycorticosteroid concentration to increase during intravertebral and intracarotid infusion of the highest dose of angiotensin (Figure 3), but the changes were not statistically significant. The lower doses of angiotensin also had no effect on vasopressin or corticoid concentrations. The highest dose of angiotensin produced significant decreases in plasma renin activity when infused into either the vertebral or carotid arteries (Figure 3). The intermediate dose also decreased plasma renin activity when infused into the carotids; intracarotid or intravertebral infusion of the lowest dose was without effect.

The cardiovascular, endocrine, and dipsogenic effects of hemorrhage are summarized in Figure 6. There was a tendency for blood pressure to decrease in some dogs, but overall, mean blood pressure did not decrease significantly. Heart rate increased from 70 ±5 to 92 ±12 beats/minute (P<0.05). Plasma renin activity increased from 3.5 ±1.9 to 14.7 4.2 ng/ml/3h (P<0.01) and this was accompanied by an increase in plasma angiotensin II concentration from 11.8 ±2.2 to 29.4 ±6.7 pg/ml (P<0.05). There was a large increase in plasma vasopressin concentration from 2.2 ±0.4 to 47.4 ±16.9 pg/ml (P<0.01) and a smaller increase in plasma corticosteroid concentration from 2.0 ±0.5 to 4.0 ±0.8 µg/dl (P<0.05). All of these changes reversed rapidly following reinfusion of the blood. All dogs drank during the hemorrhage, the mean volume consumed being 54 ±17 ml.

The present results thus confirm previous reports (Severs and Daniels-Severs, 1973) that infusion of angiotensin II into the blood supply of the brain increases arterial blood pressure. Increases in blood pressure occurred during either intravertebral or intracarotid infusion, but the responses to intravertebral infusions were more rapid in onset and greater in magnitude than the responses to intracarotid infusions. In addition, the pressor response to intravertebral angiotensin was accompanied by an increase in heart rate, whereas the response to intracarotid was not. The increases in blood pressure and heart rate produced by intravertebral angiotensin were presumably mediated via the area postrema, which receives its blood supply from the vertebral arteries (Gildenberg and Ferrario, 1977). Since the carotid arteries do not normally supply the brainstem in the dog, it is probable that the pressor response to intracarotid angiotensin was mediated via a more rostral site. The location of this site remains to be determined. It is unlikely to be the subnucleus medialis of the mesencephalon, since this area appears to

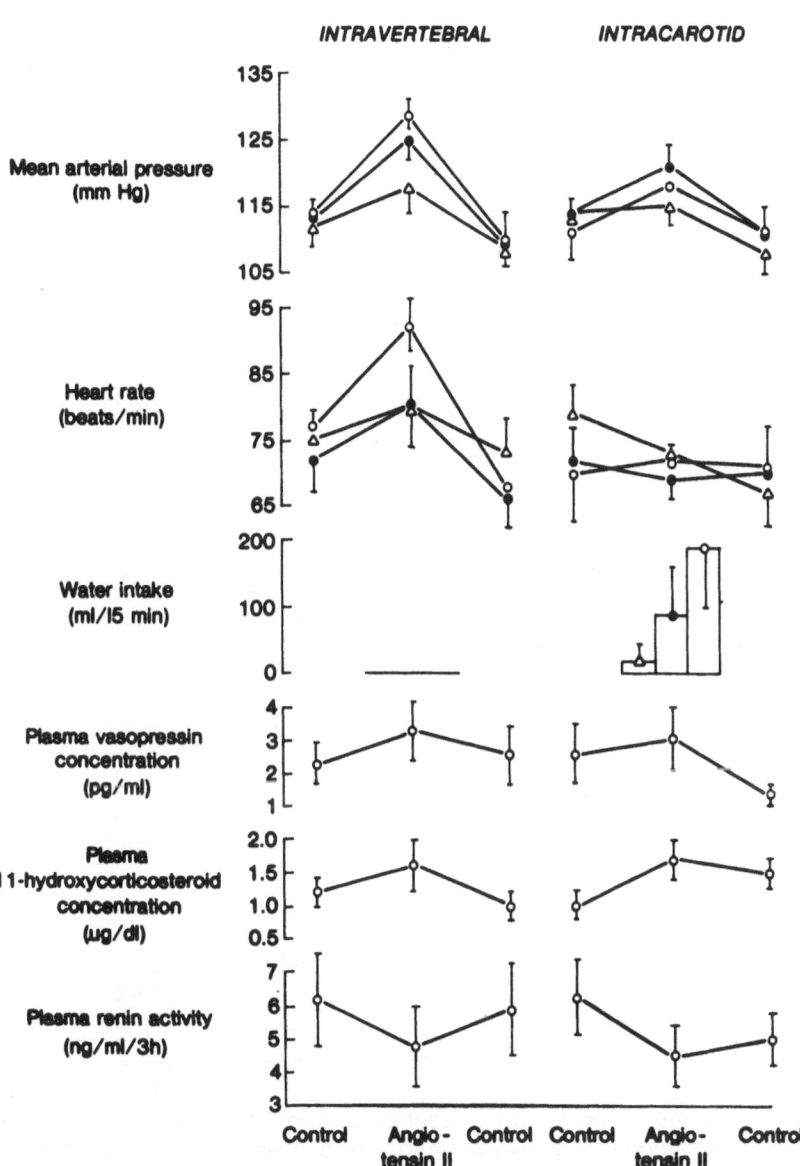

Figure 3. *Cardiovascular, dipsogenic and endocrine effects of intravertebral and intracarotid infusion of three doses of angiotensin II in conscious dogs.*

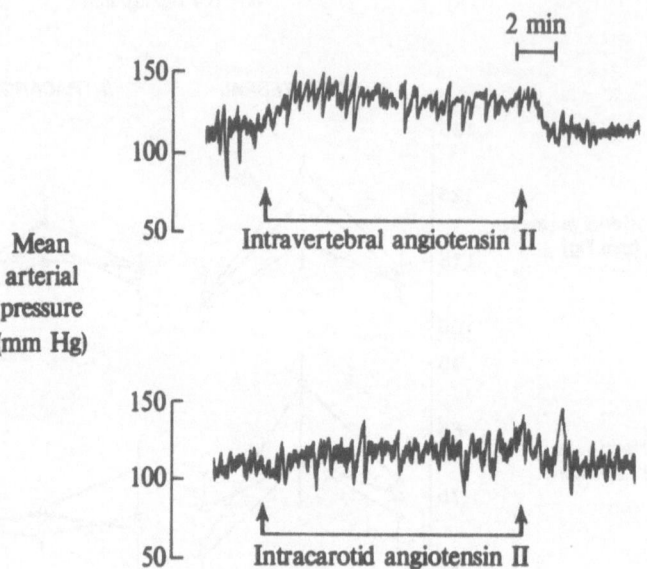

Figure 4. *Comparison of the effects of intravertebral and intra-carotid infusion of angiotensin II (1.0 ng/kg/min) on blood pressure in a conscious dog.*

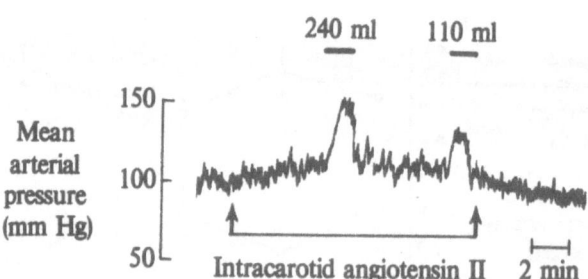

Figure 5. *Changes in blood pressure associated with drinking during intracarotid infusion of angiotensin II (1.0 ng/kg/min) in a conscious dog. Episodes of drinking are indicated by the horizontal bars.*

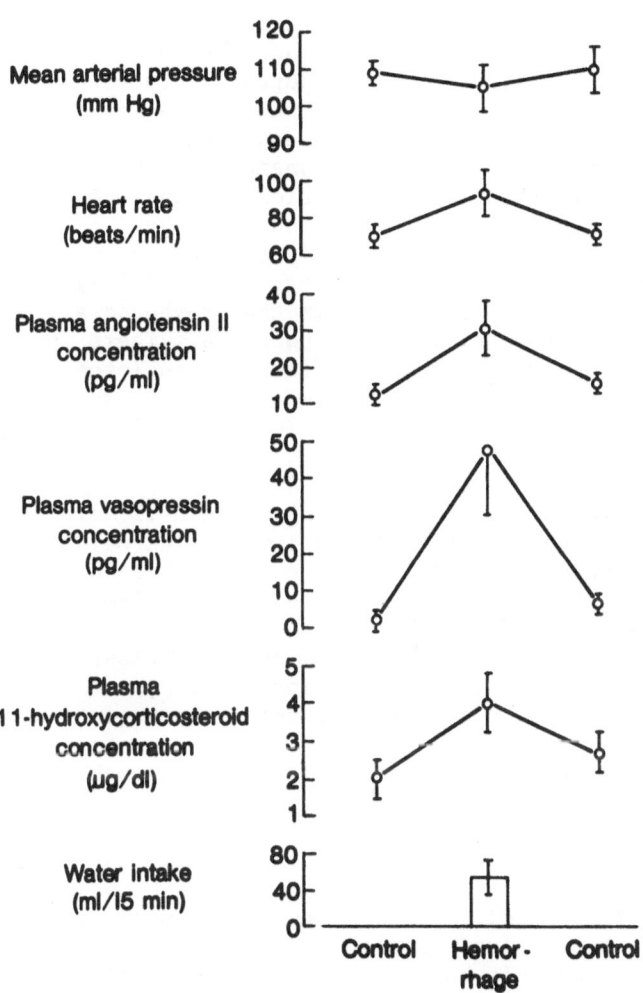

Figure 6.   Cardiovascular, endocrine and dipsogenic effects of hemorrhage (15 ml/kg) in conscious dogs.

be inside the blood-brain barrier and therefore inaccessible to angiotensin II (Severs and Daniels-Severs, 1973). As discussed earlier,
other possible sites of action include the SFO and the OVLT.

In view of the doses of angiotensin employed in the present
study and the magnitude of the blood pressure and heart rate responses which were obtained, it is probable that these central cardiovascular effects represent significant actions of circulating angiotensin II. This conclusion is supported by the studies of Scroop,
Katic, Joy, and Lowe (1971) who showed that ablation of the area
postrema reduced the increase in blood pressure produced by intravenous infusion of three doses of angiotensin. It is also likely
that the central cardiovascular actions of angiotensin contributed
to the maintenance of arterial pressure observed during hemorrhage
in the present study, and again this conclusion is supported by the
earlier report of Katic, Lavery, Joy, et al. (1971) that the cardiovascular responses to hemorrhage in the greyhound are markedly im-
paired by destruction of the area postrema. There is also evidence
that the central cardiovascular effects of angiotensin II play a
significant role in experimental renal (Scroop, Katic, Brown, et
al., 1975) and malignant (Sweet, Columbo, and Gaul, 1976) hypertension.

In the present experiments, angiotensin II elicited dose-related
increases in drinking when infused into the carotid arteries, but not
when infused into the vertebral arteries. This indicates a site of
action rostral to the brainstem, possibly the SFO or the OVLT. It
is likely that this dipsogenic action represents a physiological
effect of angiotensin, and this may have contributed to the increase
in water intake observed during hemorrhage. These results thus add
to a growing body of evidence that the renin-angiotensin system
plays a significant role in the regulation of water intake (Abdelaal,
Mercer, and Mogenson, 1976; Fitzsimons, Kucharczyk, and Richards,
1978; Severs and Summy-Long, 1975).

On the other hand, intravertebral or intracarotid infusion of
angiotensin II failed to produce a significant change in vasopressin
secretion. This finding is consistent with several other reports
that intravenous or intracarotid angiotensin does not increase vasopressin secretion (Claybaugh and Share, 1972; Cadnapaphornchai,
Boykin, Harbottle, et al., 1975) but it should be noted that positive results have been obtained by some investigators (Ramsay, Keil,
Sharpe, and Shinsako, 1978). In any case, the present studies indicate that it is highly unlikely that the renin-angiotensin system
contributed significantly to the impressive increase in vasopressin
secretion produced by hemorrhage. This conclusion is in good agreement with an earlier report by Claybaugh and Share (1972) that vasopressin secretion increases in response to hemorrhage even when
changes in renin secretion are prevented. Similarly, Morton, Semple,
Ledingham, et al. (1977) recently reported that the increase in

vasopressin secretion in dogs subjected to hypotensive hemorrhagic
shock was not prevented by the converting enzyme inhibitor,
SQ 20,881.

In the present experiments, intracarotid or intravertebral
infusion of angiotensin also failed to increase plasma corticosteroid levels, indicating that ACTH secretion was not significantly
affected by the infusions. As in the case of vasopressin, discrep-
ancies exist in the literature concerning the effects of circulating
angiotensin on ACTH secretion (Ames, Borkowski, Sicinski, and Laragh,
1965; Ramsay, Keil, Sharpe, and Shinsako, 1978). However, the
present results indicate that it is highly unlikely that the renin-
angiotensin system contributes significantly to the adrenocortical
response to hemorrhage. It is also worth noting that the elevation
of plasma angiotensin II concentration produced in response to
sodium deficiency does not appear to be associated with increased
ACTH secretion (Boyd, Adamson, Arnold, *et al.*, 1972).

Finally, intracarotid and intravertebral infusions of angiotensin suppressed plasma renin activity. The cause of this suppression was not established, but it was clearly not related to changes
in vasopressin secretion, because plasma vasopressin concentrations
did not increase (Figure 3). The decrease may have been a result
of the increase in arterial pressure produced by the angiotensin
infusions. Alternatively, it may have been mediated via the renal
nerves since Ferrario, McCubbin, and Berti (1976) have reported
that renal nerve activity decreases in response to intravertebral
infusion of angiotensin. A recent report by Lokhandwala, Buckley,
and Jandhyala (1978) provides support for this interesting possibility.

In summary, current evidence indicates that the central cardiovascular and dipsogenic actions of angiotensin II represent physiologically important mechanisms by which the renal renin–angiotensin
system participates in the regulation of arterial pressure and water
intake. On the other hand, it appears unlikely that the renin-
angiotensin system plays a significant role in the regulation of
vasopressin or ACTH secretion.

REFERENCES

Abdelaal, A. E., Mercer, P. F., and Mogenson, G. J. (1976). Plasma
    angiotensin II levels and water intake following β-adrenergic
    stimulation, hypovolemia, cellular dehydration, and water
    deprivation. Pharmacol. Biochem. Behav. 4: 317-321.
Abraham, S. F., Baker, R. M., Blaine, E. H., Denton, D. A., and
    McKinley, M. J. (1975). Water drinking induced in sheep by
    angiotensin. A physiological or pharmacological effect?
    J. Comp. Physiol. Psychol. 88: 503-518.

Ames, R. P., Borkowski, A. J., Sicinski, A. M., and Laragh, J. H. (1965). Prolonged infusions of angiotensin II and norepinephrine and blood pressure, electrolyte balance, and aldosterone and cortisol secretion in normal man and in cirrhosis with ascites. J. Clin. Invest. 44: 1171-1186.

Assaykeen, T. A., Clayton, P. L., Goldfien, A., and Ganong, W. F. (1970). Effect of alpha- and beta-adrenergic blocking agents on the renin response to hypoglycemia and epinephrine in dogs. Endocrinology 87: 1318-1322.

Bencsáth, P., Szalay, L., Debreczeni, L. A., Vajda, L., Takács, L., and Fisher, A. (1972). Denervation diuresis and renin secretion in the anaesthetized dog. Eur. J. Clin. Invest. 2: 422-425.

Bickerton, R. K. and Buckley, J. P. (1961). Evidence for a central mechanism in angiotensin-induced hypertension. Proc. Soc. Exp. Biol. Med. 106: 834-836.

Birbari, A. (1971). Effect of sympathetic nervous system on renin release. Am. J. Physiol. 220: 16-18.

Blair, M. L., Feigl, E. O., and Smith, O. A. (1976). Elevation of plasma renin activity during avoidance performance in baboons. Am. J. Physiol. 231: 772-776.

Boyd, G. W., Adamson, A. R., Arnold, M., James, V. H. T., and Peart, W. S. (1972). The role of angiotensin II in the control of aldosterone in man. Clin. Sci. 42: 91-104.

Bozovic, L. and Castenfors, J. (1967). Effect of dihydralazine on plasma renin activity and renal function during supine exercise in normal subjects. Acta Physiol. Scand. 70: 281-289.

Buckley, J. P. (1972). Actions of angiotensin on the central nervous system. Fed. Proc. 31: 1332-1337.

Buggy, J., Fink, G. D., Johnson, A. K., and Brody, M. J. (1977). Prevention of the development of renal hypertension by anteroventral third ventricular tissue lesions. Circ. Res. 40 (Suppl. 1): 110-117.

Bunag, R. D., Page, I. H., and McCubbin, J. W. (1966). Neural stimulation of release of renin. Circ. Res. 19: 851-858.

Cadnapaphornchai, P., Boykin, J., Harbottle, J. A., McDonald, K. M., and Schrier, R. W. (1975). Effect of angiotensin II on renal water excretion. Am. J. Physiol. 228: 155-159.

Capponi, A. M. and Vallotton, M. B. (1976). Renin release by rat kidney slices incubated *in vitro*. Role of sodium and of α- and β-adrenergic receptors, and effects of vincristine. Circ. Res. 39: 200-203.

Changaris, D. G., Keil, L. C., and Severs, W. B. (1978). Angiotensin II immunohistochemistry of the rat brain. Neuroendocrinology 25: 257-274.

Clamage, D. M., Sanford, C. S., Vander, A. J., and Mouw, D. R. (1976). Effects of psychosocial stimuli on plasma renin activity in rats. Am. J. Physiol. 231: 1290-1294.

Claybaugh, J. R. (1977). Evidence for a potentiating effect of circulating angiotensin in the osmotically stimulated increase in plasma antidiuretic hormone concentration. In: *Central Actions of Angiotensin and Related Hormones*. Buckley, J. P. and Ferrario, C. M. (eds.), pp. 293-306, Pergamon Press, Inc., Oxford.

Claybaugh, J. R. and Share, L. (1972). Role of the renin-angiotensin system in the vasopressin response to hemorrhage. Endocrinology 90: 453-460.

Claybaugh, J. R., Share, L., and Shimizu, K. (1972). The inability of infusions of angiotensin II to elevate plasma vasopressin concentration in the anesthetized dog. Endocrinology 90: 1647-1652.

Coote, J. H., Johns, E. J., MacLeod, V. H., and Singer, B. (1972). Effect of renal nerve stimulation, renal blood flow, and adrenergic blockade on plasma renin activity in the cat. J. Physiol. (Lond.) 226: 15-35.

Cunningham, S. G., Feigl, E. O., and Sher, A. M. (1978). Carotid sinus reflex influence on plasma renin activity. Am. J. Physiol. 234: H670-H678.

Daul, C. B., Heath, R. G., and Garey, R. E. (1975). Angiotensin-forming enzyme in human brain. Neuropharmacology 14: 75-80.

Davis, J. O. and Freeman, R. H. (1976). Mechanisms regulating renin release. Physiol. Rev. 56: 1-56.

Day, R. P. and Reid, I. A. (1976). Renin activity in dog brain: Enzymological similarity to cathepsin D. Endocrinology 99: 99-105.

Deuben, R. R. and Buckley, J. P. (1970). Identification of a central site of action of angiotensin II. J. Pharmacol. Exp. Ther. 175: 139-146.

Dorer, F. E., Kahn, J. R., Lentz, K. E., Levine, M., and Skeggs, L. T. (1975). Formation of angiotensin II from tetradecapeptide renin substrate by angiotensin-converting enzyme. Biochem. Pharmacol. 24: 1137-1139.

Epstein, A. N., Fitzsimons, J. T., and Johnson, A. K. (1974). Peptide antagonists of the renin-angiotensin system and the elucidation of the receptors for angiotensin-induced drinking. J. Physiol. (Lond.) 238: 34P-35P.

Epstein, A. N. and Ganten, D. (1977). Reciprocity of plasma and CSF angiotensin: Failure to conform. Fed. Proc. 36: 481 (abstract).

Eriksson, L. and Fyhrquist, F. (1976). Plasma renin activity following central infusion of angiotensin II and altered CSF sodium concentration in the conscious goat. Acta Physiol. Scand. 98: 209-216.

Felix, D. and Akert, K. (1974). The effect of angiotensin II on neurones of the cat subfornical organ. Brain Res. 76: 350-353.

Ferrario, C. M., McCubbin, J. W., and Berti, G. (1976). Centrally mediated hemodynamic effects of angiotensin. In: *Regulation of Blood Pressure by the Central Nervous System*. Onesti, G., Fernandes, M., and Kim, K. E. (eds.), pp. 175-182, Grune and Stratton, New York.

Fitzsimons, J. T. and Kucharczyk, J. (1978). Drinking and haemodynamic changes induced in the dog by intracranial injection of components of the renin-angiotensin system. J. Physiol. (Lond.) 276: 419-434.

Fitzsimons, J. T., Kucharczyk, J., and Richards, G. (1978). Systemic angiotensin-induced drinking in the dog: A physiological phenomenon. J. Physiol. (Lond.) 276: 435-448.

Fukiyama, K. (1972). Central action of angiotensin and hypertension. Increased central vasomotor outflow by angiotensin. Jpn. Circ. J. 36: 599-602.

Fuxe, K., Ganten, D., Hokfelt, T., and Bolme, P. (1976). Immunohistochemical evidence for the existence of angiotensin II-containing nerve terminals in the brain and spinal cord in the rat. Neurosci. Letters 2: 229-234.

Gagnon, D. J., Cousineau, D., and Boucher, P. J. (1973). Release of vasopressin by angiotensin II and prostaglandin E_2 from the rat neuro-hypophysis *in vitro*. Life Sci. 12: 487-497.

Gann, D. S. (1969). Parameters of the stimulus initiating the adrenocortical response to hemorrhage. Ann. N. Y. Acad. Sci. 156: 740-755.

Ganong, W. F. and Lopez, G. A. (1977). Control of the juxtaglomerular apparatus. Excerpta Medica Int. Cong. Ser. 402: 215-220.

Ganong, W. F., Wise, B. L., Reid, I. A., Holland, J. Kaplan, S., Shackelford, R., and Boryczka, A. T. (1978). Effect of spinal cord transection on the endocrine and blood pressure responses to intravenous clonidine. Neuroendocrinology 25: 105-110.

Ganten, D., Hutchinson, J. S., and Schelling, P. (1975). The intrinsic brain iso-renin-angiotensin system in the rat: Its possible role in central mechanisms of blood pressure regulation. Clin. Sci. Mol. Med. 48: 265s-268s.

Ganten, D., Hutchinson, J. S., Schelling, P., Ganten, U., and Fischer, H. (1976). The iso-renin angiotensin systems in extrarenal tissue. Clin. Exp. Pharmacol. Physiol. 3: 103-126.

Ganten, D., Marquez-Julio, A., Granger, P., Hayduk, K., Karsunky, K. P., Boucher, R., and Genest, J. (1971). Renin in dog brain. Am. J. Physiol. 221: 1733-1737.

Gildenberg, P. L. and Ferrario, C. M. (1977). A technique for determining the site of action of angiotensin and other hormones in the brain stem. In: *Central Actions of Angiotensin and Related Hormones*. Buckley, J. P. and Ferrario, C. M. (eds.), pp. 157-164, Pergamon Press, Inc., Oxford.

Gildenberg, P. L., Ferrario, C. M., and McCubbin, J. W. (1973). Two sites of cardiovascular action of angiotensin II in the brain of the dog. Clin. Sci. 44: 417-420.

Gutman, Y. and Benzakein, F. (1974). Antidiuretic hormone and
    renin in rats with diabetes insipidus. Eur. J. Pharmacol.
    28: 114–118.
Haack, D. and Möhring, J. (1978). Vasopressin-mediated blood pres-
    sure response to intraventricular injection of angiotensin II
    in the rat. Pflug. Arch. 373: 167–173.
Hackenthal, E., Hackenthal, R., and Hilgenfeldt, U. (1978a). Purifi-
    cation and partial characterization of rat brain acid protease
    (isorenin). Biochim. Biophys. Acta 522: 561–573.
Hackenthal, E., Hackenthal, R., and Hilgenfeldt, U. (1978b). Iso-
    renin, pseudorenin, cathepsin D and renin: A comparative
    enzymatic study of angiotensin-forming enzymes. Biochim.
    Biophys. Acta 522: 574–588.
Hirose, S., Yokosawa, H., and Inagami, T. (1978). Immunochemical
    identification of renin in rat brain and distinction from acid
    proteases. Nature 274: 392–393.
Hodge, R. L., Lowe, R. D., Ng, K. K. F., and Vane, J. R. (1969).
    Role of the vagus nerve in the control of the concentration of
    angiotensin II in the circulation. Nature 221: 177–179.
Hoffman, W. E., Schelling, P., Phillips, M. I., and Ganten, D.
    (1976). Evidence for local angiotensin formation in brain of
    nephrectomized rats. Neurosci. Letters 3: 299–303.
Horvath, J. S., Baxter, C., Furby, F., and Tiller, D. J. (1977).
    Endogenous angiotensin in brain. Prog. Brain Res. 47: 161–165.
Hutchinson, J. S., Csicsmann, J., Korner, P. I., and Johnston, C. I.
    (1978). Characterization of immunoreactive angiotensin in
    canine cerebrospinal fluid as des-Asp[1]-angiotensin II. Clin.
    Sci. Mol. Med. 54: 147–151.
Hutchinson, J. S., Schelling, P., Möhring, J., and Ganten, D. (1976).
    Pressor action of centrally perfused angiotensin II in rats
    with hereditary hypothalamic diabetes insipidus. Endocrinology
    99: 819–823.
Johnson, J. A., Davis, J. O., and Witty, R. T. (1971). Effects of
    catecholamines and renal nerve stimulation on renin release in
    the nonfiltering kidney. Circ. Res. 29: 646–653.
Joy, M. D. and Lowe, R. D. (1970). Evidence that the area postrema
    mediates the central cardiovascular response to angiotensin II.
    Nature 228: 1303–1304.
Katic, F., Lavery, H., Joy, M. D., Lowe, R. D., and Scroop, G. C.
    (1971). Role of central effects of angiotensin in response to
    hemorrhage in the dog. Lancet 2: 1354–1356.
Keil, L. C. and Severs, W. B. (1977). Reduction in plasma vaso-
    pressin levels of dehydrated rats following acute stress.
    Endocrinology 100: 30–38.
Keil, L. C., Summy-Long, J., and Severs, W. B. (1975). Release of
    vasopressin by angiotensin II. Endocrinology 96: 1063–1065.
Lokhandwala, M. F., Buckley, J. P., and Jandhyala, B. S. (1978).
    Reduction of plasma renin activity by centrally-administered
    angiotensin II in anesthetized cats. Clin. Exp. Hypertension
    1: 167–175.

Malayan, S. A., Keil, L. C., Ramsay, D. J., and Reid, I. A. (1978).
    Mechanism of suppression of plasma renin activity by centrally
    administered angiotensin II. Fed. Proc. 37: 645 (abstract).
Malayan, S. A., Ramsay, D. J., Keil, L. C., and Reid, I. A. (1978).
    Effects of vasopressin on plasma renin activity, blood pressure,
    heart rate and plasma 17-OH corticosteroid concentration in
    conscious dogs. Physiologist 21: 75 (abstract).
Malayan, S. A. and Reid, I. A. (1976). Antidiuresis produced by
    injection of renin into the third cerebral ventricle of the
    dog. Endocrinology 98: 329-335.
Mancia, G., Romero, J. C., and Shepherd, J. T. (1975). Continuous
    inhibition of renin release in dogs by vagally innervated
    receptors in the cardiopulmonary region. Circ. Res. 36: 529-
    535.
Maran, J. W. and Yates, F. E. (1977). Cortisol secretion during
    intrapituitary infusion of angiotensin II in conscious dogs.
    Am. J. Physiol. 233: E273-E285.
Morris, B. J. and Reid, I. A. (1978). A "renin-like" enzymatic
    action of cathepsin D and the similarity in subcellular
    distribution of "renin-like" activity and cathepsin D in the
    midbrain of dogs. Endocrinology 103: 1289-1296.
Morton, J. J., Semple, P. F., Ledingham, I. McA., Stuart, B.,
    Tehrani, M. A., Garcia, A. R., and McGarrity, G. (1977).
    Effect of angiotensin-converting enzyme inhibitor (SQ 20881)
    on the plasma concentration of angiotensin I, angiotensin II
    and arginine vasopressin in the dog during hemorrhagic shock.
    Circ. Res. 41: 301-308.
Mouw, D. R., Abraham, S. F., Blair-West, J. R., Coghlan, J. P.,
    Denton, D. A., McKenzie, J. S., McKinley, M. J., and Scoggins,
    B. A. (1974). Brain receptors, renin secretion, and renal
    sodium retention in conscious sheep. Am. J. Physiol. 226:
    56-62.
Mouw, D. R. and Vander, A. J. (1970). Evidence for brain Na recep-
    tors controlling renal Na excretion and plasma renin activity.
    Am. J. Physiol. 219: 822-832.
Murphy, B. E. P. (1967). Some studies of the protein-binding of
    steroids and their application to the routine micro and ultra-
    micro measurement of various steroids in body fluids by com-
    petitive protein-binding radioassay. J. Clin. Endocrinol.
    Metab. 27: 973-990.
Natcheff, N., Logofetov, A., and Tzaneva, N. (1977). Hypothalamic
    control of plasma renin activity. Pflug. Arch. 371: 279-283.
Nicoll, R. A. and Barker, J. L. (1971). Excitation of supraoptic
    neurosecretory cells by angiotensin II. Nature New Biol. 233:
    172-174.
Nolan, P. L. and Reid, I. A. (1978). Mechanism of suppression of
    renin secretion by clonidine in the dog. Circ. Res. 42: 206-
    211.

Otsuka, K., Assaykeen, T. A., Goldfien, A., and Ganong, W. F.
    (1970). Effect of hypoglycemia on plasma renin activity in
    dogs. Endocrinology 87: 1306-1317.
Passo, S. S., Assaykeen, T. A., Goldfien, A., and Ganong, W. F.
    (1971). Effect of α- and β-adrenergic blocking agents on the
    increase in renin secretion produced by stimulation of the
    medulla oblongata in dogs. Neuroendocrinology 7: 97-104.
Passo, S. S., Assaykeen, T. A., Otsuka, K., Wise, B. L., Goldfien,
    A., and Ganong, W. F. (1971). Effect of stimulation of the
    medulla oblongata on renin secretion in dogs. Neuroendocrin-
    ology 7: 1-10.
Pettinger, W. A. and Keeton, K. (1975). Altered renin release and
    propranolol potentiation of vasodilatory drug hypotension.
    J. Clin. Invest. 55: 236-243.
Pettinger, W. A., Tanaka, K., Keeton, K., Campbell, W. B., and
    Brooks, S. N. (1975). Renin release, an artifact of anes-
    thesia and its implications in rats. Proc. Soc. Exptl. Biol.
    Med. 148: 625-630.
Phillips, M. I. and Felix, D. (1976). Specific angiotensin II
    receptive neurons in the cat subfornical organ. Brain Res.
    109: 531-540.
Phillips, M. I., Phipps, J., and Knowles, D. (1978). Organum
    vasculosum: A central site of action for angiotensin II.
    Endocrinology 102: A278 (abstract).
Ramsay, D. J., Keil, L. C., Sharpe, M. C., and Shinsako, J. (1978).
    Angiotensin II infusion increases vasopressin, ACTH, and 11-
    hydroxycorticosteroid secretion. Am. J. Physiol. 234: R66-
    R71.
Rayyis, S. S. and Horton, R. (1971). Effect of angiotensin II on
    adrenal and pituitary function in man. J. Clin. Endocrinol.
    Metab. 32: 539-546.
Reid, I. A. (1977a). Effect of angiotensin II and glucocorticoids
    on plasma angiotensinogen concentration in the dog. Am. J.
    Physiol. 232: E234-E236.
Reid, I. A. (1977b). Is there a brain renin-angiotensin system?
    Circ. Res. 41: 147-153.
Reid, I. A. and Day, R. P. (1977). Interactions and properties of
    some components of the renin-angiotensin system in the brain.
    In: *The Central Actions of Angiotensin and Related Peptides*.
    Buckley, J. P. and Ferrario, C. M. (eds.), pp. 267-282,
    Pergamon Press, Inc., Oxford.
Reid, I. A., Day, R. P., Moffat, B., and Hughes, H. G. (1977).
    Apparent angiotensin immunoreactivity in dog brain resulting
    from angiotensinase. J. Neurochem. 28: 435-438.
Reid, I. A. and Jones, A. (1976). Effects of carotid occlusion
    and clonidine on renin secretion in anesthetized dogs. Clin.
    Sci. Mol. Med. 51: 109s-111s.
Reid, I. A., MacDonald, D. M., Pachnis, B., and Ganong, W. F. (1975)
    Studies concerning the mechanism of suppression of renin sec-
    retion by clonidine. J. Pharmacol. Exp. Ther. 192: 713-721.

Reid, I. A. and Moffat, B. (1978). Angiotensin II concentration
    in cerebrospinal fluid following intraventricular injection
    of angiotensinogen or renin. Endocrinology 103: 1494-1498.
Reid, I. A. and Ramsay, D. J. (1975). The effects of intracerebro-
    ventricular administration of renin on drinking and blood
    pressure. Endocrinology 97: 536-542.
Reid, I. A., Stockigt, J. R., Goldfien, A., and Ganong, W. F.
    (1972). Stimulation of renin secretion in dogs by theopylline.
    Eur. J. Pharmacol. 17: 325-332.
Richardson, D., Stella, A., Leonetti, G., Bartorelli, A., and
    Zanchetti, A. (1974). Mechanisms of renal release of renin by
    electrical stimulation of the brainstem in the cat. Circ. Res.
    34: 425-434.
Rosset, E. and Veyrat, R. (1971). Effect of vasopressin (ADH),
    aldosterone, norepinephrine (NE), angiotensin I (AI) and II
    (AII) on renin release (RR) by human kidney (HK) slices *in
    vitro*. Acta Endocrinol. 155: 179 (abstract).
Schrier, R. W., Reid, I. A., Berl, T., and Earley, L. E. (1975).
    Mechanism of suppression of renin secretion by cervical
    vagotomy. Clin. Sci. Mol. Med. 48: 83-89.
Scroop, G. C., Katic, F. P., Brown, M. J., Cain, M. D., and Zeegers,
    P. J. (1975). Evidence for a significant contribution from
    central effects of angiotensin in the development of acute
    renal hypertension in the greyhound. Clin. Sci. Mol. Med.
    48: 115-119.
Scroop, G. C., Katic, F., Joy, M. D., and Lowe, R. D. (1971).
    Importance of central vasomotor effects in angiotensin-induced
    hypertension. Brit. Med. J. 1: 324-326.
Scroop, G. C. and Lowe, R. D. (1969). Efferent pathways of the
    cardiovascular response to vertebral artery infusions of angio-
    tensin in the dog. Clin. Sci. 37: 605-619.
Severs, W. B., Changaris, D. G., Kapsha, J. M., Keil, L. C., Petro,
    D. J., Reid, I. A., and Summy-Long, J. Y. (1977). Presence
    and significance of angiotensin in cerebrospinal fluid. In:
    The Central Actions of Angiotensin and Related Peptides.
    Buckley, J. P. and Ferrario, C. M. (eds.), pp. 225-232,
    Pergamon Press, Inc., Oxford.
Severs, W. B., Daniels, A. E., Smookler, H. H., Kinnard, W. J.,
    and Buckley, J. P. (1966). Interrelationship between angio-
    tensin II and the sympathetic nervous system. J. Pharmacol.
    Exp. Ther. 153: 530-537.
Severs, W. B. and Daniels-Severs, A. E. (1973). Effects of angio-
    tensin on the central nervous system. Pharmacol. Rev. 25:
    415-449.
Severs, W. B. and Summy-Long, J. (1975). The role of angiotensin
    in thirst. Life Sci. 17: 1513-1526.
Severs, W. B., Summy-Long, J., Taylor, J. S., and Connor, J. D.
    (1970). A central effect of angiotensin: Release of pitui-
    tary pressor material. J. Pharmacol. Exp. Ther. 174: 27-34.

Shade, R. E., Davis, J. O., Johnson, J. A., Gotshall, R. W., and
    Spielman, W. S. (1973). Mechanism of action of angiotensin II
    and antidiuretic hormone on renin secretion. Am. J. Physiol.
    224: 926–929.
Simpson, J. B., Epstein, A. N., and Camardo, J. S., Jr. (1978).
    Localization of receptors for the dipsogenic action of angio-
    tensin II in the subfornical organ of rats. J. Comp. Physiol.
    Psychol. 92: 581–608.
Simpson, J. B. and Mangiapane, M. L. (1978). Comparison of angio-
    tensin actions at two sites in rat brain. Soc. Neurosci.
    Abstracts 4: 179 (abstract).
Simpson, J. B., Mangiapane, M. L., and Dellmann, H. D. (1978).
    Central receptor sites for angiotensin-induced drinking:
    A critical review. Fed. Proc. 37: 2676–2682.
Simpson, J. B., Reid, I. A., Ramsay, D. J., and Kipen, H. (1978).
    Mechanism of the dipsogenic action of tetradecapeptide renin
    substrate. Brain Res. 157: 63–72.
Simpson, J. B., Saad, W. A., and Epstein, A. N. (1976). The sub-
    fornical organ, the cerebrospinal fluid and the dipsogenic
    action of angiotensin. In: *Regulation of Blood Pressure by
    the Central Nervous System.* Onesti. G., Fernandes, M., and
    Kim, K. E. (eds.), pp. 191–202, Grune and Stratton, New York.
Starke, K. and Endo, T. (1976). Presynaptic α-adrenoreceptors.
    Gen. Pharmacol. 7: 307–312.
Sweet, C. S., Columbo, J. M., and Gaul, S. L. (1976). Central
    antihypertensive effects of inhibitors of the renin-angiotensin
    system in rats. Am. J. Physiol. 231: 1794–1799.
Taher, M. S., McLain, L. G., McDonald, K. M., and Schrier, R. W.
    (1976). Effect of beta adrenergic blockade on renin response
    to renal nerve stimulation. J. Clin. Invest. 57: 459–465.
Tanigawa, H., Dua, S. L., and Assaykeen, T. A. (1974). Effect of
    renal and adrenal denervation on the renin response to slow
    hemorrhage in dogs. Clin. Exp. Pharmacol. Physiol. 1: 325–
    332.
Tobert, J. A., Slater, J. D. H., Fogelman, F., Lightman, S. L.,
    Kurtz, A. B., and Payne, N. N. (1973). The effect in man of
    (+) - propranol and racemic propranolol on renin secretion
    stimulated by orthostatic stress. Clin. Sci. 44: 291–295.
Ueda, H., Katayama, S., and Kato, R. (1972). Area postrema.
    Angiotensin-sensitive site in brain. In: *Control of Renin
    Secretion.* Assaykeen, T. A. (ed.), pp. 109–116, Plenum Press,
    Inc., New York.
Ueda, H., Yasuda, H., Takabatake, Y., Iizuka, M., Iizuka, T., Ihori,
    M., Yamamoto, M., and Sakamoto, Y. (1967). Increased renin
    release evoked by mesencephalic stimulation in the dog.
    Jpn. Heart J. 8: 498–506.
Vander, A. J. (1968). Inhibition of renin release in the dog by
    vasopressin and vasotocin. Circ. Res. 23: 605–609.

Vander, A. J., Henry, J. P., Stephens, P. M., Kay, L. L., and Mouw,
    D. R. (1978). Plasma renin activity in psychosocial hyper-
    tension of CBA mice. Circ. Res. 42: 496-502.
Zanchetti, A. and Stella, A. (1975). Neural control of renin
    release. Clin. Sci. Mol. Med. 48: 215s-223s.
Zehr, J. E. and Feigl, E. O. (1973). Suppression of renin activity
    by hypothalamic stimulation. Circ. Res. 32-33 (Suppl. 1):
    17-26.
Zehr, J. E., Hasbargen, J. A., and Kurz, K. D. (1976). Reflex sup-
    pression of renin secretion during distention of cardiopulmo-
    nary receptors in dogs. Circ. Res. 38: 232-239.

DISCUSSION AFTER DR. REID'S PAPER

Dr. Miller
    Was that plasma renin activity and not plasma renin concen-
tration?

Dr. Reid
    Plasma renin activity.

Dr. Miller
    I just wondered whether the substrate levels might be impor-
tant there since they are probably rate limiting.

Dr. Reid
    They probably are rate limiting, but they shouldn't have
changed in fifteen minutes. I would be very surprised if they did.

Dr. Rowe
    You made no mention of central effects of angiotensin on
sodium intake. Do you not think it is important?

Dr. Reid
    You are referring to the recent reports that angiotensin
increases sodium appetite?

Dr. Rowe
    Yes.

Dr. Reid
    Yes, there certainly have been such reports, but I have had
no direct experience with this. Recently Fitzsimons reported that
sodium appetite is increased during angiotensin treatment. This
is probably yet another central effect of angiotensin.

Dr. Zehr

I discussed an observation with you yesterday, and I hesitate even to mention it here because it is so preliminary. One of my colleagues who is a central neuropharmacologist is interested in the swallowing reflex. When he applied very small amounts of angiotensin II into the forebrain, he saw an increase in the swallowing reflex in anesthetized rats. I thought that this was very interesting.

Dr. Reid

I thought about that after yesterday's conversation. I'm not sure exactly what that means.

Dr. Zehr

I don't either, but I do think that it is interesting.

Dr. Reid

You're not suggesting that is the primary effect, are you?

Dr. Zehr

No, I wouldn't think so, possibly an enhancement of some pre-existing drive on swallowing.

Dr. Jawadi

There are also reports about the effects of dopamine and phenothiazides and L-dopa on plasma renin activity. In your dog experiments, by chance have you injected these agents to see whether they have a central effect on renin release? There are conflicting data about L-dopa releasing or decreasing renin activity. That is one question. The other question is that there are some reports of somatostatin playing some role in renin release. I can recall only a handful of reports. By any chance have you injected somatostatin in your dog experiments and seen a local effect upon the CNS renin release?

Dr. Reid

In other experiments we have looked at the effect of L-dopa on renin secretion. Dr. Martha Blair did these experiments a couple of years ago, and she showed that if L-dopa is injected intravenously following inhibition of peripheral dopa decarboxylase with intravenous carbidopa, there is a decrease in renin secretion associated with a decrease in sympathetic activity. Is that what you are asking?

Dr. Jawadi

Yes.

Dr. Reid

We haven't looked at the other agents you mentioned. As for somatostatin, some people say it inhibits renin secretion; others say it doesn't. As far as I know, nobody has injected it centrally and looked at renin secretion.

Dr. Wang

You mentioned that centrally administered angiotensin II causes drinking, but in one of your slides the intravertebral infusion of angiotensin II did not cause dranking, whereas the intracarotid infusion of angiotensin II did. Do you want to make a comment on that?

Dr. Reid

Yes. There is a difference in the distribution of the carotid blood supply and the vertebral blood supply. In the dog, the carotids do not supply the midbrain, pons, or medulla; these areas are supplied primarily by the vertebral arteries. On the other hand, the carotids supply the hypothalamus and the cortex, which also receive some vertebral blood. It is a bit surprising that vertebral angiotensin did not stimulate drinking, and I guess that is what you are getting at. I assume that the reason is that the concentration of angiotensin reaching the dipsogenic sites following vertebral infusion is less than that following carotid infusion. It may be just a matter of concentration.

Dr. Peach

I can't help but ask about substrate. It seems horrendous to me that 10 or 20 percent of the CSF protein is actually angiotensinogen. If we really view it as a fairly specific protein, what in the world is a concentration like that doing floating around in the CSF? I know that Printz thinks that there are hot spot regions in the brain that contain very large concentrations of substrate. I believe they have pulled it out of a few regions and looked at it. Do you think the substrate is there to interact with circulating renin?

Dr. Reid

I've spent the last three years pondering the question of why substrate is present in the brain. I suspect that substrate is there for a reason, although I doubt that it interacts with circulating renin since renin does not cross the blood-brain barrier. As far as I know, Printz has not found hot spots, as you call them, of substrate in the brain. Substrate seems to be fairly evenly distributed throughout the brain. Our measurements suggest that nearly all, if not all, of the substrate in the brain is in the extracellular fluid rather than inside cells (Endocrinology 103: 492, 1978). Nobody knows where the substrate comes from. We have compared the properties of CSF and plasma substrates and find that they are very similar. I suspect that the substrate in the brain comes from the blood, but I don't know how it gets there.

Dr. Brooks

If there are no further questions or announcements, I would like to take this opportunity to thank you all for coming to the Fourteenth Annual Midwest Conference on Endocrinology and Metabolism. I hope to see you next year.

DISCUSSION REFERENCES

Blair, M. L., Reid, I. A., and Ganong, W. F. (1977). Effect of L-dopa on plasma renin activity with and without inhibition of extracerebral dopa decarboxylase in dogs. J. Pharmacol. Exp. Ther. 202: 209–215.

Fitzsimons, J. T. and Wirth, J. B. (1978). The renin-angiotensin system and sodium appetite. J. Physiol. (Lond.) 274: 63–80.

Morris, B. J. and Reid, I. A. (1978). The distribution of angiotensinogen in dog brain studied by cell fractionation. Endocrinology 103: 492–500.

There are no systems named below or above mentioned. I would like to ... experimentally in the laboratory to demonstrate and for their conclusions ... compares annual student conference contributions and related material to bring before next year.

LITERATURE CITED

Adams, M. J., Ford, J. R., and Shnaan, P. D. (1977). A theory of reading or flight of nignus radii activity with and without inflicted and experimental vision analysis. File to depth 1. Shnanan, Xn. Vol. m. 402: 432-11.

Birginald, F. J., and Loco, G. W. (1983). The countermeasurement system non-linear algorith ... Process IV. Chem. Phys 34 40.

Loc. Dr. ... (1964). The mechanism components ... bruh studied by FAH fractionation. Bull. method. 29 (1974).